D1535504

This is the first comprehensive treatise to be published on the subject of electrical trauma in humans. Several of the world's leading experts describe the basic mechanisms of tissue injury in victims of electrical trauma, the complex and varied manifestations of electrical trauma, and state-of-the-art clinical treatment protocols. Promising new therapies, still in the research stage, are also discussed and assessed. *Electrical Trauma* serves as a new and important resource of information from a variety of perspectives that contribute to the understanding of the electrical injury problem.

Disciplines represented include physics, engineering, biology, and clinical practice, along with a historical review of electrical accidents and their effect on society.

# ELECTRICAL TRAUMA:
# THE PATHOPHYSIOLOGY,
# MANIFESTATIONS AND
# CLINICAL MANAGEMENT

# ELECTRICAL TRAUMA:

the pathophysiology, manifestations and clinical
management

R.C. LEE

*Department of Surgery, University of Chicago, USA*

E.G. CRAVALHO

*Harvard-M.I.T. Division of Health Sciences and Technology,
and Massachusetts General Hospital, Boston, USA*

J.F. BURKE

*Trauma Services, Massachusetts General Hospital Boston, USA*

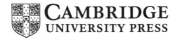

CAMBRIDGE UNIVERSITY PRESS
Cambridge, New York, Melbourne, Madrid, Cape Town,
Singapore, São Paulo, Delhi, Tokyo, Mexico City

Cambridge University Press
The Edinburgh Building, Cambridge CB2 8RU, UK

Published in the United States of America by Cambridge University Press, New York

www.cambridge.org
Information on this title: www.cambridge.org/9780521116145

© Cambridge University Press 1992

This publication is in copyright. Subject to statutory exception
and to the provisions of relevant collective licensing agreements,
no reproduction of any part may take place without the written
permission of Cambridge University Press.

First published 1992
First paperback edition 2011

*A catalogue record for this publication is available from the British Library*

*Library of Congress Cataloguing in Publication Data*

Electrical trauma: the pathophysiology, manifestations, and clinical
management / [edited by] R.C. Lee, E.G. Cravalho, J.F. Burke.
　　p.　　cm.
Includes index.
ISBN 0-521-38345-5 (hardback)
1. Electric injuries.　I. Lee, R.C. (Raphael Carl), 1949–
II. Cravalho, Ernest G.　III. Burke, John Francis, 1922–
[DNLM: 1. Electric Injuries-physiopathology.　2. Electric
Injuries–therapy.　WD 602 E38]
RD95.5.E48　1992
617.1′22-dc20
DNLM/DLC
for Library of Congress 92–3952 CIP

ISBN 978-0-521-38345-5 Hardback
ISBN 978-0-521-11614-5 Paperback

Every effort has been made in preparing this book to provide accurate
and up-to-date information that is in accord with accepted standards
and practice at the time of publication. Although case histories are drawn
from actual cases, every effort has been made to disguise the identities of
the individuals involved. Nevertheless, the authors, editors, and publishers
can make no warranties that the information contained herein is totally
free from error, not least because clinical standards are constantly changing
through research and regulation. The authors, editors, and publishers therefore
disclaim all liability for direct or consequential damages resulting from the
use of material contained in this book. Readers are strongly advised to pay
careful attention to information provided by the manufacturer of any
drugs or equipment that they plan to use.

Cambridge University Press has no responsibility for the persistence or
accuracy of URLs for external or third-party internet websites referred to in
this publication, and does not guarantee that any content on such websites is,
or will remain, accurate or appropriate.

# Contents

# Contributors

T. Bernstein, PhD, *Emeritus Professor of Electrical Engineering/Consulting Electrical Engineer, Electrical and Computer Engineering Department, University of Wisconsin-Madison, Madison, WI 53706*

D.L. Bhatt, *Laboratory for Electromagnetic and Electronic Systems, Massachusetts Institute of Technology, Cambridge, MA, 02139*

J.F. Burke, MD, *Helen Andrus Benedict Professor of Surgery, Harvard, Visiting Surgeon, Massachusetts General Hospital, Boston, MA 02114*

J. Cabanes, MD, *Directeur du Comité des Études Médicales, Electricité et Gaz de France, Paris Cedex 08, France*

M.A. Chilbert, PhD, *Assistant Professor of Biomedical Engineering, Department of Neurosurgery, Medical College of Wisconsin, Milwaukee, WI 53226*

E.G. Cravalho, PhD, *Taplin Professor of Medical Engineering, Massachusetts General Hospital, Boston, MA 02114*

R. Demling, MD, *Director, Longwood Area Trauma Center, Department of Trauma Services, Brigham and Women's Hospital, Boston MA 02115*

E. Eriksson, MD, PhD, *Professor and Chief, Division of Plastic Surgery, Department of Surgery, Brigham and Women's and Children's Hospital, Professor of Plastic Surgery, Harvard Medical School, Boston MA 02115*

D.C. Gaylor, PhD, *Massachusetts Institute of Technology, Cambridge, MA 02139*

G. Gifford Jr., MD, *Senior Associate in Plastic Surgery, The Children's Hospital, Boston MA 02115*

L. Gottlieb, MD, *Associate Professor, Section of Plastic and Reconstructive Surgery, University of Chicago, Chicago IL 60637*

B.J. Grube, MD, *Associate Director, University of Washington Burn Center, Harborview Medical Center, Seattle, WA 98104*

P.G. Hayward, MD, BS, FRCS (ED.), FRACS, *Instructor, Division of Plastic Surgery, University of Texas Medical Branch/Shriners Burns Institute, Galveston, TX 77550*

J.P. Heggers, PhD, *Professor of Surgery (Plastic), University of Texas Medical Branch, Director of Clinical Microbiology, Shriners Burns Institute, Galveston, TX 77550*

D.M. Heimbach, MD, *Director, University of Washington Burn Center, Professor of Surgery, University of Washington School of Medicine, Harborview Medical Center, Seattle, WA 98104*

P. Heroux, PhD, *Professor of Health Effects of Electromagnetic Radiation, School of Occupational Health, McGill University, Montreal, Quebec, Canada, H3A 1A3*

J.L. Hunt, MD, *Professor of Surgery, Co-Director Burn Unit, Parkland Memorial Hospital, The University of Texas Southwestern Medical Center at Dallas, Dallas, TX 75235*

C.F. Keusch, *Brigham and Women's Hospital, The Children's Hospital, Division of Plastic Surgery, Boston, MA 02115*

T.J. Krizek, MD, *Maurice Goldblatt Distinguished Service Professor of Surgery, Section of Plastic and Reconstructive Surgery, University of Chicago, Chicago, IL 60637*

R.C. Lee, MD, ScD, *Associate Professor of Surgery and Anatomy, Department of Surgery and Department of Organismal Biology and Anatomy, University of Chicago, Chicago, IL 60637*

E.A. Luce, MD, *Professor and Chief, Division of Plastic Surgery, University of Kentucky Medical Center, Lexington, KY 40536*

C. Maldarelli, ScD, *Professor of Chemical Engineering, Levich Institute and Department of Chemical Engineering, City College of New York, New York, NY 10031*

K. Prakah-Asante, MA, *Department of Electrical Engineering and Computer Science, Massachusetts Institute of Technology, Cambridge, MA 02139*

M.C. Robson, MD, *Truman G. Blocker, Jr. Professor and Chief, Department of Plastic Surgery University of Texas Medical Branch, Galveston, TX 77550*

J. Saunders, MD, *Department of Plastic and Reconstructive Surgery, University of Chicago, Chicago, IL 60637*

R. Schmukler, EngScD, *Biomedical Engineer, Center for Devices and Radiological Health, Food and Drug Administration, Rockville, MD 20857*

Kathleen J. Stebe, PhD, *Assistant Professor, Department of Chemical Engineering, The Johns Hopkins University, Baltimore, MD 21218*

M. Toner, PhD, *Assistant Professor of Surgery (Bioengineering), Massachusetts General Hospital, Harvard Medical School, Charleston, MA 02129*

B.I. Tropea, MD, *Department of Surgery, Stanford University Hospital, Stanford, CA 94305*

L. Tung, PhD, *Assistant Professor, Department of Biomedical Engineering, The Johns Hopkins University, Baltimore, MD 21205*

J.C. Weaver, PhD, *Senior Research Scientist and Associate Director Biomedical Engineering Center, Harvard–MIT Division of Health Sciences and Technology, Cambridge, MA 02139*

# Preface

This book was motivated by the need to consolidate and review information on tissue injury in victims of electrical trauma so that the pathophysiology and clinical manifestations might better be understood and integrated. The physiological manifestations of electrical trauma range from the simple to the complex and from the innocuous to the fatal. This variation relates to large differences in victim exposure to many factors, including contact voltage, contact duration, presence of clothing in the current path, and the direction of the circuit path through the victim. These differences along with a limited knowledge of the pathophysiology contribute to the present state of confusion that exists among medical staff caring for victims of electrical shock. As a result, progress toward a rational approach to electrical trauma has been relatively slow.

Over the past half-century, survival following major trauma has steadily improved as the capability to perform vital physiologic support has increased; however, little progress has been made in improving the survival of damaged tissue. Limb amputation rates among victims experiencing direct electrical contact are quite high and have remained at a near constant level over the past several decades. At least 85% of victims who survive this ordeal are left disabled. We hold the view that rational therapy to salvage damaged tissue must be based on a detailed understanding of the responsible cellular derangements which ultimately lead to arrest of cell function. Thus, the first purpose of this book is to review the underlying physicochemical mechanisms responsible for tissue damage in electrical injury victims.

We believe this to be the first comprehensive book on electrical trauma. We have organized this multi-authored text in a fashion to make it most useful. Subjects covered in this book range from molecular biophysics of thermal and pure electrical membrane damage to the cellular pathophysiologic consequences to potential strategies for the clinical management of these injuries. An up-to-date review of research in electrical trauma is also presented with the goal of providing sufficient background to those entering the field to facilitate a rapid assimilation of existing knowledge.

This book is intended for both clinicians and laboratory scientists interested in electrical trauma. Unfortunately, it was impossible to avoid the problems created by combining information from one intellectual discipline with information from another without sacrificing comprehensiveness. Undoubtedly, some clinicians may not be able to interpret some of the mathematical statements, and conversely some physical scientists will not fully conceptualize all of the clinical aspects. None the less, considerable effort has been made to present this information in an interpretable manner.

*R.C. Lee*
*E.G. Cravalho*
*J.F. Burke*

# Acknowledgements

The authors are grateful for the contributions of many who have assisted in the preparation of this text. First and foremost have been Georgina Teare, Teresa Raffaelli, and Diane Rudall, who have served as editorial assistants in the preparation of this book. The staff of Cambridge University Press have been a valuable source of support and inspiration in the organization of the book. Many of the contributors to this book met in Chicago in July, 1989 to confer on the subject of electrical trauma. This conference was sponsored by the Electrical Power Research Institute and the Pacific Electric and Gas Company of San Francisco. Administrative support for the conference and the book was generously provided by Dr J. Derek Teare, Director of the Electrical Utility Program of the Energy Laboratory of the Massachusetts Institute of Technology.

*R.C. Lee*
*E.G. Cravalho*
*J.F. Burke*

# Part I:

## Introduction

# 1

# Electrical burns: a historical review

THEODORE BERNSTEIN

The medical practitioner who is interested in electrical trauma should have an understanding of the engineering aspects of the system which caused the injury. It is also important that the electrical parameters which determine the severity and consequences of the shock also are understood.

### History

Prior to Edison's development of the electric lamp in 1879, electrical shock, except from lightning, was a rare phenomenon because there were few electrical devices available which could provide a shock. The explosive growth in the use of electrical systems from 1880 to 1900 led to many cases of electrical shock and to subsequent studies as to how electricity kills or causes injuries. Some of these studies were applied in designing the electric chair for the first legal electrocution at Auburn Prison, New York, in 1890. By about 1900, it was finally determined that the usual mode of death in electrocution was ventricular fibrillation.

All electric chairs used for electrocuting criminals use a head and calf electrode. The application cycle for the electricity is not standardized between states. In Alabama, a 60 Hz sinusoidal voltage is applied as follows: 1800 V for 22 seconds, a voltage reduction to 700 to 800 V in 12 seconds, an increase in voltage to 1800 V in 5 seconds, and then the power is turned off. There is a current of about 7 A when the 1800 V is applied.

### Electrical terminology

There are various electrical terms which must be understood in order to follow any discussion of the engineering aspects related to the cause of electrical trauma.

3

### Voltage

Voltage, with the units of volts, is a measure of the electrical potential difference between any two points. It is important to note that the voltage at a point must always be measured with respect to some other point. One cannot express the voltage at a point without expressing or implying a second point from which this voltage is measured. The voltage is important because it is the voltage difference between two points that is a factor in determining the current that will be in a given electrical path between these points. As an example, the voltage on a bare conductor might be 7200 V with respect to ground; a squirrel running on the conductor or a bird on the conductor would not be shocked because each of its feet is at the same 7200 V with respect to ground, while the voltage difference across its body is zero.

The voltage also determines whether the electricity will break down insulation between the two points. The higher the voltage between points, the thicker is the given insulating material required to prevent dielectric breakdown. Thus, voltage determines insulation requirements and the magnitude of the current in a given circuit.

### Current

The current in a conductor is measured in amperes and is a measure of the rate of motion of charge carriers in the conductor. Current is important in that it is related to conductor heating and determines the required size of the conductor, whereas the circuit voltage determines the insulation required for the conductor. The continuous current rating, ampacity, for a conductor depends on the temperature rise permitted for the conductor and its insulation since heat in a conductor is related to the square of the current in the conductor.

### Frequency

The current and voltage supplied by power companies are usually alternating sinusoidally. The current or voltage alternates between positive and negative peak amplitudes in a regular fashion at a rate of 60 cycles per second. The unit of cycle per second is called the hertz and is abbreviated as Hz. The usual frequency supplied by power companies is 60 Hz in North America and 50 Hz in Europe.

### Resistance

The resistance of a given circuit, measured in ohms, is used to determine the current in a circuit for a given voltage difference across the circuit. For direct current circuits, such as from a battery, or alternating current circuits with resistance loads, dividing the voltage difference across the circuit by the circuit resistance gives the current in the circuit. This relationship is called Ohm's Law.

The resistance for a given size conductor is inversely proportional to the conductivity of the conductor material. This conductivity has a very large range of values from about $10^7$ S/m (siemens per meter) for copper, 1 S/m for the human body, $10^{-3}$ S/m for earth, and $10^{-14}$ S/m for porcelain insulators. The human body has about the same conductivity as saltwater or a semiconductor such as silicon or germanium.

### Power

The power, measured in watts, is related to the product of the current in a circuit and the circuit voltage. For a resistance load, power exactly equals the product of current and voltage. Heating of a device is related to the power since power is the rate of energy use or dissipation, joules per second. The higher the power, the greater is the rate of energy use or dissipation. For a given power transmission, raising the voltage will reduce the required current. This explains why power transmission lines operate at high voltage so that the current in the lines will be reduced and smaller diameter conductors can be used for the long distance transmission.

### Heating

It is easiest to understand the relationship between power dissipation and heating by an example. Suppose the power dissipated is 100 watts. If this power were dissipated in a volume smaller than that of a 100-watt lamp, the smaller volume would tend to be higher in temperature than if the power were dissipated in the volume occupied by the 100-watt lamp. If 100 W were dissipated in a volume larger than that for the 100-watt lamp, the volume would tend to be cooler than that of the 100-watt lamp; so the heating effect is a function of the power dissipation, the volume in which the dissipation takes place, and the cooling action within or around the volume.

### Grounding

The earth itself has a low conductivity, but it has such large physical dimensions that there is practically a zero resistance for currents in the earth. There can be considerable resistance at the grounding electrode where the current has to enter the earth through the relatively small area of the buried conductor in contact with the earth.

Power electrical circuits used for transmission, distribution, and in homes and plants, are usually grounded. This means that one conductor in the circuit is connected to an electrode buried in the ground. One reason for grounding is to provide a path to ground for lightning currents. The usual connection to the earth is provided by connection to a system of buried conductors, with as much surface area as possible in contact with the earth to reduce the resistance of the grounding electrode. Some common grounding electrodes are a buried municipal water system or multiple ground rods.

The normal electrical currents in a grounded circuit are not in the grounding electrode or earth, as the currents are in the metallic circuit conductors. There will be currents injected into the ground when lightning strikes the circuit or if there is a connection between one of the ungrounded, energized conductors and the earth as when a crane resting on the ground contacts a power-line.

### The electric arc

The electric arc can be a cause of severe burns. The temperature of an electric arc is on the order of 2000 °C to 4000 °C (3600 °F to 7200 °F).

The breakdown strength for air that can initiate an arc through air depends on the shape of the electrodes and the waveshape of the applied voltage. A typical value used is 30 kV/cm or 76.2 kV/in (1 kV = 1000 volts). This means that there must be a voltage difference of 30 000 volts for each centimeter of gap length or 76 200 volts for each inch of gap length to initiate an arc through air. There is a fundamental property relating to arc initiation that, no matter how small the air gap is made between conductors, there can be no breakdown across an air gap if the voltage is below approximately 300 volts. After the arc is initiated, only 20 V/cm or 50.8 V/in is required to maintain the arc; thus, once the arc is initiated it will be maintained over a much larger air gap length than the original initiation distance. The arc voltage is practically independent of arc current and primarily depends on the arc length.

As an example using arc properties, an arc welder with 80 V open circuit voltage cannot initiate an arc across an air gap; but, when the electrodes touch and are separated, an arc is initiated by the spark at separation so that the output voltage, with load, of 40 V can now maintain an arc about an inch long. Another example helps refute the assertion that sometimes is made that a crane was a foot or two away from a 7200 V line when the electricity arced through air to the crane; the crane had to be within 0.1 inch of the line or more likely touched the line and the arc came about when the crane boom pulled away and the arc was initiated by the separation of the contact.

Arcs can be initiated at lower voltages across insulating material, well below 300 V, when there is current tracking across a surface or through the material. This can heat the material and allow an arc to be initiated. Other arcs can be initiated at low voltages when a worker bridges energized conductors with a screwdriver or metal tape.

Burns are caused by arcs when the individual is in the current path and the electricity arcs to his body. Another type of burn occurs when there is a large arc in some equipment and the worker is burned by the intense heat of the arc near his body.

### Electrical shock parameters

The electrical parameters important in electrical injury depend on the waveform of the electrical source, such as alternating current, direct current, pulse, or lightning discharge. Alternating current shock effects depend on the magnitude, frequency, and duration of the current with the voltage only being important in determining the current. For 60 Hz sinusoidal currents, the approximate thresholds are 0.5 mA for startle reaction, where a shock may be perceived but there will be no severe muscular reaction; 5 mA for let-go current, where current through a hand and arm may cause the hand to involuntarily close and remain closed so that the energized conductor cannot be released; and 500 mA for shock durations less than 0.2 second or 50 mA for shock durations longer than two seconds for ventricular fibrillation. For alternating current frequencies above 1 kHz or for direct current, the current thresholds for a given effect are higher than for 60 Hz. Direct current shock thresholds are about three times higher; however, there doesn't seem to be a let-go phenomenon. An individual can let go of an energized circuit if he or she is willing to suffer the intense shock when the circuit is broken. With lightning or pulse type shocks, it is the energy in the shock and the timing in relation to the heart cycle that is significant. Pulse shocks during the T wave of the heart cycle can lead to ventricular fibrillation and are most hazardous. Pulse shocks with an energy content of 50 J can be lethal while shocks below 0.25 J are disagreeable but probably not hazardous. The annoying electrostatic shock produced when walking across a carpet is of the order of 10 mJ.

The voltage of the electrical system involved in an accident case is important as the voltage and resistance or impedance in the path of the shock will determine the current. The human body has a minimum resistance of about 500 to 1000 ohms hand-to-hand or hand-to-foot if skin and contact resistance are neglected. The actual resistance will be larger depending on the type of contact, area of contact, and condition of the skin. Low voltage, shocks below 600 V, lead to ventricular fibrillation. Burns can occur, though not always, depending on the type of contact, current, and duration of the shock. Higher voltage shocks with currents over one ampere will usually cause burns, particular if arcing is involved. The mode of death for these higher current shocks is often asystole rather than ventricular fibrillation. Unlike ventricular fibrillation, a blow or fall may convert asystole to a normal heart rhythm in some cases. It is not surprising to find that a lineman may survive after a high voltage, high current shock with serious burns while another person is dead, because of ventricular fibrillation, with no burn marks on the body after a low current, 120 V shock. Lightning, with its high, brief peak median current of 30 000 A, can also cause asystole.

### The 60 Hz transmission and distribution system

Power is often generated by utilities at voltages of 10 to 20 kV as three phase, 60 Hz power. The term three phase indicates that there are three conductors associated with the system with the nominal voltage indicated being the rms voltage between any two of the three conductors. The effective or root mean square, rms, voltage is the usual value read on an ac voltmeter and is used for circuit calculation. It is the peak value of the voltage divided by the square root of 2. When a value is given for a sinusoidal, alternating voltage or current, it is usually the effective value and not the peak value. Thus, a 12.47 kV, three-phase system has an effective alternating voltage of 12.47 kV between any two of the three conductors. The reason this is called three phase is that there is a time difference between the times when each of the three possible alternating voltages between conductors reaches a peak – the peaks do not occur at the same instant. A voltmeter which reads the voltage between any two of the three phases would not show this time or phase difference between the phases. The phase conductors usually are not grounded. Many systems use a Y connection with a fourth wire, the neutral, grounded so that the voltage between any phase conductor and ground is the phase to phase voltage divided by the square root of 3. A 12.47 kV, three-phase system has a voltage of 7.2 kV to ground. Three phase is used to provide more efficient transmission of larger powers. Large motors run more smoothly and with greater efficiency when they are operated from three phase.

The utilities may generate electricity at voltages of 10 to 20 kV. The upper limit on voltage is determined by insulation requirements in the generator. Lower generated voltages would require larger conductors in the generator. This voltage is raised, using transformers, to three-phase line-to-line voltages, such as 69, 115, 138, 230, 345, or 500 kV for transmission over great distances where the lower currents required for transmitting power allow the use of smaller conductors. The voltage is then stepped down to voltages, such as 4.16, 12.47, 13.2, 24.94, or 34.5 kV line-to-line, or 2.4, 7.2, 7.62, 14.4, or 19.9 kV line to ground for distribution. The conductors that supply the transformer that reduces the distribution voltage for final use are called the primary conductors. Common primary voltages in rural or residential areas are 7.2 or 2.4 kV, line to ground, the latter used for older systems.

The primary conductors are frequently involved in accident cases. *These conductors are usually bare, without insulation, and obtain their insulation by insulators at the power poles or by air.* It is these bare, primary conductors that are involved in cases when a crane contacts a power-line, or someone with a television antenna or aluminum ladder contacts the primary conductor. It is the phase voltage to ground that is important in power-line contact accidents because the current path is from a phase conductor to ground. The phase conductor to ground voltage determines the current that will be in a given ground fault resistance.

An accident that occurs frequently is one which results when a child climbs a tree in which there is a power-line. The power-line, supplying a transformer for nearby homes, is usually a primary conductor with a voltage to ground of 7200 or 2400 volts. The child either contacts the primary feeder directly or pushes a limb onto the bare feeder. The current then goes from the conductor through the child and tree to ground either through the living tree which is a fair conductor or through a bare, grounded conductor also in the tree foliage.

A child climbing on a power tower can contact the power-lines and the tower at the same time to provide a path between the line and grounded tower through his body.

In boom or ladder contacts to power-lines, the boom or ladder is energized with the line-to-ground voltage so that arcing can occur at any point where there is some failure of insulation between this voltage and ground – such as the tire of a truck upon which the boom is mounted. Persons, standing on the ground, contacting a crane, that, in turn, is contacting a power-line can be electrocuted as the crane is at the same voltage as the line. The crane operator on the metal crane, however, is rarely injured as there is negligible voltage drop across any part of the crane, so he is like a bird on a power-line with high voltage on his body to ground, but little voltage difference across his body.

The circuit protection for the power-line cannot prevent injury to persons contacting the line or damage to equipment as the protection can only protect the power-lines and power system from damage by the excess current caused by a fault. Because of the high resistance at the contact to earth, the current in an object contacting the line and the earth will usually be limited to a value below the line circuit current protection setting. If the current path to ground is through a person, the current is further reduced by the body resistance. It would be virtually impossible to have a functioning power system that could prevent injury or damage to any object that faults the power lines. The operating values for circuit protection devices are well above the human hazard level.

## The 60 Hz, 120/240 V electrical system

Single-phase power enters a premises utilizing a three-wire system, with one of the conductors being grounded at the service entrance. The three-wire system is called the secondary wiring as it comes from the secondary of a transformer supplied by the high voltage primary conductors. The grounded secondary conductor, also called the neutral conductor, always has a white colour for its insulation when routed inside the premises. The other two conductors, called the ungrounded conductors, have an insulation colour other than white or green – often black or red. The voltage between the ungrounded conductors, used for larger loads, such as electric ranges or clothes dryers, is nominally 240 V. The voltage between either the ungrounded conductor and the neutral or ground is 120 V. The nominal 120 V is sometimes referred to as 110 V or 115 V.

### Plugs and receptacles

Wall outlet receptacles rated 120 V, 15 A or 20 A, installed after 1962 are of the grounding type with sockets for the two parallel blades and a grounding pin on the attachment plug. The larger parallel blade socket is connected to the white, grounded conductor at silver or white coloured terminals. The smaller parallel blade socket is connected to the ungrounded conductor at brass or copper coloured terminals. The grounding pin socket is grounded by a green insulated wire, a bare wire, or by the grounded conduit.

The three-prong attachment plug used to energize equipment provides 120 V power between the two parallel blades when plugged into a receptacle. The equipment grounding pin on the plug is connected, by a green wire, to all exposed metal parts on the equipment. Under normal operating conditions, there is no current in this third, equipment grounding pin. In the event of an insulation failure in the equipment such that the exposed metal parts of the equipment are energized, the equipment grounding conductor provides a path for electricity so that there will be sufficient current to actuate the fuse or circuit breaker protecting the ungrounded conductor. The equipment is then de-energized because of the fault. The equipment grounding conductor carries no current and plays no part in the normal operation of the equipment, but is an important safety feature. Without the equipment grounding conductor, a fault in the equipment that energizes the exposed metal case, may, or may not, cause the circuit breaker of fuse to operate depending on whether there is a sufficiently low resistance path to ground from the exposed metal parts. Equipment with such a fault resting on a wooden table would not have sufficiently low resistance path to ground from exposed metal parts to cause the overcurrent protection to operate. The equipment could continue to function normally with its exposed metal parts at a voltage of 120 V. Someone touching both this exposed energized metal and a grounded object such as a faucet or grounded tool could provide a path for current and receive a lethal shock. The equipment grounding pin can be considered something like a safety valve and its function should never be defeated by breaking off the equipment grounding pin or using an adapter for conversion from a three-prong to two-prong plug without properly grounding the adapter to the grounded screw in the receptacle face plate.

### *Fuses and circuit breakers*

The conventional 120 V system is energized by an ungrounded and a grounded conductor with 120 V between these conductors. The ungrounded conductor is protected by a fuse or circuit breaker that primarily protects the wires in the wall from overheating because of overcurrent. The rating of the fuse or circuit breaker depends on the current carrying capacity of the wire it is protecting. The fuse or circuit breaker is designed so that it will operate in the event there is excessive current in the ungrounded conductor such that the wire insulation will be overheated. It is important to note that a fuse or circuit breaker has an inverse current–time operating relationship. This means that the higher the current, the more rapid the operation. A fuse or circuit breaker protecting an outlet is designed to protect the wiring in the wall from being overheated. The fuse or circuit breaker will carry its rated current indefinitely. A 15 A or 20 A circuit breaker will actuate in less than 1 hour at 125% of rating and in less than 2 minutes at 200% rating. At 300% breaker rating, the usual trip time is 5 to 35 seconds.

Because of the high values for operating current, fuses or circuit breakers offer no primary protection from electrical shock.

### Ground fault circuit interrupter

A device that can prevent lethal electrical shocks is the ground fault circuit interrupter (GFCI). The GFCI operates as a device to interrupt power in the event there is an accidental low current path to ground other than through the grounded conductor. Most electrocutions occur when an individual contacts energized defective equipment and a ground, other than the grounded conductor. The GFCI detects the low current ground fault and opens the circuit.

Currents of the order of 0.1 A can be hazardous to humans. A conventional circuit breaker operating at 15 to 20 A could never provide any protection for such low current shocks, while a GFCI can provide protection as it can trip at currents to ground as low as 5 mA. The GFCI compares the current in the ungrounded lead to that in the grounded conductor for conductors routed to receptacles. If there is a difference in current of 5 mA, the circuit for that line is opened. The basic concept is that the unbalance in current is caused by a ground fault – an unintended path to ground. This ground fault could be a person touching the energized conductor. The 5 mA level was determined as the level of shock which might cause an individual to be 'frozen' to the circuit and not be able to let go of an energized conductor.

### Double insulation

Double insulation, when referring to electrical tools and appliances, implies that the insulating system between internal energized conductors and any possible point of external contact consists of both a functional and protecting insulation, with the two physically separated. The protecting insulation must survive the functional insulation and protect against electric shock in case the functional insulation fails. The functional insulation is insulation necessary for the proper functioning of the appliance, such as the winding insulation of a motor or transformer. The protecting insulation is an independent insulation that provides protection in case of failure of the functional insulation. An enclosure of insulating material is an example of protective insulation.

Double insulated appliances are identified as such on the nameplate. They have and only require a two-bladed plug. Any exposed metal parts have protecting insulation inside; for example, an exposed metal chuck on a drill has protecting insulation, such as internal insulating material, isolating the metal chuck from the metal parts of the motor which might become energized because of a fault.

### *Intended or expected electrical shocks*

The design of most electrical equipment ensures that an individual should rarely contact energized parts and be subjected to electric shock. For such equipment, electrical safety is provided primarily by insulation or guarding to prevent contact and by suitable grounding. Any contact with energized parts is considered hazardous. There are other equipment where, even though it may not be intended, contact with energized parts is expected; electrical safety must be provided by ensuring that any possible electric shock will not be hazardous or lethal. Examples of such electrical devices are the electric fence, gun, welder, cattle prod, and fly electrocuter. Safety is provided by limiting the current output or by using frequencies for the current that will be in the safe range.

### Lightning

A lightning stroke has a unidirectional current that peaks in about 10 microseconds and decays in about 100 microseconds. Peak currents have been measured up to 270 kA, though the median peak current measured is about 30 kA. This current is a more or less constant current, which means the resistance in the path has no effect on the current. Very large voltages are developed when the current passes through a high resistance such as a tree or person. An individual struck by lightning often is injured by the arcing across his body produced when the high voltage across his body exceeds breakdown levels. The high current pulse can cause asystole rather than ventricular fibrillation in some cases.

Most people are killed or injured by lightning when outdoors. Standing next to a tree is foolhardy, since the probability of being struck by lightning is related to the square of the height. The tree's height increases the probability of its being struck while its high resistance causes a large voltage to be developed by the lightning current along the trunk. This voltage can cause sideflash to an individual standing near the trunk.

**General references**

1 Bernstein, T. (1973). Effects of electricity and lightning on man and animals, *Journal of Forensic Sciences*, **18** (1), 3–11.
2 Bernstein, T. (1973). A 'grand success'. The first legal electrocution was fraught with controversy which flared between Edison and Westinghouse,' *IEEE Spectrum*, **10**, (2), 54–8.
3 Bernstein, T. (1975). Theories of the causes of death from electricity in the late nineteenth century, *Medical Instrumentation*, **9**, (6), 267–73.
4 Bernstein, T. (1983). Electrocution and fires involving 120/240 V appliances, *IEEE Transactions on Industry Applications*, IA–19, (2), 155–9.
5 Bernstein, T. (1985). Safety criteria for intended or expected non-lethal electrical shocks. In *Electrical Shock Safety Criteria. Proceedings of the First International Symposium on Electrical Shock Safety Criteria.* Bridges, J.E., Ford, G.L., Sherman, I.A. & Vainberg, M. eds, pp. 283–93, Pergamon Press, New York.
6 Biegelmeier, G. & Lee, W.R. (1980). New considerations on the threshold of ventricular fibrillation for a.c. shocks at 50–60 Hz. *Proceedings, Institution of Electrical Engineers*, **127**, 103–10.
7 Bridges, J.E. (1981). An investigation on low-impedance low-voltage shocks, *IEEE Transactions on Power Apparatus and Systems*, **PAS–100** (4), 1529–37.
8 Dalziel, C.F. & Mansfield, T.H. (1950). Effect of frequency on perception currents, *AIEE Transactions*, **69, (2)**, 1162–8.
9 Dalziel, C.F. & Massoglia, F.P. (1956). Let-go currents and voltages, *AIEE Transactions*, **75, (2)**, 49–56.
10 Dalziel, C.F. & Lee, W.R. (1968). Reevaluation of lethal electric currents, *IEEE Transactions on Industry Applications*, **4**, 467–76.
11 Dalziel, C.F. (1971). Deleterious effect of electric shock. In *Handbook on Laboratory Safety*, 2nd edn. Steere, N.V. pp. 521–7, Chemical Rubber, Cleveland.
12 Geddes, L.A., Bourland, J.D. & Ford, G. (1986), The mechanism underlying sudden death from electric shock. *Medical Instrumentation*, **20 (6)**, 303–15.
13 IEC Report Publication (1984). *Effects of Current Passing Through the Human Body, Part 1: General Aspects*, Publication 479–1, 2nd edn, Geneva: International Electrotechnical Commission.
14 Lee, W.R. (1977). Lightning injuries and death. In *Lightning, Vol 2 Lightning Protection*, pp. 521–43. Academic Press, New York.

# 2

# Industrial electrical accidents and their complications observed by Electricité de France (EDF)

JEAN CABANES

Passage of an electric current through a living organism releases a certain amount of energy which may have two effects: a transient change in the physiology of an organ or of the entire body translated either by a reaction of inhibition or by excitation; heating, the extent of which is defined by Joule's law.

Three clinical situations arise as a result of the first process: inhibition, an acute and transient event, commonly referred to as 'electrical shock'; respiratory arrest; and especially, circulatory arrest, usually related to ventricular fibrillation which is the basic cause of immediate fatalities.

Electrical burns are the result of the second process, and their topography, extent and later consequences are related to the pathway of the electric current through the body and to the parameters in Joule's equation: voltage, intensity and the duration of passage of the current.

Electrical accidents observed at Electricité de France, the national electric company which is virtually the sole producer, transporter and distributer of electricity in France have been the object of continuous study by the Committee on Medical Studies of EDF for almost 40 years. Its statistical and clinical results have been published in many papers [1-16].

The latest statistical analysis involved a ten-year period and 1231 accidents, representing an average of 125 accidents per year in a total workforce of some 120 000 employees.

As in previous studies, the present study was made possible solely through a collaborative effort by all of the medical departments of EDF: on the one hand, with the Department of Occupational Safety and on the other hand, with the Department of Medical Assessment which provided the majority of medical information.

For investigation of sequelae, reports were provided by the Medical Committee on Disabilities, which is in charge of determining the medical and social cost of sequelae.

Finally, with respect to the technical aspect of an accident, information was provided by the Department of Prevention and Occupational Safety of the EDF which completed the technical data: voltage, intensity, and especially duration of passage of the current through the body.

### General characteristics of electrical accidents

First a few general characteristics relating to electrical accidents are discussed.

#### *Etiology*

Electrical accidents primarily affect young male workers on the job; electrical linemen appear to constitute the most exposed group of workers. The causes of these types of accidents are dominated by human error; equipment failure is less to blame because of continuing vigilance by the Department of Prevention and Safety.

#### *Immediately caused death*

In 29 cases out of 1231 accidents (2.4%), electrical injury caused immediate death of the victim. Cases where the victim died immediately were, in the majority of instances, caused by passage of an electrical current through the body and most probably result from ventricular fibrillation; in only one case was death caused by trauma. Ventricular fibrillation, which is not spontaneously reversible in man, can only occur under very specific conditions of current intensity and duration of passage of the current.

The curves defined by the International Electrotechnical Commission in publication No. 479, provide the probabilities for this incidence according to these two parameters (Fig. 2.1). Curve $c_1$ gives the limit (probability 0), curve $c_2$ defines a 5% probability, and curve $c_3$ provides a 50% probability.

#### *Apparent death: intensive care*

Out of 1202 accidents which were not immediately fatal, victims lost consciousness in 86 cases (7.2%). These cases of apparent death are related to inhibition of major bodily functions: respiration, consciousness, but usually they did not involve cardiovascular arrest. This type of inhibition is an acute and transient event which, clinically, is generally referred to as 'electric shock'. Respiratory arrest may be caused either by contracture of

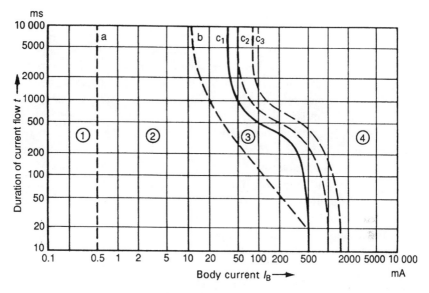

Fig. 2.1. Curves taken from publication 479 of the I.E.C. showing thresholds of action of 50–60 cycle alternating current, according to intensity and duration of passage of the current.

| Zones | Physiological effects |
|---|---|
| Zone 1 | Usually no reaction effects. |
| Zone 2 | Usually no harmful physiological effects. |
| Zone 3 | Usually no organic damage to be expected. Likelihood of muscular contractions and difficulty in breathing, reversible disturbances of formation and conduction of impulses in the heart, including arterial fibrillation and transient cardiac arrest without ventricular fibrillation increasing with current magnitude and time. |
| Zone 4 | In addition to the effects of Zone 3, probability of ventricular fibrillation increasing up to about 5% (curve $c_2$), up to about 50% (curve $c_3$) and above 50% beyond curve $c_3$. Increasing with magnitude and time, pathophysiological effects such as cardiac arrest, breathing arrest and heavy burns may occur. |

*Notes*

1. As regards ventricular fibrillation, this figure relates to the effects of current which flows in the path 'left hand to feet'.

2. The point 500 mA/100 ms corresponds to a fibrillation probability in the order of 0.14%.

muscles involved in respiration, or by inhibition of central nervous system centres which control respiration when contact with cerebral structures occurs. Respiratory arrest and loss of consciousness are reversible if intensive care measures are instituted before development of irreversible lesions in the nerve control centers occurs with subsequent cardiovascular arrest. In this study involving 58 cases (67%), intensive care was administered spontaneously. In 28 other cases, intensive care measures resulted in a favourable outcome, which suggests that these cases involved respiratory arrest alone without cardiovascular arrest. If these 28 cases which had a favourable outcome are compared with the 29 cases where death occurred immediately, it appears that intensive care measures were effective in about half of the cases, a figure which corresponds to results observed in previous investigations and to those reported in many similar studies in other European countries.

### Initial lesions

Apart from immediate fatalities and loss of consciousness, electrical accidents cause initial lesions and a certain number of progressive complications. Initial lesions observed may be summarized as consisting primarily of trauma and electrical burns. Trauma was observed in 70 cases (6% of accidents). It involved mainly head injuries and traumatic injuries of the spinal cord and limbs. Burns are certainly the most frequently observed type of lesion observed, since these were reported in 1142 cases (93% of accidents).

#### Arc burns

*Arc burns* are the most frequently observed burns (77%). Most often they involve a very small area (less than 1% of body area) and are caused by low-voltage shock. Small burns occur on the hands or face in the vast majority of cases. Intermediate size burns (1 to 10% of body surface) occur less frequently but involve the same areas of the body as small burns. Extensive burns, which sometimes are exacerbated because the victim's clothing catches fire, are more often the result of accidents involving high voltage. Lastly, ocular burns, or ocular arc injuries, account for one-third of arc burns. They are most often caused by low voltage. Frequently occurring alone, ocular burns may also be associated with other types of burns, especially of the face.

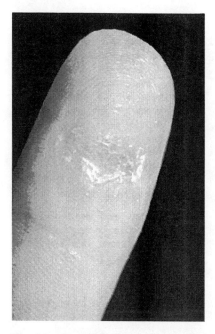

Fig. 2.2. Electric mark on the pad of the ungual phalanx of the index finger. (Photograph Lebeaupin)

### Electrothermal burns

*Electrothermal burns* caused by passage of an electric current occur more rarely (15% of burns). They too, often have a very limited extent and occur as the result of low-voltage shock. The most extensive burns occur rarely (10% of electrothermal burns) but may be serious because of the depth of tissue involved along the pathway where the current flowed.

### Mixed burns

*Mixed burns* which associate the two processes are the least frequent of all: 6% of burns. They most often are caused by high-voltage shock. Unlike the preceding types, they often are extensive, with multiple sites of involvement. This category includes the majority of serious burns with severe, progressive effects and which cause major sequelae (Figs 2.2–2.7). Although burns involving the lips and tongue occur primarily in children and are never observed in the industrial setting, photos of these are also presented (Figs 2.8, 2.9).

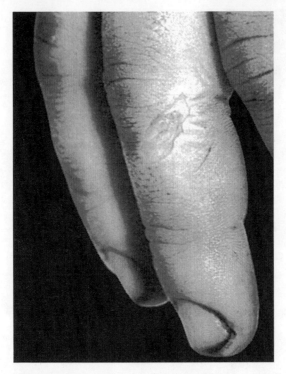

Fig. 2.3. Electrothermal burn, of middle finger on right hand. (Photograph Lebeaupin)

### Clinical course – delayed-onset fatalities

The clinical course of electrical injuries often involves the onset of cardiovascular, neurological and especially renal complications which play a major role in the development of sequelae and are the cause of eventual fatal outcome. Fatalities which occurred later on were observed in 12 cases. In seven cases, fatal outcome was caused by the *extent of the burns* complicated by kidney failure. *Three cases which resulted in eventual fatalities* were due to *trauma*; two other deaths appear to have been caused by onset of cardiovascular disorders. If these 12 delayed-onset deaths are added to the 29 immediately caused fatalities, there is a total of 41 deaths, with an *overall mortality rate of 3.3%*. This mortality is slightly less than that observed in the last investigation where overall mortality was 3.9%, but it is very much lower than in previous investigations where mortality exceeded 5%.

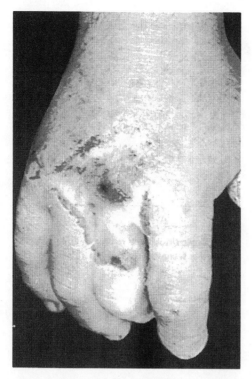

Fig. 2.4. Burn on right hand with large lesions on the middle finger that will require amputation. (Photograph Lebeaupin)

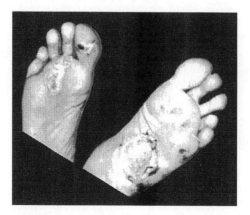

Fig. 2.5. Electrothermal burns on the foot with multiple contact points (hobnailed shoe). (Photograph Lebeaupin)

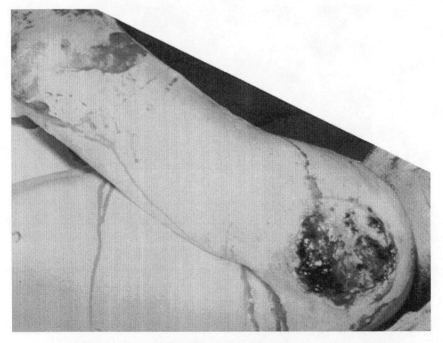

Fig. 2.6. Serious high-voltage electric accident involving multiple burns. Appearance of upper left arm with deltoid contact point and strong deep lesions along the entire limb which will necessitate its amputation. (Photograph Lebeaupin)

### *Sequelae*

Sequelae resulting from electrical injuries are frequent and differ from one patient to another. Indeed, they have been observed in 290 cases or 24% of non-fatal accidents. Occasionally occurring in combination in the same victim (408 sequelae in 290 patients who developed sequelae), they often are the source of partial disabilities (21% of non-fatal accidents).

### *Sequelae caused by burns*

The most frequent sequelae are those resulting from electrical burns. They have been observed in 231 cases or 19% of non-fatal accidents. Most often they involve ugly and/or disabling scars (212 cases) and as for burns, these scars are located on the upper limbs primarily, in particular on the victims' hands. In 13 cases or 1.1% of nonfatal accidents, one or more amputations had to be performed because of the effects of deep electrothermal burns caused by passage of the electric current.

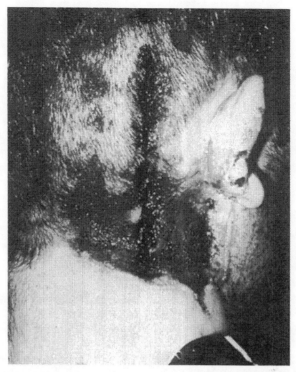

Fig. 2.7. Composite burn on the nape and on the neck. (Photograph Lebeaupin)

### Neurological and psychological sequelae

87 accident victims (7.3%) experienced *neurological* and/or *psychological* sequelae. These sequelae include headache, dizziness, physical or psychological lassitude, mood and personality disturbances. In 11 cases, there were *dissociated cerebral sequelae (incomplete post-concussional syndromes)* (Table 2.1).

In those cases where post-concussional syndrome was subtle or incomplete, headache and dizziness were the most frequently observed symptoms. The electroencephalogram was normal in most cases.

In 12 cases, *true post-concussional syndrome* was observed, which was similar to that reported following head injury (Table 2.2). In a third of cases, psychological and neurotic symptoms were observed in combination. In almost half of cases, the electroencephalographic tracing was abnormal. Finally, tests of vestibular function were disturbed in half of cases. Possibly these post-concussional syndromes are the result of passage of the electric

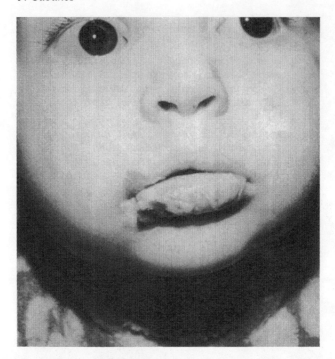

Fig. 2.8. Burn on lower lip resulting from sucking on a live extension cord. (Photograph by Dr Marchac)

current, but more probably they may be trauma-related, since, in almost half of cases, head injury was noted or they may be due to initial anoxia since here too, in close to half of cases, the victim initially appeared to be dead.

*Psychological or neurovegetative sequelae* These occur more rarely than cerebral sequelae and only involved about 1% of cases. Symptoms and their intensity were highly variable (Table 2.3). In three cases, there were true neurotic disturbances. Electroencephalographic abnormalities occurred more rarely than in the case of post-concussional syndromes, and, on an aetiological basis, head injury may only have played a part in a third of cases.

*Peripheral neurological sequelae* These sequelae were noted in 51 cases or in 4.3% of victims. They consisted primarily of sensory, motor, vasomotor and trophic disturbances and involved the upper limbs in particular.

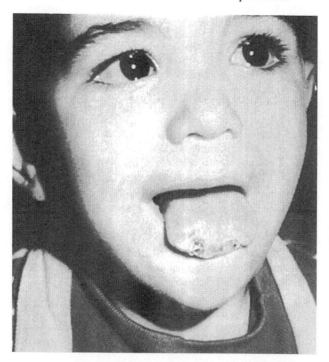

Fig. 2.9. Tongue burn resulting from sucking on a live extension cord. (Photograph by Dr Marchac)

*Spinal cord injuries* Only a single case was observed: this involved sensory-motor paraesthesia, perhaps resulting from the direct effect of electrocution.

### Sensory sequelae (ocular and auditory)

Sensory sequelae were observed in 43 cases or in 3.6% of nonfatal accidents. Ocular sequelae were of two types: effects of ocular arc injuries and cataracts.

*Ocular arc injuries* Sequelae of these were the most frequent (25 cases) or close to 8% of arc injuries observed (300). Most often these involved simple cases of chronic conjunctivitis. More rarely, effects of corneal burns (four cases) or burns of the retina (four cases), both may cause decreased visual acuity.

*Cataracts* These occur rarely. Only three cases were observed. One case

Table 2.1. *Dissociated cerebral sequelae*

| Case | Age | Voltage (volts) | Pathway of current | HI | LC | Type of post-concussional sequelae | EEG | Vestibular tests |
|---|---|---|---|---|---|---|---|---|
| 1 | 41 | 15 000 | LUL–RUL | – | + | Headache | N | |
| 2 | 50 | 10 000 | RUL–LLL | + | – | Headache | N | |
| 3 | 23 | 15 000 | Arc | + | – | Headache, dizziness | N | Abnormal |
| 4 | 35 | 220–380 | Arc | – | + | Headache, dizziness | ? | |
| 5 | 30 | 220 | RUL–? | + | + | Headache, dizziness | N | |
| 6 | 50 | 220–380 | Head–LUL– | – | + | Headache, memory and sleep disturbances, lassitude | N | Abnormal |
| 7 | 33 | 10 000 | RUL–RLL | – | + | Headache, sleep disturbances irritability, lassitude | | |
| 8 | 43 | ? | Arc | – | – | Headache, memory disturbances | N | |
| 9 | 49 | 380 | RUL–? | + | + | Disturbances of balance, memory and behaviour | Abn. | |
| 10 | 31 | 6600 | Arc | – | – | Dizziness, post-traumatic neurosis | N | |
| 11 | 46 | 220–380 | Head–RUL | + | + | Headache, irritability, depression | Abn. | |

*Notes:*
RUL = right upper limb; LUL = left upper limb; HI = head injury; RLL = right lower limb; LLL = left lower limb; N = normal;
Abn = abnormal; LC = loss of consciousness.

Table 2.2. *Post-concussional syndrome*

| Case | Age | Voltage (volts) | Pathway of current | HI | LC | Type of post-concussional sequelae | EEG | Vestibular tests |
|---|---|---|---|---|---|---|---|---|
| 1 | 26 | ? | Arc | − | − | post-concussional syndrome | N | |
| 2 | 39 | 20 000 | RUL–LLL | + | + | post-concussional syndrome | Abn | Abnormal |
| 3 | 42 | ? | Arc | − | − | post-concussional syndrome | ? | Abnormal |
| 4 | 21 | ? | RUL–? | + | + | post-concussional syndrome | ? | |
| 5 | 25 | lightning | ? | − | − | post-concussional syndrome | Abn | |
| 6 | 26 | 380 | RUL–LUL | − | − | post-concussional syndrome | N | |
| 7 | 25 | ? | ? | + | − | post-concussional syndrome | Sub-Nor. | Abnormal |
| 8 | 43 | ? | Arc | + | − | post-concussional syndrome | N | Abnormal |
| 9 | 44 | ? | RUL–RLL–LLL | − | − | post-concussional syndrome, neurosis | Abn | |
| 10 | 35 | ? | RUL–? | + | + | post-concussional syndrome, neurosis | N | Abnormal |
| 11 | 48 | lightning | ? | − | + | post-concussional syndrome, neurosis | N | Abnormal |
| 12 | 43 | 15 000 | Head–RUL–LLL–RLL | + | + | post-concussional syndrome, neurosis | Abn | Abnormal |

*Notes:*
RUL = right upper limb; LUL = left upper limb; RLL = right lower limb; LLL = left lower limb; HI = head injury; LC = loss of consciousness.

Table 2.3. *Psychological and neurovegetative sequelae*

| Case | Age | Voltage (volts) | Pathway of current | HI | LC | Description of psychological and neurovegetative sequelae | EEG |
|---|---|---|---|---|---|---|---|
| 1 | 42 | 20000 | RUL–LLL–RLL–LLL | – | – | Depression | |
| 2 | 31 | 135000 | RUL–LLL | – | + | Memory disturbances, mixed neurotic disturbances | Sub-N |
| 3 | 29 | 90000 | RUL–LLL | – | – | Insomnia, lassitude, joint pain, neurotic disturbances | ? |
| 4 | 37 | 15000 | RUL–RUL | – | + | Disturbances of memory and concentration | N |
| 5 | 47 | 15000 | Arc | + | – | Insomnia, nervousness | Abn |
| 6 | 23 | 63000 | RUL–? | + | – | Personality disturbance, anxiety, intolerance to noise | ? |
| 7 | 32 | 20000 | RUL–LUL | + | + | Memory disturbances | ? |
| 8 | 34 | 150 | LUL–RUL | + | + | Intolerance to noise | Abn |
| 9 | 22 | ? | ? | – | + | Nervousness | N |
| 10 | 50 | 20000 | Arc | – | + | Memory disturbances, slowed cognition, anxiety | N |
| 11 | 32 | ? | RUL–RLL | – | + | Fainting, anxiety | |
| 12 | 50 | 1000 | LUL–RLL | – | + | Neurovegetative dystonia, causalgia | ? |
| 13 | 40 | 127–220 | ? | – | + | Sensation of suffocation upon exertion, paraesthesia | N |

corresponding to the conventional description of electrical-injury cataracts: an accident caused by electrical contact with the head, with development of a cataract 6–8 months after the accident. The second case followed phototrauma alone without passage of the current, similar to the type we published a description of[17]. The third case is less certain regarding the causal relationship with the electrical accident, although possible.

*Auditory sequelae* These were observed in 15 cases or in 1.3% of accidents. Most often (12 out of 15 cases), these involve cochlear lesions in combination with vestibular disturbances. In a few cases, there was vestibular damage alone (Table 2.4). The history of head injury was a rather frequent finding (6 out of 15 cases); that of electrical contact with the victim's head was noted in three cases. Arc-induced explosion injuries are sometimes the sole cause of auditory damage.

### Cardiovascular sequelae

Cardiovascular sequelae occur rarely; eight such cases were observed: four dysrhythmias associated with conduction disturbances; two cases of ECG changes which may correspond to myocardial damage; and two cases of sequelae of phlebitis.

We did not observe any coronary artery disturbances such as those previously reported[18].

### Trauma-related sequelae (excluding head injuries)

These sequelae corresponded to various clinical manifestations and were observed in 23 cases or in 2% of accidents.

### Permanent disabilities (PD)

Sequelae were the cause of permanent types of disability in 253 cases, or in 21% of non-fatal accidents. Figure 2.10 lists the distribution of permanent disabilities according to their percentage impairment. Rates for permanent disabilities most often were less than 10%. If the 41 fatalities are added to these 253 cases of permanent disability, the figure of 294 serious accidents or 24% is obtained. The same percentage had already been observed in each of the three previous investigations.

**References**

1 François, R.Ch. & Cabanes, J. (1962). Etude des accidents électriques ayant entrainé le décès ou une incapacité permanente partielle des accidentés parmi le personnel d'Electricité de France pendant la

Table 2.4. *Auditory sequelae*

| Case | Age | Voltage (volts) | Pathway of current | HI | LC | Description of auditory damage |
|------|-----|-----------------|--------------------|----|----|-------------------------------|
| 1 | 24 | 220–380 | Arc | – | – | Tinnitus, bilateral partial hearing loss |
| 2 | 35 | 220–380 | Arc | – | + | Bilateral partial hearing loss |
| 3 | 37 | 200–600 | Arc | – | – | Left partial hearing loss |
| 4 | 46 | 220–380 | Head–RUL | + | + | Aggravation of existing bilateral partial hearing loss |
| 5 | 28 | 90 000 | Arc | + | + | Tinnitus, bilateral partial hearing loss |
| 6 | 41 | 20 000 | Arc | – | – | Tinnitus, slight bilateral hearing loss |
| 7 | 50 | 20 000 | Arc | – | + | Tinnitus, bilateral partial hearing loss |
| 8 | 42 | ? | Arc | – | – | Bilateral partial hearing loss, right vestibular hypoexcitability |
| 9 | 44 | 15 000 | ? | + | + | Bilateral partial hearing loss and hypoexcitability, dizziness |
| 10 | 43 | 15 000 | Head–RUL–LLL–RLL | + | + | Tinnitus, right deafness, dizziness, right vestibular hypoexcitability |
| 11 | 50 | 220–380 | Head–LUL–RUL | – | + | Bilateral partial hearing loss, central vestibular damage |
| 12 | 48 | Lightning | ? | – | + | Slight bilateral auditory damage, bilateral hypoexcitability |
| 13 | 22 | 200–600 | RUL–LUL | – | + | Bilateral vestibular hyperexcitability |
| 14 | 34 | 150 | LUL–RUL | + | + | Right vestibular hyperexcitability |
| 15 | 43 | ? | Arc | + | – | Dizziness, bilateral vestibular hypoexcitability |

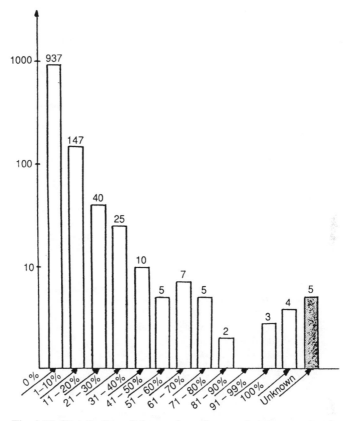

Fig. 2.10. Distribution of the number of cases of permanent disabilities (PD) according to their percentage impairment for 253 cases out of 1190 non-fatal accidents.

période 1949–1958. Comité Médical E.D.F.–G.D.F. paru dans *Arch. Mal. Prof., no 3, Séance du 9 Octobre 1961 de la Société de Médecine et d'Hygiène du Travail*, pp. 118–122.

2 François, R.Ch. & Cabanes, J. (1962). L'utilisation des statistiques d'accidents électriques dans l'étude des conséquences médicales qu'ils entrainent. *Arch. Méd. Chir. Normandie*, Juin-Juillet, no 119.

3 François, R.Ch. & Cabanes, J. (1968). Résultats obtenus par les méthodes de réanimation d'urgence pratiquées à l'occasion des accidents électriques à E.D.F. *Journées de Réanimation Méd.-Chir.*, Nancy, 25–27 Avril.

4 François, R.Ch., Paris, J., Le Loc'h, H. & Cabanes, J. (1969). Soins d'urgence et indication d'évacuation des brûlés électriques *16ème Congrès. Int. de Méd. du Travail*, Tokyo, 22–27 Septembre.

5 François, R.Ch. & Cabanes, J. (1969). Etude des accidents électriques observés à E.D.F. pendant la période 1959–1964. *Arch. Mal. Prof., 30, 12, Société de Médecine et d'Hygiène du Travail*, Séance du 10 Mars.

6 Cabanes, J. (1974). Etude des accidents électriques observés à E.D.F. pendant une période de 5 ans. *Table ronde A.I.S.S.*, Paris, 19–21 Mars.

7 Cabanes, J. (1975). Accidents oligoanuriques au cours de l'évolution des accidents électriques. *Colloque A.I.S.S.*, Marbella, Octobre.

8 Le Loc'h, H. & Cabanes, J. (1975). Etude des accidents électriques observés à E.D.F. pendant une période de 5 années. *Arch. Mal. Prof.*, 36, 10–11, 608–615.

9 Cabanes, J. (1977). Etude des accidents électriques observés à E.D.F. sur une période de 5 années. *Société Française de Médecine Préventive et Sociale*, Paris, 26 Novembre.

10 Cabanes, J. (1977). Recensement et évaluation des accidents électriques en France. *Wissenchaftliche Tagung Forschungsstelle für Elektropathologie*, Fribourg i Br., 13–14 Octobre.

11 Cabanes, J. (1978). Etude comparative des accidents électriques observés à E.D.F. sur deux périodes de 5 années. *Congrès International de Médecine du Travail*, Dubrovnik, 25–30 Septembre.

12 Cabanes, J. (1981). Les accidents oligo-anuriques au cours de l'évolution des accidents électriques à Haute Tension. *Journées de la Forschungsstelle für Elektropathologie*, Fribourg i Br., 17–18 Septembre.

13 Cabanes, J., Cabane, J.P. & Gourbière, E. (1985). Etude des brûlures électriques observées à E.D.F. sur une période de 10 années. *6ème Congrès de la Société Française d'Etude et de Traitement des Brûlures*, Toulouse, 20–21 Septembre.

14 Gourbière, E. (1986). Etude des brûlures électriques à E.D.F. sur une période de 10 ans. Thèse, Paris.

15 Cabanes, J. (1987). Electrical injuries observed in employees of E.D.F. *Forschungsstelle für Elektropathologie*, Fribourg i Br., 11 Septembre.

16 Cabanes, J. (1987). Etude des brûlures électriques à E.D.F. sur une période de 10 ans *1st. Meeting of Mediterranean Burns Club*, Paler, 18–20 Juin.

17 François, R.Ch. & Cabanes, J. (1963). A propos d'un cas de cataracte en rapport probable avec un phototraumatisme par arc électrique sous passage direct du courant *Arch. Mal. Prof.*, 24, 535.

18 François, R.Ch., Cabanes, J. & Dagneaux, M. (1966). Traumatismes électriques et lésions coronariennes *Journées de Réanimation Médico-Chirurgicale de Nancy*, 6–8 Mai.

# 3

# The pathophysiology and clinical management of electrical injury

R.C. LEE

## Introduction

It is estimated that 4% of all United States hospital burn unit admissions are for electrical trauma[1]. High-voltage electric shock can produce devastating damage that often leaves the survivor with permanent injuries. More than 90% of these injuries occur in males between the ages of 20 and 34 and are work related. Mortality rates from electrical trauma range from 3% to 15%, more than 1000 deaths per year in this country alone.

These injuries are generally quite complex. Extensive skeletal muscle, neural and vascular tissue injury is characteristically scattered in its distribution along the current path. Major limb amputation rates have been reported to be as high as 71%[2]. These statistics represent several thousand injured young adults each year. An incomplete understanding of the pathophysiology of tissue injury and an inability to accurately diagnose the extent of electrical injury at the time of admission seriously impede effective clinical management. Furthermore, the variable circumstances of accidental electrical shock make it nearly impossible to formulate valid empirical guidelines for predicting the extent of tissue damage.

Over the past two decades, the clinical outcome for the electrical trauma victim has not improved substantially. To some extent, this has resulted from the slow progress in understanding the underlying pathophysiology of tissue injury. Unfortunately, fundamental misconceptions about the nature of electrical trauma, arising from the complex interdisciplinary nature of the underlying pathophysiology of electrical injury, have obscured the basic issues and have complicated the problem. In order to understand this subject fully, the physics of joule heating, thermal damage to cells, dielectric breakdown of materials, electroporation, in addition to cellular and organismal physiology must be taken into account. The standard practices of surgical debridement and early reconstruction could also be enhanced by promptly applying appropriate therapy designed to reverse the damage to fatally injured although transiently viable tissue. This therapy must, however, account for all of the complex pathophysiological interactions which accompany electrical shock.

Electric fields established in tissues during high voltage electrical shock produce cell damage either through joule heating of tissue to supraphysiological temperatures[1,3], cell membrane breakdown by strong electrical forces (electroporation)[4,5] or some combination of the two. The role of joule heating in damaging tissue has long been recognized[6], but only recently has its direct electrical effect on the cell been identified[4]. The relative contribution of these two mechanisms must be determined because each carries important implications for the pattern of injury and, hence, treatment[4,5]. Moreover, the kinetics of joule heating in humans still has not been measured, a shortcoming which must be remedied if appropriate therapeutic strategies are to be developed[7].

This introductory chapter is a concise overview of the present state of the biophysical and clinical understanding of electric trauma; the following chapters contain considerable additional detail. The complexity of the subject is clearly reflected by the divergent opinions expressed by the various authors represented in this book. Clearly, many questions remain to be answered.

## Relevant biophysics and physiology

### Electrical conduction (ohmic)

By definition, electrical current arises from the flux of electrical charges; the type of the charge carrier (electron or ion) depends on the material. Although current in metallic conductors is carried by electrons, the charge carriers in aqueous solutions are ionized salts. During electrical shock, electrons are converted to ions by electrochemical reactions across the metal–skin interface (Fig. 3.1), a process with a rate dependent on the magnitude of the potential drop across the interface[8]. These reactions generate heat and toxic chemical by-products which may alter tissue oxygen and pH and may contribute to local tissue injury.

Pure water is ten thousand times more resistive than physiological saline to electric current. The presence of salts provides mobile ions which raise the conductivity of saline to approximately 1 siemens (S)/m. 1 siemens = 1/ $\Omega$(ohm), 1 V (volt) = 1 A (ampere) × 1$\Omega$. Because saline is such a good electrical conductor, the human body in contact with a 60 Hz power source

Electrical injury mechanisms

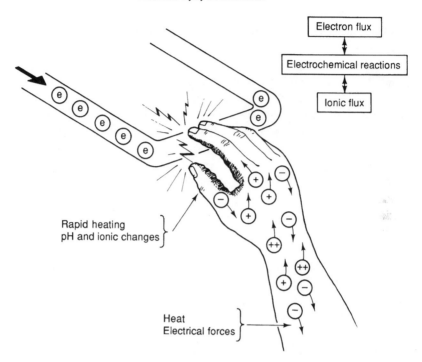

Fig. 3.1. Sketch of some of the effects of the electrochemical conversion at the body surface during electrical shock.

behaves like a pure resistive load, which means that almost all current flow results from ion movement rather than from oscillating electric fields (i.e. displacement or capacitative current).

When current passes through the human body, the epidermal layer and metal–skin surface contact impedances dominate the initial electrical impedance. In most areas, the epidermis is a 100 to 500 $\mu$m layer of fused, squamous epithelial cells which cover the body surface, forming a thin, electrically insulated, closed shell. Depending on the state of epidermal hydration, the resistance of 1 sq. cm of epidermis may range from $5 \times 10^4$ to $5 \times 10^5$ $\Omega$. In the palms of the hands and the soles of the feet, the epidermis can build up to double or triple that thickness, resulting in two to three times greater resistance. There is little difference in the measured resistance between adjacent fingers on one hand and between two fingers on opposite hands because the epidermis dominates the electrical resistance to current passage throughout the body.

Current conduction within subcutaneous tissues is affected by the density, shape, orientation and size of cells. Because cell membranes are good insulators, electrical current tends to pass around and between them, effectively diminishing the tissue area available for ion flux, and makes tissues less conductive than physiologic saline. Resistance to current flow generally increases with cell density, but as cell size increases the membrane has less influence on cellular electrical properties because the membrane itself does not change. Cell orientation and shape also mediate current conduction. Thus, the conductivity of muscle parallel to the long axis of the muscle cells is greater than the conductivity perpendicular to the major axis. As a cell becomes larger than its space constant $\lambda_m$, its properties are dominated by the cytoplasm, resembling those of physiologic saline. Table 3.1 lists the electrical conductivity of the most abundant human tissues.

### *Dielectric breakdown: 'arcing'*

When the electric field strength within a material exceeds the critical value above which the field pulls the electrons out of their orbital shells, the material becomes ionized and highly conductive. This event is called dielectric breakdown and is manifested by a bright flash (arc) as electrons give off photons; lightning is a common example. The dielectric strength of a material is the maximum electric field strength a material will withstand before breakdown. Air's breakdown strength is approximately $2 \times 10^6$ V/m; values for other materials appear in Table 3.2. However, no matter how small the air gap, dielectric breakdown generally will not occur unless there is at least a 300 V potential difference across the gap. Nevertheless, the exact arc initiation voltage depends on the temperature and the geometry of the two charged surfaces and, after an arc is initiated, only $2 \times 10^3$ V/m is required to maintain the arc.

Arc burns frequently occur on the skin of high voltage shock victims. However, even though temperatures for arcs range between 2000 and 4000 °C, a brief arc transmits only enough heat energy to cause a superficial (partial thickness) skin burn because the density of air is only slightly greater than that of water (0.001). At the time of contact with a power source, more than 95% of the imposed voltage drop initially occurs across the insulating epidermis. Thus, a typical 10 kV contact would generate an electric field of $10^6$ to $10^8$ V/m within the epidermal layer. As a result, the epidermal layer instantly reaches temperatures in excess of 1000 °C and vaporizes almost instantaneously. Consequently, for exposure times greater than the epidermal breakdown time (perhaps 1 ms), the body

Table 3.1. *Typical tissue values*

| Symbol | Parameter | Units | Value | Reference |
|---|---|---|---|---|
| $\Gamma$ | Frequency factor in damage integral | 1/s | $3.1 \times 10^{98}$ | 14 |
| | | | $2.9 \times 10^{37}$ | 22 |
| | | | $9.09 \times 10^{36}$ | 19 |
| B | Energy of activation | J/mole | 628,000 | 14 |
| | | | 244,000 | 22 |
| | | | 249,000 | 19 |
| h | Empirical heat transfer coefficient | W/°C | $10^{-4}$ | 52 |
| $c_b$ | Specific heat of blood | joule/°C | $3.3 \times 10^3$ | 65 |
| $c \cdot \rho$ | Heat capacity | joule/m$^3$ °C | | 51,66,67 |
| | (a) skin | | $3.4 \times 10^6$ | |
| | (b) fat | | $1.98 \times 10^6$ | |
| | (c) muscle | | $4.14 \times 10^6$ | |
| | (d) bone | | $4.14 \times 10^6$ | |
| $\sigma$ | Electrical conductivity | S/m | | 8,17,51 |
| | (a) skin | | $3.8 \times 10^{-4}$ | |
| | (b) fat | | $5 \times 10^{-4}$ | |
| | (c) muscle | | $4 \times 10^{-3}$ | |
| | (d) bone | | $1 \times 10^{-3}$ | |
| $\omega_b$ | Blood flow in tissues | ml/6 kg s | | 68,69 |
| | (a) skin | | 9.8 | |
| | (b) fat | | 3.75 | |
| | (c) muscle | | 2.71 | |
| | (d) bone | | 1.35 | |
| k | Thermal conductivity | W/m °C | | 51,65,67 |
| | (a) skin | | 0.36 | |
| | (b) fat | | 0.2 | |
| | (c) muscle | | 0.385 | |
| | (d) bone | | 1.1 | |
| $T_b$ | Temperature of blood | K | 310 | |
| $T_s$ | Temperature of ambient air | K | 298 | |

behaves as a 500 to 1000 $\Omega$ resistive load[6,9,10]. Since voltage is equal to the current multiplied by the resistance, it is reasonable to expect that a 10 kV contact would produce peak currents between 10 to 20 A[10].

### Sensory and neuromuscular responses

Many cells, such as muscle and nerve, utilize electricity as a control signal, producing cellular effects which are unrelated to joule heating. Applying weak fields from a non-physiologic source can, therefore, interfere with cell

Table 3.2. *Breakdown strength*
*(E$_{max}$) of a few materials*

| Material | $E_{max}$ (V/m) |
|----------|------------------|
| Glass | $9 \times 10^6$ |
| Nylon | $19 \times 10^6$ |
| Polyethylene | $18 \times 10^6$ |
| Air (at STP) | $2 \times 10^6$ |

function[12] or, if the field is strong enough, cause direct cell damage. As the current passing through tissues is increased, several distinct thresholds may be observed which are frequency dependent. These thresholds are compared in Table 3.3 and are valid for fields with frequencies below 1 kHz. At the commercial power frequency of 60 Hz (US), the threshold for human (male) perception of current passed hand-to-hand is approximately 1.0 mA. If the current is raised to 16 mA, the muscles in the forearm are stimulated to contract, causing involuntary spasms. Because the flexors are more powerful, the hand assumes the closed fist position and the person cannot voluntarily let go of an object in the palm. This is called the 'let-go' threshold and represents a physiological response to the induced trans-membrane potential depolarization by the applied current. At a current of 60 mA, the heart in 30% of victims will begin to fibrillate in 30 s. Based on *in vitro* studies, a current of 1500 mA is required to produce skeletal muscle cell damage solely by electrical forces (no heat-inflicted damage).

### Joule heating

Current flux in a material dissipates energy in the material as moving charges collide with the molecules of the material. This energy dissipation is measurable as heat. Heating via electrical current is called joule heating. The heat energy dissipation in a unit volume of material per unit time is the power dissipation density ($P$, watts/m$^3$) of the material. Mathematically, it is equal to the product of the current density ($J$, A/m$^2$) and the electric field strength ($E$, V/m), that is,

$$P = J \cdot E. \tag{1}$$

Because Ohm's law states that the current density is related to the electric field by the conductivity of the material ($\sigma$), that is,

Table 3.3. *Thresholds for effects of commercial electrical power*

| Response | Threshold current* |
|---|---|
| Perception | 1.0 mA (M[§]) |
| | 0.5 mA (F) |
| 'Let-go' | 16 mA (M) |
| | 11 mA (F) |
| Cardiac: Arrhythmia | 60 mA |
| Ventricular fibrillation | 100 mA |
| Disruption of skeletal muscle membranes | 1500 mA [20] |

*Notes:*
* Assumes current path in the upper extremity.
§ (M): Males, (F): Females.

$$J = \sigma E, \tag{2}$$

and thus we can express the power dissipation density in the form of joule heating as:

$$P = \sigma |E|^2. \tag{3}$$

This expression can be used to calculate the rate of temperature rise in tissues when the electric field or current density distribution is known. If the duration of current passage and the thermal properties of the tissue are also known, the temperature rise itself can be calculated.

The biological significance of joule heating in electrical trauma can be estimated by first determining the tissue temperature as a function of time. Lee and Kolodney[4], and later Tropea and Lee[12], numerically simulated the joule heating response using a finite element method to solve the bioheat balance equation[13]. This equation states that the heat energy entering a point in the tissue $(\rho c \frac{dT(t)}{dt})$ is equal to the sum of the heat energy diffusion into the point $(\kappa \nabla^2 T(t))$, the heat energy carried by blood flow $(\rho_b c_b \omega_b (T_b - T(t)))$, the heat energy generated by cellular metabolism $(q_m)$ and the heat energy generated by joule heating $(P)$. This 'bioheat' equation is written:

$$\rho c \frac{dT(t)}{dt} = \kappa \nabla^2 T(t) + \rho_b c_b \omega_b (T_b - T(t)) + q_m + \sigma E^2 \tag{4}$$

where $\rho$ is the tissue density, $c$ is the heat capacity, $\kappa$ is the thermal conductivity (Table 3.1), $T_b$ is the blood temperature, $\rho_b$ is the blood specific density, $c_b$ is the heat capacity of blood, and $\omega_b$ is a constant proportionally

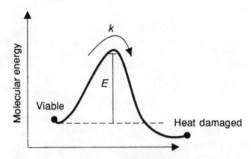

Fig. 3.2. Single barrier model of a two-state rate process representing heat damage to tissue. The rate of conversion from normal to heat damaged tissue is $k$. The process is not spontaneously reversible.

related to the tissue perfusion rate per gram of tissue (Table 3.1). For the range of temperatures which appear to be relevant to subcutaneous tissue injury the dependence of $\sigma$ on temperature is negligible.

### *Cellular response to supraphysiological temperatures*

Cells can respond to supraphysiological temperatures in many ways; the precise nature of the response, however, depends on temperature and heat kinetics. The probability of cell injury depends on the duration of the exposure to temperatures above 43 °C, making the process of injury rate dependent. Thus, thermal injury can be modeled using a damage rate equation based on the concept of activation energy[14]. The activation energy ($B$) for a reaction is the critical amount of energy required for the reaction to take place (Fig. 3.2). Therefore the reaction rate will be proportional to the fraction of the system constituents which have an energy at least equal to the activation energy. From the Maxwell–Boltzman energy distribution law, this fraction is $e^{-B/RT}$, where $R$ is the gas constant and $T$ is the temperature in Kelvin. For the case of a population of cells exposed to supraphysiological temperatures, the rate of cellular damage accumulation ($k$) can be defined by the activation energy ($B$) and the rate of damage accumulation ($\Gamma$) as temperature ($T$) approaches infinity, as indicated by:

$$k = \Gamma e^{-B/RT} \tag{5}$$

For convenience, we can define a damage parameter $X$ which is the fraction of the cell population which is heat damaged. As indicated above, the rate of damage accumulation $dX/dt$ is equal to $k$. Because $X$ is a function of $t$ we write $X(t)$. The statistical function $X$ can meaningfully vary from 0 to 1, representing a range from no cellular injury to all cells damaged, respectively. Thus, the damage in the region of interest is completed when $X = 1$. The Arrhenius relation can be integrated to predict the lethal damage time ($LT$) for arbitrary temperature elevations $T(t)$:

$$X(t) = \int_0^{LT} \Gamma e^{-\frac{B}{RT(t)}} \mathrm{d}t \tag{6}$$

Several experimental studies have demonstrated that thermal damage accumulation in biological systems can be described by Equation (6). In one of the earliest studies, Moritz and Henriques[15] performed experiments on pig skin by directly exposing the surface of the skin to a rapidly flowing stream of hot liquid (water or oil) at temperatures ranging from 44 to 100 °C for durations of between 1 s and 7 h. Exposures were designated as subthreshold or suprathreshold based on whether or not they were sufficient to cause complete transepidermal necrosis. Similar exposures were made on medical student volunteers. Moritz and Henriques' results indicated that there is little or no quantitative difference in the susceptibility of human and porcine skin to thermal injury. Furthermore, they demonstrated that the probability of significant tissue damage depended on temperature and duration of exposure. Figure 3.3 compares their data with that predicted by the model based on Equation (6); the similarities between the shape of the two curves is convincing. By fitting the experimental data to the Arrhenius equation, Henriques estimated the activation energy for damage to the epithelium to be 150 kcal/mole. By comparing this value to the known activation energies of several biological processes, he concluded that the mechanism of damage was probably thermal alteration to proteins.

Henriques[15] also observed that the earliest histological signs of skin damage (first-degree burn) corresponded to an $X = 0.53$ and that the epidermis was completely damaged (second-degree burn) when $X = 1.0$ at the skin surface. Separately, Diller and Hayes[16] and Palla[17] coupled this mathematical description of cellular heat damage kinetics, Equation (5), with a multidimensional numerical solution of the bioheat equation to predict the distribution of burn injury to skin and subcutaneous tissues caused by heating the skin surface. These applications provided important insight into the parameters which govern the severity of burns.

To gain insight into the energetics of heat injury to cells, Mixter *et al.*[18] studied the effects of elevated temperatures (between 45 and 65 °C) on human fibroblasts. Cells bathed in a nutrient solution containing eosin Y stain were subjected to a prescribed temperature exposure regime. Since eosin Y stains necrotic cells, they measured damage by counting the stained

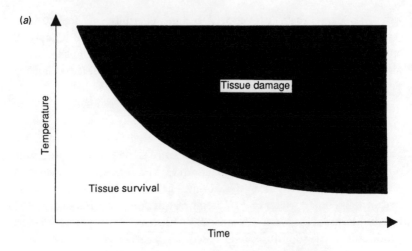

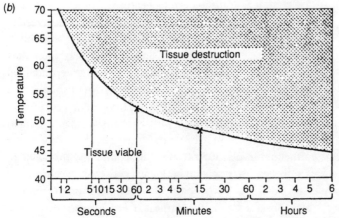

Fig. 3.3. The time–temperature dependence of thermal injury as predicted by Equation (6) is sketched (*a*) above and agrees with the measurements of heat tolerance in human epidermis[15] as shown in the graph (*b*) below.

cells. The time required for 50% of the cells to die ($X = 0.5$, hereafter referred to as $LT_{50}$) at a given temperature was set to the Arrhenius equation, yielding an activation energy for fibroblast necrosis of approximately 80 kcal/mole, a value that is substantially less than that for intact epithelium.

The effects of elevated temperatures on human fibroblasts were studied later and independently by Moussa *et al.*[19], using the appearance of irreversible morphological changes in the cells (blebs) to indicate cell damage. Using constant temperature protocols for values between 44 and 68 °C, they calculated the activation energy to be 59.5 kcal/mole. Moreover, for temperature protocols involving a linear rate of heating, the lethal damage time could be predicted using Equation (6). Further studies by Moussa *et al.*[20] addressed the rate of haemolysis of red blood cells exposed to elevated temperatures. They performed experiments similar to the earlier fibroblast experiments using temperatures between 44 and 60 °C. Two models were used to examine the data. The first method assumed that the damage kinetics involved two first-order processes, a double energy barrier model, consisting of a reversible alteration followed by irreversible damage. The first step was found to have an activation energy of 60 kcal/mole, and the second, 31 kcal/mole. The second approach assumed that the number of cells damaged at any given time was normally distributed. This statistical model fitted the data better, but the kinetic model provided more practical information about the damage energetics which could readily be used in a conceptional model such as Diller's[16].

Most important to our understanding of the pathophysiology of heat injury to cells, Gershfeld and Murayama[21] addressed the mechanism of red blood cell lysis at supraphysiological temperatures. Noting that haemolysis can occur at even slight temperature elevations above the physiological level, they proposed that different mechanisms govern haemolysis at different temperatures because the processes commonly thought to be involved (denaturation of structural proteins, inactivation of enzymes) do not occur below 45 °C. They postulated that haemolysis occurring below this temperature took place because the membrane lipid bilayer was transformed. Gershfeld and Murayama have also shown that this bilayer lipid assembly occurs spontaneously only at a critical temperature: the growth temperature of the particular cell. The critical temperature is a function of the types of phospholipids forming the membrane and thus varies among membranes of different compositions. Above the critical temperature, a certain amount of instability in the lipid membrane occurs. In this instance, assuming cell surface area remains constant and no lipid synthesis occurs, regions of the membrane are transformed, becoming lipid deficient, and resulting in leakage. These types of membrane transformation, in turn, can nucleate cell lysis.

In the Gershfeld and Murayama study, haemolysis was studied for the temperature range of 4 to 50 °C. Below 37 °C, no significant haemolysis occurred, but above 45 °C, haemolysis occurred with an activation energy of about 80 kcal/mole, which is consistent with the activation energies required to denature protein. Between 38 and 45 °C, haemolysis also occurred, but with a lower activation energy of 29 kcal/mole, a value considered too low to enable protein denaturation. However, this activation energy was sufficient to allow bilayer lipid membrane transformation.

We have measured the energetics of heat damage to skeletal muscle cell membranes[22]. Skeletal muscle cells were loaded with a fluorescent dye, fluorescein diacetate, which is split by cellular enzymes to pure fluorescein which is membrane impermeable. Dye leakage out of the cell following the application of electric pulses was used to determine the extent of membrane damage at different temperature levels. These studies demonstrated that supraphysiological temperatures damaged membranes at a rate which was temperature dependent. The data, presented in Fig. 3.4, indicate that, when cells are at supraphysiological temperatures, cell membrane lysis is probably the initial destructive event.

### Electroporation

Two types of membrane electrical breakdown have been experimentally demonstrated[23-25] to result from applied electric fields. The first, membrane rupture by electroporation, occurs in bilayer lipid membranes when transmembrane potentials between 200 to 500 mV are applied for longer than 0.1 ms. In the other, a breakdown process similar to dielectric breakdown appears in pure bilayer lipid membrances when transmembrane potentials exceed 800 mV[19]. For dielectric breakdown to occur the membrane voltage must be raised to the breakdown potential more rapidly than pores can form[23]. Dielectric breakdown manifests itself through a transient drop in the electrical resistance of the membrane.

Electroporation is thought to occur when strong electrical forces drive polar water molecules into molecular scale defects in the lipid bilayer component of the cell membrane (Fig. 3.5), causing the defect to enlarge[5,25]. If the pores become large enough, they continue to expand until the membrane ruptures. This process can happen in less than 100 $\mu s$[25]. Rupturing a soap bubble by pricking it with a pin is a familiar example of this[26]. However, in cell membranes, large proteins may act to stabilize the lipid bilayer and prevent the spread of pores beyond specific lipid domains of the membrane. This may explain why quasistable defects can be produced in cell membranes which spontaneously reseal soon afterwards.

Taylor and Michael[26], in a classic report, suggested that axisymmetric holes in thin sheets of fluid where surface tension forces predominate will expand if their initial radii are larger than the thickness of the sheet, while

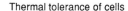

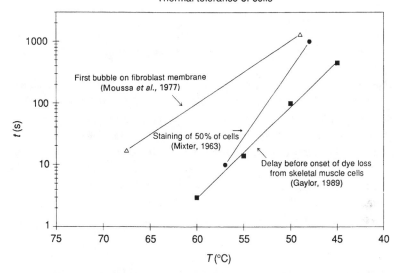

Fig. 3.4. Results of time delay until irreversible morphological changes in the cell occur. Mixter[18] used staining of damaged cells to indicate damage while Moussa *et al.*[19] used the appearance of the first bubble on the cell membrane. The damage criterion for the muscle cells experiments performed in our laboratories, as reported by Gaylor,[22] was the change in permeability of the cell membrane to fluorescein.

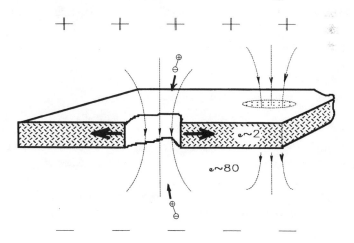

Fig. 3.5. Electric current lines are sketched as the current density increases in the aqueous pores of the cell membrane. The electric field is strongest in the pore. Water molecules are drawn into the pore from both sides because they are bipolar.

holes with radii smaller than that will close. This effect reflects the interfacial tension, which reduces the surface area. An applied $V_m$ lowers the critical pore radius to the point beyond which mechanical forces at the pore's edge cannot restrain the pore from expanding until the membrane is ruptured.

Several investigators have developed theories which use similar assumptions to explain electroporation. Powell and Weaver[25] based their model on the work of Litster[27], who introduced the idea that the Brownian motion of molecules in the membrane caused transient molecular defects or pores to form in bilayer lipid membranes. These defects are restrained by the interfacial forces at the pore's edge. The energy $\Delta\zeta$ needed to create a pore of radius $r$ is the increase in energy associated with the creation of the edge of the defect minus the eliminated surface area. If the defect was cylindrical, then:

$$\Delta\zeta = 2\pi\gamma r - \pi\psi r^2 \tag{7}$$

where $\psi$ is the interfacial energy per unit area of the membrane and $\gamma$ is the strain energy per unit length of the membrane pore edge. Powell and Weaver then added a term to this energy equation to include electrostatic energy effects which are associated with the transmembrane potential $V_m$:

$$\Delta\zeta = 2\pi\gamma r - \pi r^2(\psi + aV^2_m) \tag{8}$$

where $a$ is a positive parameter dependent on the dielectric permittivity of the membrane and the intracellular and extracellular fluids and on the membrane thickness $\delta_m$. Thus $V_m$ tends to decrease the stability of the membrane against thermal fluctuations by decreasing the amount of energy required to form a pore.

### Induced transmembrane potential by electric fields

Normally, the intracellular and extracellular fluids have nearly equal concentrations of mobile ions and thus their conductivities are very similar. Cell membrane conductivity, however, is characteristically $10^6$–$10^8$ fold less than the intracellular fluid. The cell can therefore be viewed as an insulating shell with a highly conductive interior. Because of the structure and electrical properties of cells, the magnitude of the transmembrane potential imposed by an electric field is dependent on cell size and shape. Consequently, currents established in the extracellular space by such low-frequency fields are shielded from the cytoplasm by the electrically insulating cell membrane. This shielding leads to large, induced transmembrane potentials in certain membrane regions. For a nonspherical cell, the maximum induced transmembrane potential depends on the cell's orientation with respect to the electric field. The largest induced potentials are reached in the ends of the cell when the major axis of the cell is parallel to the direction of the electric field. To predict the tissue electric field strength that puts a cell at risk of electrical breakdown, the induced transmembrane potential as a function of tissue field strength must be known.

Major electrical trauma frequently involves the upper extremities, setting up electrical current pathways as qualitatively depicted in Fig. 3.6. In such instances, the long axes of most skeletal muscle cells are oriented approximately parallel to the direction of the electric field lines. The potentials induced in the ends of these cells are significantly larger than those experienced by skeletal muscle cells in any other orientation or experienced by smaller cell types such as fibroblasts (Fig. 3.7). Thus, skeletal muscle is expected to be particularly susceptible to damage by the mechanism of membrane electroporation. The same argument holds for peripheral nerves which are also long, cylindrically shaped cells. In addition, cells that are surrounded by other cells can be expected to be more vulnerable than cells on the muscle surface because they experience a larger imposed transmembrane potential (see Chapter 4 p. 86). Similarly, it is plausible that muscle damage adjacent to cortical bone is explained by the higher resistivity of cortical bone.

## Pathogenesis of tissue injury

The extent of tissue injury manifested in electrical trauma victims is highly variable, dictated primarily by the circumstances of injury. For those who survive the possibility of cardiac arrhythmia, the remaining damage can range from a minimal skin contact burn with some transient neurological damage (Fig. 3.8) to extensive vaporization and charring of tissue (Fig. 3.9). The goal of this section is to interpret the clinical manifestations of electrical shock in terms of the previous discussion of the biophysical mechanisms associated with electrical trauma.

The extensive amount of muscle damage frequently manifested in victims of major electrical trauma has been likened to a crush injury[36,37]. Over the past two decades, considerable evidence has accumulated suggesting that rhabdomyolysis and peripheral nerve injury are important distinguishing features of electrical injury. The characteristic release of myoglobin from muscle cytoplasm[2] into the circulation of shock victims is well documented and is compelling evidence of rhabdomyolysis. However, the pathogenic

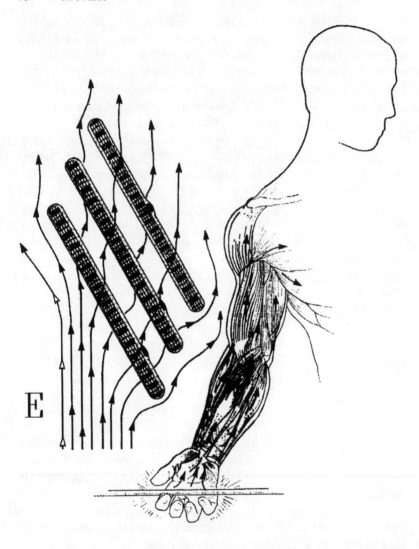

Fig. 3.6. Illustration of the current path through the upper extremity during electrical contact. The expanded view demonstrates electric field lines around muscle cells when the cells are almost parallel to the major axis of the skeletal muscle cells.

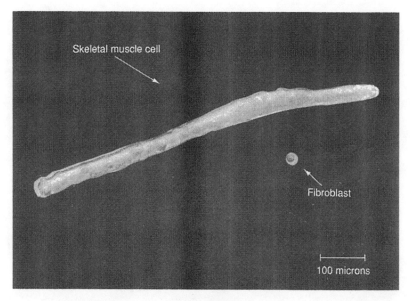

Fig. 3.7. The relative size of a single skeletal muscle cell versus that of a fibroblast can be appreciated from this photomicrograph of an 800 $\mu$m-long rat skeletal muscle cell adjacent to a 25 $\mu$m-diameter fibroblast in cell culture.

mechanisms responsible for rhabdomyolysis and neurolysis have not been specifically demonstrated by clinical studies. Joule heating had been commonly believed to be the only cause of tissue injury in electrical trauma; this has recently been called into question because the shock victim so often presents few external signs of thermal injury despite extensive underlying muscle and nerve damage[38]. Additionally, Lee and Kolodney[3] postulated that electroporation may contribute to rhabdomyolysis in electrical trauma victims.

### *The relative role of thermal versus nonthermal effects*

Many high voltage contacts establish electric fields between 1 and 10 kV/m in tissues. Examples include the field in the lips of a child who has bitten into a 110 V power cord and that in the upper extremity of a utility lineman in contact with a 10 kV power line. But in order to weigh the relative importance of membrane electrical breakdown and joule heating to the cellular damage occurring in electrical trauma, the magnitude and time dependence of the electric field and temperature exposures must be known.

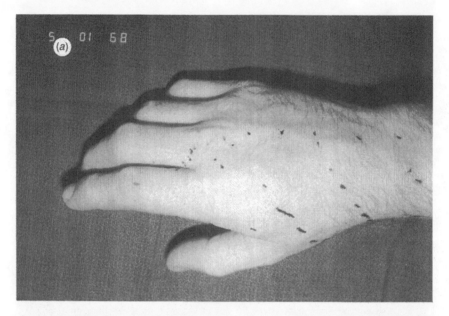

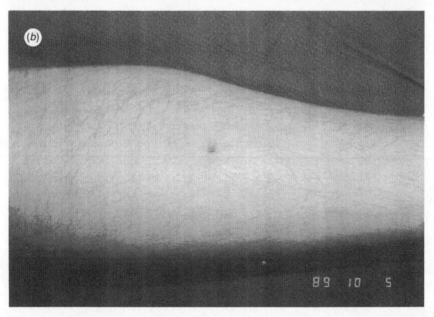

Fig. 3.8. 37 year-old electrician who briefly touched a 208 V line with the right index finger while his right leg brushed against grounded pipe. (a) Illustration of the skin contact point on index fingers and area of sensory loss in radial sensory nerve distribution. (b) Contact point on right leg.

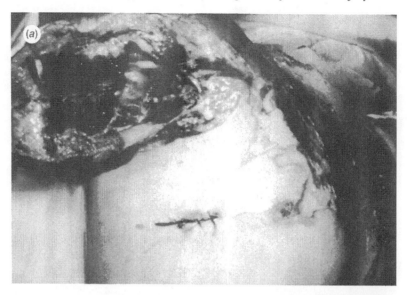

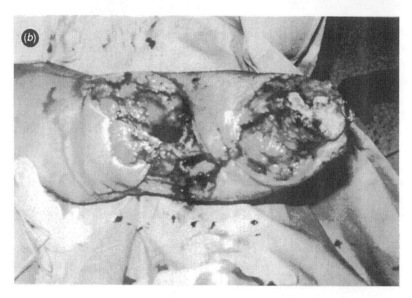

Fig. 3.9. 18 year-old college student who grasped a fallen tree limb which had come to rest on a power-line. (*a*) Remaining right arm which had been mostly vaporized from prolonged contact. (*b*) Loss of left hand and left forearm. (*c*) Forearm and hand prosthesis in place after amputation at the shoulder of the right upper extremity was performed.

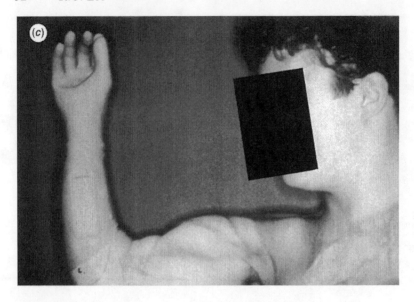

Usually, only the voltage contacted by the victim is known accurately; statistics from the Edison Electric Institute[39] indicate that contacts in the range of 6000 to 10 000 V are the most common cause of nonfatal injuries. The duration of the contact usually can only be estimated. Hence, the spatial distribution of both the electric field and the temperature attained in affected tissues are very difficult to determine. However, a few experimental and theoretical studies have been performed to attempt to address these issues.

Chilbert *et al.*, from the Medical College of Wisconsin, performed experiments on hogs to measure the amount of current flowing into various tissues during simulated electrical trauma[40,41]. They found that, while the artery and nerve exhibit the largest current densities because of their high conductivity, muscles carry the highest percentage of current due to their large cross-sectional area. They also noted that, because of its high resistivity, bone passes the least amount of current.

A second research group, Zelt *et al.* from the Microsurgical Research laboratories of Royal Victoria Hospital in Montreal, developed a high-voltage electrical injury model which used primates[42,43]. A computer-controlled system applied a predetermined amount of energy hand-to-hand, and the temperature, current, and voltage drop were monitored at various locations throughout the arm. In agreement with Sances' results[41], this group of researchers found that the muscle carried the highest percentage of the current. However, they measured a significantly larger current in the bone than the Sances team. The highest temperatures were measured in the muscles with the smallest cross-sectional area and at the wrists and elbow, where highly resistive bone predominates. Also of interest was the observation[43] of a 'central core of damage' in the muscles, even though measured voltage drops varied little over the muscle cross-section[44].

In a subsequent investigation, Chilbert *et al.*[45] passed electrical current through the hind limbs of dogs until the temperature of the gracilus muscle reached 60 °C. The muscle was removed and both electrical impedance measurements and cellular histology analysis were performed. Their results indicated a strong correlation between increases in the extent of cellular damage and decreases in electrical impedance. While this study clearly demonstrated that rhabdomyolysis was an important component of electrical trauma, it was not designed to discriminate between thermal and nonthermal mechanisms of injury.

To address the question of whether electroporation could account for the type of muscle disruption demonstrated by Chilbert *et al.*[45], a series of *in vitro* studies were performed[24] using rat *biceps femoris* muscle. Electric field pulses between 30 V/cm and 150 V/cm that lasted between 0.1 to 10 ms were applied to a muscle preparation consisting of intact 2 cm long muscles placed parallel to the applied field. The impedance of the muscle was measured after 0, 10, 30 and 60 field pulses (Fig. 3.10), which were spaced 30 s apart to allow thermal relaxation. The exposure chamber and muscle tissue were kept at 10 °C for the entire duration of the two hours of the experiment. The maximum temperature rise for the largest combination of pulse width and electric field amplitude was 8 °C, a clearly nonpathologic temperature peak ( $< 20$ °C).

Consequently, it was found that muscle cell disruption and the resulting drop in impedance was caused solely by electroporation. The probability of the muscle cell membrane rupture by electroporation was found to increase with the square of the electric field strength[24] and to be proportional to the duration of cell exposure to the field. Field strengths greater than 60 V/cm and field exposure durations greater than 0.1 ms were required to cause membrane damage. Experiments indicated that membrane rupture was caused directly by the imposed transmembrane potential and was not spontaneously reversible. Furthermore, it was demonstrated that the histological pattern of skeletal muscle disruption characteristic of electrical shock could be reproduced in this model of electroporation injury (Fig. 3.11); scanning electron microscopy also revealed membrane damage (Fig.

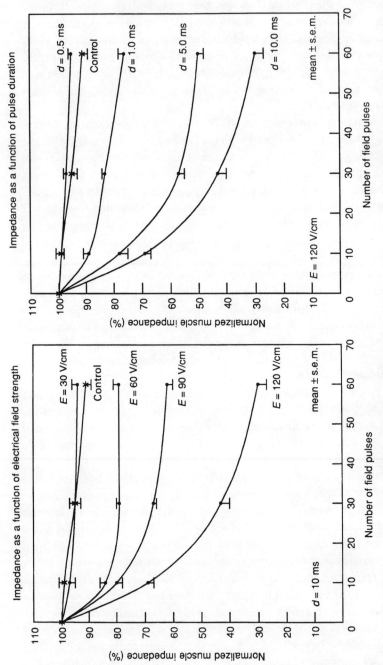

Fig. 3.10. Muscle impedance drop caused by exposure to short duration ($d$), high-intensity electric field pulses ($E$). Pulses were separated by 10 seconds. Impedance measurements were normalized to the initial value before field pulses were applied. Each point represents the mean and standard error of the mean for five muscle samples.

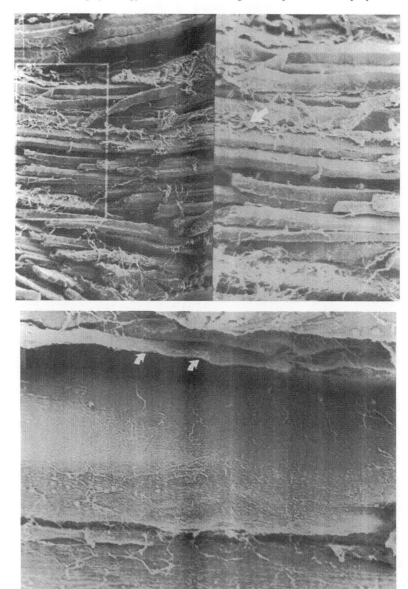

Fig. 3.11. Scanning electron micrograph (SEM) showing organization of control (*above*) and field-exposed (*below*) skeletal muscle explants. Each photograph is of a split view showing calibrated (80x) (*left*) and magnified (*right*) views. The magnified view corresponds to the white box on the calibrated view. Note the twisting of the muscle cell bundle (*larger arrow*) and the loss of parallel organization in the field-exposed cells, indicating cellular disruption. The control did not receive electric shock.

56    R.C. Lee

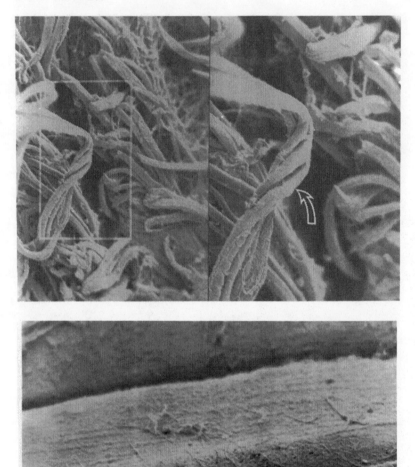

Fig. 3.12. High magnification (2000x) SEM view of the muscle surface in control (*above*) and shocked (*below*) muscles. Note the structural defects in the membrane of the shocked muscle cell. The crack (*large arrows*) may represent a coalescence of smaller defects (*small arrows*). Arterioles in the control view (*curved arrow*) are not to be confused with muscle cells.

3.12). It is entirely possible that the cellular disruption found by Chilbert *et al.* was due to electroporation. Human cells can be expected to be even more susceptible because they are characteristically larger than the muscle cells used in these experiments.

In order to address the specific questions relating to the contribution of heat injury, a better understanding of heat kinetics is needed. To accomplish this, Tropea and Lee[12] undertook a computer simulation of electrical shock involving the upper extremity. This work is presented in Chapter 3, p. 36. The simulation is based on data accumulated by the Edison Electric Institute[39] indicating that the majority of contact voltages for surviving electric utility linemen range from 1 to 10 kV. The data emanated from that model provide some useful insights into the tissue temperature dynamics in major electrical trauma victims. From this, it was apparent that the duration of contact was the most important parameter governing the mechanism of tissue injury.

### *Duration of contact*

The most meaningful insight into the pathogenesis of tissue injury in electrical trauma can be gained by evaluating the predictions of the damage accumulation expression equation (6), given the tissue temperature–time curves calculated by Tropea and Lee[12]. For the distal forearm, more than 0.5 s are required before most of the cells are heat damaged when the hand-to-hand contact voltage is 10 kV. However, another response is important to consider. Within 10 to 100 ms (the excitation–contraction response time of human skeletal muscles), muscles located in the current path will contract. Depending on the relative hand-conductor position, this can either induce the victim to improve the mechanical contact by grasping the conductor or propel the victim away from the contact. Judging from eyewitness reports, the latter is more common, perhaps because most victims experience generalized muscle contractions. Under these circumstances it therefore seems reasonable to predict contact durations on the order of 100 ms or less. The most abundant information regarding duration of contact for accidental electrical shock is from eyewitness reports, although this is probably the least reliable source. The most common report is that the victim was instantly 'blown' or 'knocked' away from the contact. Until more precise clinical data are available, the relative role of heating versus electroporation cannot be answered. Additional cellular pathological studies may be the only way to address these issues.

### Central role of the cell membrane

The results from the author's research as well as that by others indicate that both heat and electroporation damage the cell membrane. This evidence suggests that *the loss of normal integrity of the cell's plasma membrane appears to be the most important event in the pathogenesis of electrical trauma.* While supraphysiological temperatures can lead to denaturation of macromolecules throughout the cell, the weight of the evidence indicates that the cell membrane is the structure most susceptible to damage[18,21,22,54]. Of course, under conditions relevant to this discussion, electroporation only takes place at the cell membrane. In Fig. 3.13, experimental data from the experiments[22] is presented which illustrate leakage of membrane impermeable dye from rat skeletal muscle cells. The cell membranes were permeated either by exposure to supraphysiological temperatures or by exposure to strong field pulses and the amount of dye remaining in the cytoplasm measured and plotted. These experiments document that skeletal muscle membrane damage can be caused either by exposure to supraphysiological temperatures or by electroporation.

## Clinical manifestations and treatment guidelines

As a consequence of the confusion regarding the mechanisms of electrical injury, many empirically established guidelines exist. While major improvements in survival following electrical trauma over the past two decades have resulted, primarily from advances supporting organismal physiology in trauma victims in general, few advances have been made towards reversing tissue necrosis. The goal of this section is to place the foregoing discussion of electrical trauma and our experimental results into a clinically relevant context. In addition, an effort will be made to provide some insight into the rationale for treatment.

### Classification of injury

The prevailing practice is to classify electrical injuries as 'high voltage' if the contact voltage was 1000 V or more, or 'low voltage' if the contact voltage was less than 1000 V. This classification is irrelevant to the pathophysiology of electrical injury because it is the electric field (the spatial gradient of voltage) which is the significant parameter. The difference between the electric cord injury to an infant's lips and a lineman in contact with 10 000 V is not the field strength or pathophysiology of tissue injury, it is the volume and site of tissue injured.

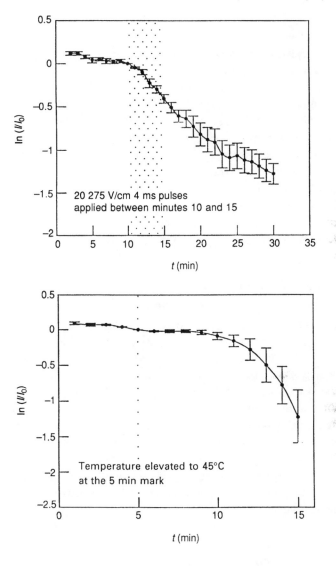

Fig. 3.13. Results from two experiments conducted in one laboratory[22] demonstrating that either electroporation or exposure to supraphysiological temperatures could damage adult rat skeletal muscle cell membranes. Rapid loss of fluorescein dye from the cytoplasm indicated injury. (*left*) Plot of intracellular dye content before ($I_0$) and after ($I$) the application of electric shocks to muscle cells oriented perpendicular to the applied field. (*right*) Before and after step temperature changes from 37 to 45 °C. The increased rate of dye loss reflects membrane damage. The fact of perpendicular orientation explains the magnitude of the field strength required to produce damage.

Because the vast majority of injuries are caused by contact with commercial electrical power, no attempt has been made to discuss the role of frequency as an influential parameter. In practice this becomes a problem only when injuries from lightning are discussed. With respect to the charging time of cells, the duration of lightning pulses is very short ( $<$ $<$ 1 $\mu$s), meaning that lightning should be considered as a very high frequency current. These currents are not amplified by the cell membrane, since the membrane is no more vulnerable to electrical breakdown than are other cellular structures. With respect to lightning injury, it is very unlikely for someone to survive a direct strike by lightning. The heat and mechanical stress from thermo-acoustic effects are strong enough to split trees. Survivors are usually those who were near a strike and most of their resultant injuries lie on the skin surface and resulted from complex electromagnetic interactions.

### General considerations

Following current practice, victims of major electrical trauma should be admitted to a hospital intensive care unit staffed by a multidisciplinary team. Factors such as the length of contact, the contact voltage, the circuit paths, clothing worn, and protective circuitry give important insight into the severity of the injury and should be recorded as accurately as possible; often the victim sustains a fall after contact which can cause major skeletal and internal organ injuries as well. It is crucial to evaluate the patient for blunt trauma before concentrating on the treatment of electrically injured tissue. Also, because of tetanic contractions induced by electric current, skeletal fractures and joint dislocations are common. Cardiac arrest can also be caused by the electric current. Since a victim may have suffered from cardioversion in a fall, cardiac injury should be suspected in all electrical accident survivors.

While the current path in electrical shocks are predictable, in very high voltage shocks (i.e. voltage $<$ 50 kV), several entry and exit points are possible since current paths are established through multiple arcs. Moreover, standard commercial current (60 Hz ac) reverses direction 120 times a second; a skin contact therefore can simultaneously serve as both an entry and exit point. That this is not readily understood explains the common mistake of trying to classify all skin wounds on victims injured by commercial electric power as either entrance or exit wounds.

Any organ in the current path can be damaged by the joule heating and/ or electroporation resulting from electric shock. In the majority of cases,

Table 3.4. *Basic clinical management principles*

| | |
|---|---|
| Initial | Support vital organ systems<br>Access other injuries: fractures, haemorrhages, etc.<br>Correct pH and electrolyte imbalances<br>Fluid volume resuscitation |
| Early | Fasciotomies<br>Operative debridement<br>Urine alkalysation ⟶ { Second look procedure:<br>Treat cardiac muscle<br>damage |
| Intermediate | Begin surgical reconstruction<br>Nutritional support<br>Correct electrolyte disorders<br>Musculoskeletal splinting<br>Neurophysiological studies |
| Late | Rehabilitation<br>Manage neurological sequelae |

the clinical picture is dominated by direct injuries to skin, nerve, skeletal muscle, bone and organs in the cardiovascular system. While secondary problems often develop in the lung and kidney, this essay focuses on the organs which are primarily affected in electrical trauma.

Hunt *et al.* reviewed the widely practised management guidelines for electrical trauma victims in 1980[60]. These have not changed significantly since they were first published. These guidelines are summarized in Table 3.4. Because of the variation in deep or occult tissue damage, and our inability to predict accurately the amount of tissue loss, standard fluid management guidelines based on the surface wound size cannot be established. Intravenous fluid requirements are often massive and the volume of resuscitation fluid should be guided by the urine output and the presence of myoglobulinuria. Thus, maintaining adequate perfusion pressure and monitoring acid–base balance are important. While these guidelines provide for the initial overall management of the patient, they are not specific to preventing ongoing tissue loss nor reversing myonecrosis.

### *Cutaneous injury*

The high-voltage electrical trauma victim usually presents with charred skin craters at the contact sites and an adjacent area of inflamed, oedematous skin (Fig. 3.14). However, there is no correlation between the

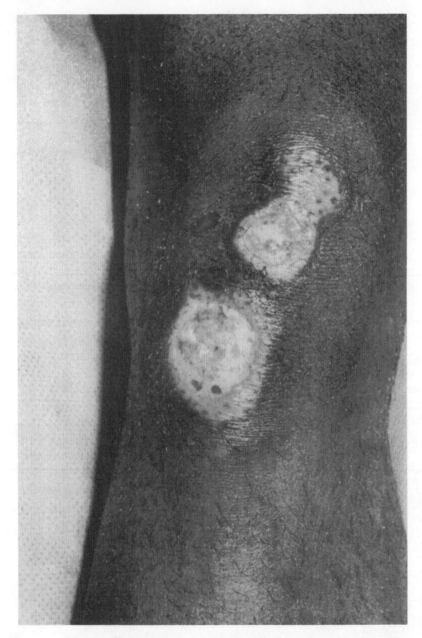

Fig. 3.14. Sharply demarcated wound on the knee of a shock victim who was kneeling during contact.

size of the contact skin injury and the actual total extent of all injuries. The total extent of injury to the victim is nearly always more extensive than is apparent. Frequently, there is charred tissue surrounding the skin craters which requires debridement. Flame burns are frequently found in association with electric shock because clothing was ignited by an arc. Several clinical reports list electrical injury victims according to the percentage of the skin surface area burned. Clearly, there is not much value in this other than to record the extent of flame burn as a comorbid factor.

As stated above, an ambient air temperature of a 3000 °C electrical arc is enough to cause substantial skin injury, even when no current actually passes through the victim. The depth of such a burn is related to the duration of exposure and may be predicted from models published by Diller[16] and Palla[17]. Occasionally, injured victims will arrive at the emergency room covered by a black coating. This can result from the metallic contacts being vaporized by the arc, followed by metal condensation on the epidermis (Fig. 3.15), an effect which can give the illusion of an eschar. The most important concept to realize is that victims of arc burns do not suffer the same injuries as those whose injuries result from current flow through the body. Instead, arc burns should be treated as thermal burns.

### Nerve injury

When the victim makes direct contact with a current, acute peripheral and central nerve damage almost invariably occurs and must be identified. Even when the victim has experienced relatively minor trauma, some peripheral nerve injury is common (Fig. 3.8). In fact, in many instances where only a brief shock without other system injuries had occurred, peripheral nerve dysfunction is often the only manifestation of the injury. The relatively high vulnerability of nerves is consistent with the fact that their space constant ($\lambda_m > 1$ mm) is quite large compared to the small size of other cells. Thus, theoretically, peripheral nerves should be highly vulnerable to damage by electroporation.

Peripheral nerve damage may be manifested by paraesthesia, dysaesthesia or anaesthesia, or as a motor nerve dysfunction. If abnormalities are found on physical examination, nerve conduction measurements of peripheral nerves must be made to assess quantitatively the extent of damage and precisely localize the conduction blockade. Patients with peripheral nerve damage may regain sensory and motor functions spontaneously in a matter of several weeks if the surrounding tissue is healthy and if there has not been a large thermal component in the injury.

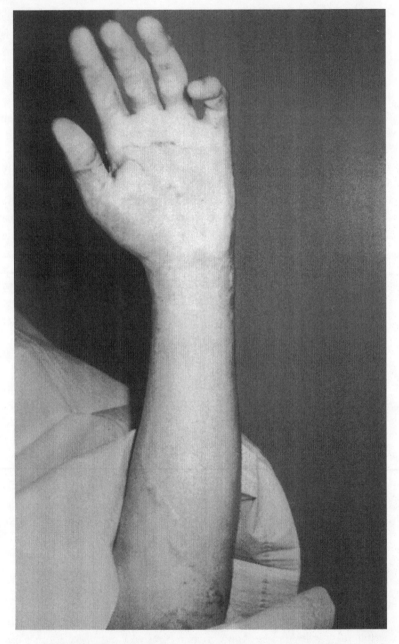

Fig. 3.15. The left upper extremity of an electrician whose wrench contacted two conductors in a circuit breaker box. The wrench was partially vaporized, leaving a black coating on the burned epidermis. The skin received mostly partial thickness burns.

These clinical findings support our theoretical hypothesis that peripheral nerves are the tissues most vulnerable to injury. Therefore, repeated clinical and neuro-physiological examinations are essential for establishing a prognosis as well as for guiding the therapeutic course.

Particularly in cases in which nerve injury is the only form of damage (other than with skin contact burns), the evidence points to electroporation as the prominent mechanism of injury. It is unlikely for the peripheral nerve to reach substantially higher temperatures than surrounding tissues, although the relative susceptibility of nerves to heat injury is not clinically established. However, it does not seem likely that peripheral nerve membranes would be more vulnerable to heat injury than other mammalian cell membranes. If contact duration is long enough to produce high temperatures, heat injury will also be a factor. The conductivity of peripheral nerve tissue is between 20 and 50% higher than surrounding tissues. Because the rate of joule heating is proportional to the conductivity, as shown in Equation (4), the temperature change in nerves could be somewhat higher than in the surrounding tissues. But since nerves are usually less than 1 cm in diameter, heat conduction to surrounding tissues will buffer this effect.

### Skeletal muscle injury

Injury to skeletal muscle tends to dominate the clinical picture of electrical trauma[36,37]. Fixed, contracted muscle in the rigor state is one of the clinical hallmarks of major electrical trauma, resulting, as it does, from muscle cell disruption. By virtue of their large size, skeletal muscle cells are certainly more vulnerable to injury than smaller cells in other tissues (with the exception of peripheral nerves). Although it seems unlikely, they may also be more vulnerable to injury from exposure to supraphysiological temperatures, for reasons discussed on pp. 34–6[14,15,18,22].

The importance of this is underscored by the common finding of nonviable muscle covered by viable fascia, tendons, and other subcutaneous tissues. In fact, muscle layers adjacent to bone seem to be more vulnerable to electrical injury than more superficial muscles. This certainly could not be predicted by the temperature dynamics shown in the chapter by Tropea and Lee[14]. The findings of Zelt *et al.*, increased injury in the central core of muscles, are also enigmatic in light of this data. The inconsistency between the pattern of injury and that predicted by the solution to the bioheat equation suggests that an alternate mechanism of injury, such as electroporation, may be acting synergistically.

Because of the nonuniform pattern of damage to skeletal muscle and because of the inability to detect visually changes in electroporated muscle tissues, methods for localizing the damaged muscle are needed. The resistivity of electrically injured muscle decreases proportionately to the extent of cell membrane lysis[24,45]. Thus, identifying instances of this damage is crucial if we are to distinguish between apparent and actual viable muscle tissue. We have found that technetium-99m stannous pyrophosphate (Tc-PYP) radionucleotide scanning is useful in localizing nonviable muscle in electrical trauma victims because it is sensitive enough to map large areas of damaged muscle[60]. The isotope is administered intravenously and the scan is performed 2 h later.

Compartment syndrome and compression neuropathies are other common manifestations of an electrically traumatized extremity. Within minutes after injury, tissue oedema begins to increase due to increased vascular permeability and release of intracellular contents into the extracellular space. If peripheral sensory nerves are intact, pain with passive flexion and extension may, if present, be useful as an early finding of compartment syndrome. The most common compartments affected are those of the forearm and the leg which have two and four compartments, respectively. When one compartment is damaged, the adjacent ones also must be decompressed.

Escharotomy and fasciotomy may be required anywhere on the body and should be performed even if compartment syndrome is only slightly suspected (Fig. 3.16). Tense compartments may be recognized by palpation, and compartment pressures should be documented. Compartment fluid pressures in excess of 30 mm Hg are abnormal and indicate the need for fasciotomy. However, measurements of fluid pressures in smaller compartments, such as the intrinsic muscles of the hand, are notoriously unreliable, and fasciotomy should be performed empirically whenever the high voltage trauma involves the hand.

Releasing of intracellular muscle contents into the circulation can cause significant electrolyte derangements. Elevated temperatures lyse red blood cells in the current path, releasing nephrotoxic-free haemoglobin in the serum and acute anaemia. Blood assays including haematocrit, haemoglobin, serum electrolytes ($Na^+$, $K^+$, $Cl^-$, $HCO_3^-$ and $Ca^{2+}$), and arterial blood gases should be obtained immediately. Additional studies including blood and urine myoglobin, plasma-free haemoglobin and isoenzymes of creatinine phosphokinase levels should also be obtained to guide therapy. Peripheral pulses and arterial pressures should be accurately determined by Doppler assay to rapidly diagnose significant vascular compromise. We have found arteriography to be only rarely helpful; moreover, Clayton *et*

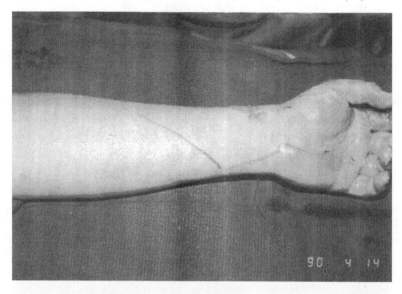

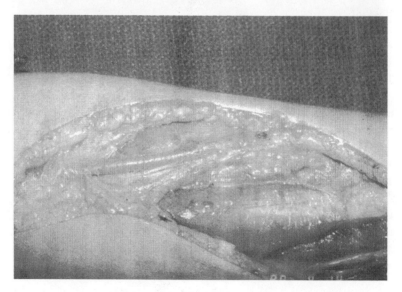

Fig. 3.16. Wide forearm fasciotomy in a male electric shock victim. Note the bulging muscles and the widely gaping skin edges. The muscle appears viable at this point, approximately 4 hours after injury. Several days later, some forearm muscle was debrided before final skin grafting.

al.[59] have found in a large study that major arteries usually remain patent after electric shock.

After initial resuscitation, patients with high-voltage electrical injuries requiring decompression of their extremities should be taken to the operating theatre without delay. Escharotomies may be performed at the bedside, whereas fasciotomies should be performed in an operating room environment. Decompression of compressed compartments is one of the most important steps for treatment. Fasciotomy may salvage an otherwise moribund muscle group. The superficial and deep muscle compartments must be opened and frequently it is helpful to release the epimysium which may also cause constriction. Frequently, the release of a muscle compartment is followed by massive bulging of muscle and a readily observed increase in tissue perfusion. When the electrical current path is through the hand, the intrinsic muscles of the hand should be similarly decompressed. Similarly, the nerves must be released from any potential sites which may cause compression, i.e. carpal tunnel, Guyon's canal and the cubital tunnel. Well-fashioned splints are essential to maintain joints in a position of function and to protect vascular perfusion.

Deciding at the initial operation what muscle tissue is irretrievably injured and requires debridement is a difficult problem. Electrically damaged muscle is often normal in appearance at initial exploration, unless there has been severe heat exposure. Even muscle which incorporates Tc-PYP may appear normal on first inspection. The most widely practised surgical approach is to reinspect the wound and debride obviously necrotic tissue every 48 h. Between debridements, allograft is applied to decompressed, exposed viable muscle, and mafenide (Sulfamylon) is applied to marginal tissue every 6–8 h. Mafenide is the topical antimicrobial of choice due to its penetrating power and its action against *Clostridium perfringens*. Closure should wait until a wound is in bacteriological balance and free of all dead and/or marginal tissue. Whether the recognition of additional nonviable tissue at each of the serial debridements represents 'progressive necrosis' or 'progressive recognition' of fatally damaged tissue remains an unresolved question.

### Skeletal injury

Skeletal injury often accompanies major electrical trauma. Cortical bone has a much higher heat capacity than surrounding soft tissues; consequently, it takes longer to cool. Because the periosseus muscles are more vulnerable to injury than more superficial muscle groups, it is commonly believed that joule heating is responsible for the bulk of heat damage to the surrounding tissue. This explanation would only be valid in circumstances where both bone and muscle are electrically in series rather than in parallel. The latter seems to be most prevalent. Based on our theoretical model, we have shown that the temperature of muscle rises more quickly than bone. Thus, the belief that muscle injury results from bone heating is unlikely.

The most common skeletal injuries are related to powerful tetanic contractions by the muscle which lead to long bone fractures, joint dislocations and cervical spinal features. These should be managed according to standard procedures. Management of electrically damaged bone obeys rules for other types of skeletal trauma of which the basic tenets are debridement and early coverage with vascularized soft tissue. Prolonged exposure and subsequent drying should be carefully avoided. Late problems such as heterotopic ossification of tissues and skeletal growth disorders in injured adolescents often require surgical correction.

### *Rehabilitation*

Sensory and motor functions in injured extremities may be severely impaired, requiring extensive postoperative therapy and functional reconstruction including tendon transfers and nerve grafting. The decision to salvage an electrically injured extremity should be carefully weighed against the potential for significant morbidity and mortality, especially when a cold, insensate, stiff extremity will be less useful to a patient than a functional prosthesis. This decision should be made as soon as possible to minimize the risks as well as the physical and psychological effort invested in salvaging an extremity that will be amputated eventually.

The late sequelae of electrical injury are generally the consequence of acute tissue loss or damage; the extent of tissue damage may not be recognized immediately. Neuromuscular problems usually result from muscle fibrosis and peripheral neuropathies, coupled with loss of tissue from debridements and joint stiffness. Sensorimotor neuropathies, paraesthesias, dysaesthesias, and reflex sympathetic dystrophy may persist long after the wounds have healed. Cold intolerance may persist for 2 to 3 years, and growth disturbances producing skeletal deformities in children are frequent long-term sequelae.

The aetiology of many of the late sequelae of electrical trauma is unknown. Cataracts occur in 1–2% of victims even though the current path obviously did not involve the head or the neck. A full spectrum of central neurologic disorders has been described as late sequelae of electrical shock[61]. Paraplegia and tetraplegia have been reported to appear even 5 years after the injury[7]. Subtle mental status and personality changes may severely affect the patient's motivation and participation in the rehabilitation programme that is crucial to regaining optimum function.


### Horizons in management

The weight of existing evidence suggests that the underlying pathophysiology of electrical trauma is concentrated at the level of the cell membrane. This is of paramount importance. Conceptually, if the cell membrane is resealed soon after rupture, the cell may survive. In fact, cells are known to survive transient membrane permeabilization. Electroporation has been used for two decades in research involving the exchange of proteins between cells and for inducing a membrane impermeable agent into the cytoplasm during research. Mechanical disruption of cells by scraping them from the culture plate is another widely used technique for loading fluorescent probes into cells. However, these techniques are successful only if the cell survives. Many investigators report informally that cells survive transient permeabilization that lasts for up to 45 minutes. Whether cells *in vivo* will survive transient membrane permeation requires further investigation.

Several years ago, we began studies designed to identify physiologically tolerable agents which can seal permeated cell membranes. Recently several synthetic macromolecules were found that appear to fulfill this objective. Among these agents, a water soluble, electrically amphipolar poloxamer 188 (an 8 kD reverse tri-block co-polymer may be useful clinically in reversing areas of tissue loss.

In a series of cell culture experiments utilizing poloxamer 188, adult rat skeletal muscle cells were harvested as described above[35] and maintained under standard culture conditions. The cells were then loaded with the fluorescent dye carboxyfluorescein diacetate. Cytoplasmic enzymes cleave the diacetate groups which render the dye membranes impermeable. Next, cells were subjected to a single, 4 ms duration, 400 V/cm electric field pulse while under epifluorescent imaging. The amount of dye remaining in the cytoplasm was measured by video image analysis. The effect of the co-polymer on membrane integrity was measured by adding 8 mg/ml of the co-polymer to one group of cells 3 min after the shock while the control group received phosphate-buffered saline instead of the co-polymer. Data from individual control and co-polymer treated cells are shown in Fig. 3.17 and indicate that the presence of the co-polymer reversed the membrane damage. Preliminary results from a second series of experiments suggest

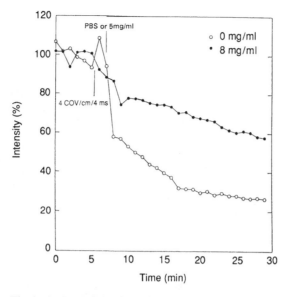

Fig. 3.17. Normalized intracellular carboxyfluorescein content before and after delivery of a single 400 V/cm, 4 ms duration electric field pulse while the cell is oriented perpendicularly to the field. Note the effect of adding PBS (the control, represented by open circles) or the R-21 co-polymer (treated cells, closed circles) 3 minutes after applying the electric field on the rate of dye loss.

that the co-polymer will reseal cell membranes damaged by exposure to temperatures up to 50 °C. Further study of this effect is currently in progress. Pre-incubating cells in media containing the co-polymer also seems to stabilize the membrane against electroporation injury[62].

Other potential strategies for resealing the membrane include using naturally occurring fusagenic proteins (Table 3.5) and relatively unstable lysosomes comprised of lyso-phospholipids and either DMSO or cholesterol (Fig. 3.18)[63]. Another approach for improving cell survival is the use of pharmacologic agents to block ion channels on the remainder of the intact membrane. Research along both of these possibilities is progressing.

### Summary and conclusions

The pathogenesis of electrical injury is more complex than was once thought. The cellular membrane damage evidenced by myoglobin release may occur by either heating or electroporation. The relative contributions of heat and electroporation depend on the duration of electric current

Table 3.5. *Bilayer lipid membrane fusion promoters*

| Promoter | Source |
| --- | --- |
| Synexin | Membrane intercalating–calcium binding protein ubiquitous in secretory cells |
| Calelectrin | From the electric organ of electric fish |
| Lectins | *(a)* Wheat germ agglutinin<br>*(b) Ricinus communis* agglutinin<br>*(c)* Soybean agglutinin |
| Clathrin | Ubiquitous protein in almost all cells |
| Sperm proteins | *(a)* Bindin<br>*(b)* Lysin |

passage, the orientation of the cells in the current path, their location and other factors. If the contact time is brief, nonthermal mechanisms of cell damage will be most important but when contact time is much longer, heat damage predominates. The time before heat damage becomes significant is a function of the electric field strength in the tissue. When heat damage predominates, the injury may no longer be limited to the plasma membrane alone. If other intracellular membranes are involved, damage is likely to be irreversible. These parameters also determine the pattern of injury. Damage by joule heating is not known to be dependent on cell size, whereas larger cells are more vulnerable to membrane breakdown by electroporation. Cells do survive transient plasma membrane rupture under appropriate circumstances. So, if electroporation is the primary mechanism of damage, then injured tissue may be salvageable and the challenge for the future is to identify a technique to promptly reseal the damaged membranes.

Current therapy requires a fully staffed and well-equipped intensive care unit, available operating suites and the full range of available medical specialists. Major teaching hospitals are usually the prime candidates for operating an electric trauma unit. After the initial resuscitation, efforts should be directed primarily towards preventing additional tissue loss mediated through the compartment syndrome, compressive neuropathies or the presence of necrotic tissue. Renal and cardiac failure due to the release of intracellular muscle contents into the circulation must be prevented. Attention can then be directed towards maximizing tissue salvage and preventing late skeletal and neuromuscular complications. Finally, complex reconstructive procedures are needed to optimize the

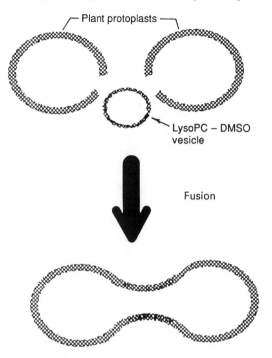

Fig. 3.18. Spontaneous resealing of electroporated plant protoplasts by the addition of Lyso-PC lysosomes (vesicles) to the bath as demonstrated by Nea *et al.*[63]

functional value of the remaining tissue. These goals should be borne in mind throughout the acute care of the patient.

In the future, new guidelines for treating electrical trauma will be based on a clearer picture of the relevant pathophysiology. These strategies will rely on improved diagnostic imaging and on reversing the fundamental problem of cell membrane damage. Moreover, complex biochemical and organ system pathophysiologic interactions will have to be carefully managed[64]. Research is presently directed towards improving understanding of these basic issues. If successful, these efforts should tremendously improve the prognosis of victims following electrical trauma.

**Acknowledgements**

The author is indebted to the editorial assistance of Anthony Steinhoff, Philip River and Pravin Patel, MD, without which this manuscript would not have been completed. The research presented here has been partly

74      *R.C. Lee*

supported by: The Electric Power Research Institute; Empire State Electric
Research Corporation; EUA Service Corporation; Northeast Utilities
Service Corporation; Pacific Gas & Electric Company; Pennsylvania
Power & Light Company; The Public Service Company of Oklahoma and
The Public Service Electric and Gas Company of New Jersey.

**References**

1 DiVincenti, F.C., Moncrief, J.A. & Pruitt, B.A. Jr. (1969). Electrical
   injuries: a review of 65 cases. *Journal of Trauma*. 9: 497. (1978).
2 Rouse, R.G. & Dimick, A.R. (1978). The treatment of electrical injury
   compared to burn injury: A Review of pathophysiology and
   comparison of patient management protocols. *Journal of Trauma*, **18**,
   43.
3 Lee, R.C. & Kolodney, M.S. (1987). Electrical injury mechanisms:
   dynamics of the thermal response. *Plastic and Reconstructive Surgery*,
   **80**, 663.
4 Lee, R.C. & Kolodney, M.S. (1989). Electrical injury mechanisms:
   Electrical breakdown of cell membranes. *Plastic and Reconstructive
   Surgery*, **80**, 672. 1987.
5 Lee, R.C., Gaylor, D.C., Bhatt, D.L. & Israel, D.A. (1988). Role of cell
   membrane rupture in the pathogenesis of electrical trauma. *Journal of
   Surgical Research*, **44(6)**, 709.
6 Jaffé, R.H. (1928). Electropathology: A Review of the pathologic
   changes produced by electric currents. *Archives of Pathology*, **5**, 837.
7 Farrell, D.F. & Starr, A. (1968). Delayed neurological sequelae of
   electrical injuries. *Neurology*, **18**, 601.
8 Geddes, L.A. & Baker, L.E. (1967). The specific resistance of biological
   material – a compendium of data for the biomedical engineer and
   physiologist. *Medical and Biological Engineering*, **5**, 271.
9 Hunt, J.L., Mason, A.D., Masterson, T.S. & Pruitt, B.A. (1976). The
   Pathophysiology of acute electrical injuries. *Journal of Trauma*. **16(5)**,
   335.
10 Sances, A., Larson, S.J., Myklebust, J. & Cusick, J.F. (1979). Electrical
   injuries. *Surgery, Gynecology & Obstetrics*, **149**, 97.
11 McLeod, K.J., Lee, R.C. & Ehrlich, H.P. (1987). Frequency
   dependence of electrical field modulation of fibroblast protein
   synthesis. *Science*, 236, 1465.
12 Tropea, B.I. & Lee, R.C. Determinants of heat-mediated injury in
   electrical trauma victims, this volume.
13 Pennes, H.H. (1948). Analysis of tissue and arterial blood temperatures
   in the resting human forearm. *Journal of Applied Physics*, **1**, 93.
14 Henriques, F.C. (1947). Studies of thermal injury V: The Predictability
   and the significance of thermally induced rate processes leading to
   irreversible epidermal injury. *Archives of Pathology*, **43**, 489.
15 Moritz, A.R. & Henriques, F.C. (1947). Studies of thermal injury II:
   The relative importance of time and surface temperature in the
   causation of cutaneous burns. *American Journal of Pathology*, **23**, 695.
16 Diller, K.R. & Hayes, L.J. (1983). A finite element model of burn
   injury in blood-perfused skin. *Transactions ASME Journal of
   Biomechanical Engineering*, **105**, 300.

17 Palla, R.L. (1981). A heat transfer analysis of scald injury. *US Dept. of Commerce NBSIR* 81-2320.
18 Mixter, G., Jr, Delhery, G.P., Derksen, W.L. & Monahan, T.I. (1963). The influence of time on the death of HeLa cells at elevated temperatures. In *Temperature: its measurement and control in science and industry*. pp. 177–82, New York: Reinhold.
19 Moussa, N.A., McGrath, J.J., Cravalho, E.G. & Asimacopoulos, P.J. (1977). Kinetics of thermal injury in cells. *Journal of Biomedical Engineering*, **99**, 155.
20 Moussa, N.A., Tell, E.N. & Cravalho, E.G. (1979). Time progression of hemolysis of erythrocyte populations exposed to supraphysiological temperatures. *ASME Journal of Biomechanical Engineering*, **101**, 213.
21 Gershfeld, N.L. & Murayama M. (1968). Thermal instability of red blood cell membrane bilayers: Temperature dependence of hemolysis. *Journal of Membrane Biology*, **101**, 67.
22 Gaylor, D.G. (1989). *Physical Mechanisms of Cellular Injury in Electrical Trauma.* PhD Thesis, Massachusetts Institute of Technology (supervised by R.C. Lee).
23 Zimmerman, U. (1986). Electrical breakdown: electropermeabilization and electrofusion. *Review in Physiology Biochemistry & Pharmacology*, **105**, 176.
24 Bhatt, D.L., Gaylor, D.C. & Lee, R.C. (1990). Rhabdomyolysis due to pulsed electric fields. *Plastic and Reconstructive Surgery*, **86**, 1.
25 Powell, K.T. & Weaver, J.C. (1986). Transient aqueous pore in bilayer membranes: a statistical theory. *Bioelectrochemistry and Bioenergetics*, **15**, 211.
26 Taylor, G.I. & Michael, D.H. (1973). On making holes in a sheet of fluid. *Journal of Fluid Mechanics*, **58(4)**, 625.
27 Litster, J.D. (1975). Stability of lipid bilayers and red blood cell membranes. *Physics Letters*, **53(A)**, 193.
28 Gaylor, D.G., Prakah-Asante, K. & Lee, R.C. (1988). Significance of cell size and tissue structure in electrical trauma. *Journal of Theoretical Biology*, **133**, 223.
29 Adrian, R.H. (1983). Electrical properties of striated muscle. In *Handbook of Physiology, Section 10: Skeletal Muscle.* pp. 275–300, Bethesda, MD: American Physiological Society.
30 Jack, J.J.B., Noble, D. & Tsien, R.W. (1975). *Electric Current Flow in Excitable Cells*, London: Oxford University Press.
31 Milton, R.L., Mathias, R.T. & Eisenberg, R.S. (1985). Electrical properties of the myotendon region of frog twitch muscle fibers measured in the frequency domain. *Biophysical Journal*, **48**, 253.
32 Cooper, M.S. (1986). Electrical cable theory, transmembrane ion fluxes, and the motile responses of tissue cells to external electrical fields. In *Bioelectric Interactions Symposium, IEEE/Engineering in Medicine and Biology Society, 7th Annual Conference*. Chicago, IL.
33 Bekoff, A. & Betz, W.J. (1977). Physiological properties of dissociated muscle fibers obtained from innervate and denervated adult rat muscle. *Journal of Physiology*, **271**, 25.
34 Bekoff, A. & Betz, W.J. (1977). Properties of isolated adult rat muscle fibers maintained in tissue culture. *Journal of Physiology*, **271**, 537.
35 Bischoff, R. (1986). Proliferation of muscle satellite cells on intact myofibers in culture. *Developmental Biology*, **115**, 129.

36  Schanne, O.F. & Ceretti, E.R.P. (1978). *Impedance Measurements in Biological Cells*. New York: John Wiley & Sons.

37  Artz, C.P. (1974). Changing concepts in electrical injury. *American Journal of Surgery*, **128**, 600.

38  Baxter, C.R. (1970). Present concepts in the management of major electrical injury. *Surgical Clinics in North America*, **50**, 1401.

39  Vimont, A.B. & Rich, W.B. (Kentucky Utilities Company) (1977). Non-fatal, Contact Electric Shock and Burn Accidents. Edison Electric Institute Safety and Industrial Health Committee Summary Report. The Edison Electric Institute: Washington, DC.

40  Sances, A., Jr., Mykelbust, J.B., Larson, S.J. *et al.* (1981). Experimental electrical injury studies. *Journal of Trauma*, **21**, 589.

41  Sances, A. Jr., Myklebust, J.B., Szablya, J.F. *et al.* (1983). Current pathways in high-voltage injuries. *IEEE Transactions in Biomedical Engineering*. BME-30, 118.

42  Daniel, R.K., Ballard, P.A., Heroux, P., Zelt, R.G. & Howard, C.R. (1988). High-voltage electrical injury: acute pathophysiology. *Journal of Hand Surgery*, **13(A)**, 44.

43  Zelt, R.G., Ballard, P.A., Heroux, P. *et al.* (1986). Experimental high voltage electrical burns: the role of progressive necrosis. *Proceedings of the 55th Annual Scientific Meeting American Society for Plastic and Reconstructive Surgery*, **9**, 222.

44  Tropea, B.I. (1987). A Numerical Model for Determining the Human Forearm Thermal Response to High Voltage Injury. SB Thesis, Massachusetts Institute of Technology (supervised by R.C. Lee).

45  Chilbert, M., Maiman, D., Sances, A., Jr *et al.* (1985). Measure of tissue resistivity in experimental electrical burns. *Journal of Trauma*, **25(3)**, 209.

46  Sekins, K.M., Dundore, D., Emery, A.F., Lehmann, J.F., McGrath, P.W. & Nelp, W.B. (1980). Muscle blood flow changes in response to 915 MHz diathermy with surface cooling as measured by Xe133 clearance. *Archives of Physical Medicine Rehabilitation*, **61**, 105.

47  Russell, H.E., Hartford, C.E., Boyd, W.C. & Barnes, R.W. (1975). Muscle blood flow in circumferentially burned extremities. *Surgical Forum*, **26**, 71.

48  Bard, A.J. & Faulkner, L.R. (1980). *Electromechanical Methods: Fundamentals and Applications*. New York: John Wiley & Sons.

49  Carter, A.O. & Morley, R. (1969). Effects of power frequency voltages on amputated human limb. *British Journal of Industrial Medicine*, **26**, 224.

50  Peterson, R.R. (1980). *A Cross-sectional Approach to Anatomy*. Chicago: Yearbook Medical Publishers, Inc.

51  Poppendieck, H.F., Randall, R., Breeden, J.A., Chambers, J.E. & Murphy, J.R. (1966). Thermal and electrical conductivities of biological fluids and tissues. Reports under Contract No. ONR 4095(00), Geoscience Ltd., Solana Beach, California, specifically: DDC No. Ad 630712.

52  Henriques, F.C. & Moritz, A.R. (1947). Studies of thermal injury I: the conduction of heat to and through skin and the temperature attained therein. *American Journal of Pathology*, **23**, 531.

53  Dickson, J.A. & Calderwood, S.K. (1980). Temperature range and

selective sensitivity of tumors to hyperthermia: a Critical review. *Annals of the New York Academy of Sciences*, **335**, 180.

54 Rocchio, C.M. (1989). The Kinetics of Thermal Damage to an Isolated Skeletal Muscle Cell. SB Thesis, Massachusetts Institute of Technology (supervised by R.C. Lee).

55 ADINAT (Automatic Dynamic Incremental Nonlinear Analysis of Temperatures) (1984). Report ARD 84–2. Massachusetts: ADINA Engineering.

56 Bingham, H. (1986). Electrical burns. *Clinics in Plastic Surgery*, **13**, 75.

57 Chen, M.M. (1985). The tissue energy balance equation. In *Heat Transfer in Medicine and Biology*, Shitzer, A. & Eberhard, R.C. (eds), vol. I. pp. 153–62, New York: Plenum Press.

58 Weinbaum, S. & Jiji, L.J. (1985). A new simplified bioheat equation for the effect of blood flow on local average tissue temperature. *ASME Journal of Biomechanical Engineering*, **107**, 131.

59 Clayton, J.M. & Hayes, A.C., Hammel, J., Boyd, W.C. Hartford, C.E. & Barnes, R.W. (1977). Xenon-133 determination of muscle blood flow in electrical injury. *Journal of Trauma*, **17**, 293.

60 Hunt, J.L., Sato, R.M. & Baxter, C.R. (1980). Acute electric burns: current diagnostic and therapeutic approaches to management. *Archives of Surgery*, **115**, 434.

61 Grube, B.J. & Heimbach, D.M. Acute and delayed neurological sequelae of electrical injury. (this volume).

62 Ji, L. & Lee, R.C. (1990). An 8 kD reverse tri-block co-polymer inhibits electroporation of skeletal muscle cells *in vitro*. *Journal of Cell Biology*, **111(4)**, Part II, Abst. ASCB.

63 Nea, L.J., Bates, G.W. & Gilmer, P.J. (1987). Facilitation of electrofusion of plant-protoplasts by membrane-active agents. *Biochemical et Biophysical Acta*, **897**, 293.

64 Robson, M.C., Murphy, R.C. & Heggers, J.P. (1983). A new explanation for progressive necrosis in electrical burns. *Plastic and Reconstructive Surgery*, **73**, 437.

65 Melcher, J.R. (1980). *Continuum Electromechanics*, Chap. 10. Cambridge, MA: MIT Press,.

66 Sances, A., Szablya, J.F., Morgan, J.D., Myklebust, J.B. & Larson, S.J. (1981). High voltage powerline injury studies. *IEEE Transactions Power Apparatus and Systems*. PAS-100, 552.

67 Bowman, H.F., Cravalho, E.G., & Woods, M. (1975). Theory, measurement and application of thermal properties of biomaterials. *Annual Review in Biophysics & Bioengineering*, **4**, 43.

68 Eberhard, R.C. (1985). Thermal models of single organs. In *Heat Transfer in Medicine and Biology*, Shitzer, A. & Eberhard, R.C. (eds), vol. I, pp. 261–73, New York: Plenum Press.

69 Bowman, H.F. (1985). Estimation of tissue blood flow. In *Heat Transfer in Medicine and Biology*, Shitzer, A. & Eberhard, R.C. (eds), vol. I, pp. 193–205, New York: Plenum Press.

# Nomenclature

## Terms

$X =$ arbitrary damage accumulation function
$\tau_e =$ duration of tissue exposure to damaging supraphysiologic temperatures
$\sigma =$ electrical conductivity
$\Phi =$ electrical potential function
$\lambda_m =$ electrical space constant of the cell membrane
$\zeta =$ energy required to open a membrane pore
$\psi =$ interfacial energy per unit area of cell membrane
$\rho =$ mass density
$\delta_m =$ membrane thickness
$\alpha =$ proportionality constant
$\xi(t_h) =$ pulse for $t_h$ seconds
$\Gamma =$ rate of cell membrane damage at temperature equal to infinity
$\Omega =$ resistance in ohms
$\nabla =$ spatial derivative
$\kappa =$ thermal conductivity
$\omega_b =$ volume rate of perfusion
$A =$ amperes
$B =$ energy of activation barrier height
$c =$ specific heat
$c_m =$ membrane capacitance per unit length of cell
$E =$ electrical field
$F =$ capacitance in farads
$G_e =$ conductance of a portion of the membrane at the end of the cell
$g_m =$ membrane conductance per unit length of cell
$h =$ empirical heat transfer coefficient
$I =$ total current
$J =$ current density
$k =$ forward reaction rate constant
$L =$ cell half-length
$LT_{50} =$ contact time needed to cause injury to 50% of a population of cells
$P =$ power distribution density
$q =$ heat metabolism
$q_s =$ heat flux at skin–air interface
$R =$ universal gas constant

$r_i$ = cytoplasmic resistance per unit length of cell
$r_o$ = extracellular space resistance per unit length of cell
$S$ = siemens (mho)
$t$ = time
$T$ = tissue temperature in K
$T_{air}$ = temperature of the air
$T_b$ = temperature of blood
$T_s$ = temperature of surface skin
$u(t)$ = step function
$V$ = volts
$V_c$ = voltage drop across the full length of cell
$V_m$ = transmembrane potential
$W$ = watts
$x, y$ = Cartesian coordinates of transverse cross-section
$z$ = longitudinal coordinate

## Subscripts

air = air
b = blood
c = conduction
h = heating phase
m = membrane
n = node
s = surface
t = tissue

# Part II:

Clinical manifestations and management

# 4

# Soft tissue patterns in acute electric burns

## JOHN L. HUNT

> As regards the United States of America where electricity is very extensively
> employed, I have been unable to find any statistical records. One must remember
> that in America life is held very cheap, and that safeguards and protective
> legislation tend to be regarded as undue restrictions upon industry and commerce.
> *Jex-Blake (1913). Death by electric currents and lightning. British Medical
> Journal, 3.*

Electric burns represent a unique form of thermal injury. While flame burns
have obviously occurred since antiquity, commercial electrical injuries are
relatively recent in origin. Prior to the introduction of commercial
electricity in the later part of the nineteenth century, lightning, no doubt,
was responsible for the morbidity and mortality associated with electricity.

In 1982, in the United States, lightning was responsible for approximately 250 deaths, more than by any other natural disaster[1,2]. Lightning
injuries account for very few admissions to burn units: there have been only
seven patients, ages ranged from 11 to 35 years with a mean total body
surface area (TBSA) of 12%, admitted to the Parkland Memorial Hospital
(PMH) burn unit. No patient required a burn operation, and there were no
deaths.

Electrical burns constitute approximately 5% of all admissions to major
burn units in the United States[3]. At the PMH burn unit, 463 patients were
admitted with an acute electric burn over a 13-year period, including 75
patients whose injury was due to an electric arc and therefore no flow of
electricity through the body. The other 388 patients had electricity enter
and leave their body. The mean age of the latter group was 28 years with a
range of less than 1 year to 82 years (Fig. 4.1) and their average total body
surface area burn was 11% (range 1–68) (Fig. 4.2). The injury most often
involved a white male (only 7% were females), usually over 20 years (77%),
often injured while at work (85% of all high-voltage injuries), with contact
sites on one or more extremities (85%), and often on the dominant
extremity. The mean hospital length of stay was 21 ± 24 days, range 1–196,
and a mode of 1 day, significantly greater than for all nonelectric burns with
a similar mean burn size – 12 days. Of 302 operative procedures, performed
in 101 patients, the mean was 3 with a range of 1–10. Seventy-one patients

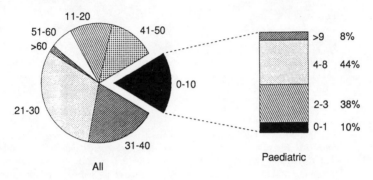

Fig. 4.1. An analysis of electric burns with age (Parkland Hospital 1975–
1988). 388 patients.

had fourth-degree (involving muscle) burns and twenty-five patients had
multiple amputations. Once discharged, intensive physical and occupational rehabilitation was required in many patients with high-voltage injuries.
The ultimate result was often unsatisfactory because of functional
impairment (contractures, amputations, neurologic impairment, cataracts), cosmetic disfigurement and psychological disability. The majority of
victims with a major amputation did not return to their previous
occupation[4].

A number of factors, both electrical and physical, interact when the
victim comes into contact with electricity[5-7]. In order to diagnose and treat
the variety of soft tissue patterns associated with electric burns, a basic
understanding of the relationships between amperage, voltage and tissue
resistance is important. In most accidents, only the voltage is known,
amperage and resistance are virtually impossible to determine. Both the
length of time and the area of contact with the electrical source are
important determinants of the depth and extent of the injury[8]. Although
skin resistance at the contact sites initially acts as a barrier to the flow of
current, it does so for only a short time, and once resistance is overcome,
current flows. The thick skin on the palm of the hand and sole of the foot or
wet surfaces such as the lips are examples of local wound conditions that
affect current flow. For practical purposes, contact sites in high-voltage
accidents offer no significant barrier to the flow of current.

There is no longer controversy as to whether only heat is responsible for
the tissue necrosis in electrical burns; recent experimental studies have
identified high concentrations of various metabolites of arachidonic acid,
specifically thromboxane A2 and prostaglandins, in areas of muscle
necrosis[9]. Lee *et al.* presented experimental evidence that cell damage is
caused by short-term nonthermal effects of electric fields[10,11].

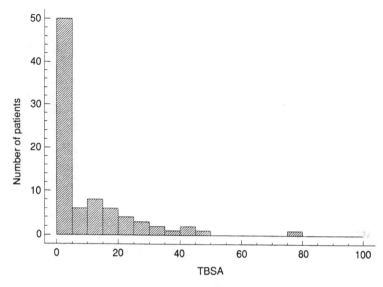

Fig. 4.2. An analysis of electric burns in 50 patients 1975–1988.

Electrical injuries are arbitrarily divided into high and low voltage, the former being any injury due to more than 1000 volts[12]. Electrical burns are caused by one or both of the following mechanisms: either the current passes through the body or the electricity arcs[13]. The former causes cutaneous and deep tissue injury both locally and distant from the contact sites. An arc is composed of ionized particles which heat the surrounding gasses to as high as 3000 °C.[14] A cutaneous burn occurs and, if the clothes are ignited, a large surface area may be burned deeply. Local deep soft tissue will be burned because of the very high temperature, but no remote muscle damage occurs.

Amperage plays an important part in the pathophysiology of the injury, and this will be discussed in more detail in a subsequent chapter. Current of less than 0.2 mA evokes a startle reaction from the victim. While this does not result in any cutaneous injury, it may cause the victim to lose balance and fall thereby sustaining associated physical trauma. If 0.6 mA is contacted, the victim usually is not able to let go of the electrical source. This produces a very painful experience, but no major tissue damage. A current of 100 mA causes respiratory paralysis presumably due to a direct effect on the respiratory centre in the brain. As little as 1.5 A causes ventricular fibrillation and sudden death, often with no evidence of a cutaneous burn.

Low-voltage accidents usually occur in and around the home and are often associated with young age-groups[15]. Only 5% of patients below the age of 19 and less than 2% under the age of 10 sustained a high-voltage injury in the PMH series of patients admitted to the hospital. Electric burns occurring in the home are usually from 120 volts 60 cycle current, and usually result in minor cutaneous burns and minimal-to-no soft tissue damage. There are some home power tools and industrial machines that use 220 and 440 volts; although not classified as high voltage, they are none the less capable of causing significant superficial and deep tissue burns. A notorious low-voltage household injury that can cause serious functional and cosmetic sequelae occurs when the victim, usually less than 5 years of age, bites on an electrical cord[16-17]. Contact points typically occur at one or both angles of the mouth and result in coagulation necrosis of the oral commissure (Fig. 4.3). The gum and tongue may be burned, and, if the latter is severe, rapid intra-oral oedema can cause airway compromise early after the injury. Conservative therapy is recommended with close follow-up for 6 to 10 days after the accident because spontaneous haemorrhage may occur from the coagulated branch of the facial artery or vein. Various devices and techniques are used to minimize scarring. The contracture often results in some degree of microstomia[18] and reconstruction is delayed until the scar is mature.

Direct-current injuries are infrequent, but include encounters with lightning, automobile batteries (very high amperage and low voltage), electroplating, and the power supply for some public transportation systems. There were no patients admitted with direct current injuries in the PMH series.

When electrical energy is converted to thermal energy, coagulation necrosis of tissue occurs at the point(s) of contact. Electric contact sites are typically areas of third or fourth degree burns, have discrete borders, and very often are not surrounded by second degree burn[19] (Fig. 4.4). The central part of the contact is depressed, brown–black, charred, dry and insensate.

In the medical literature, and in the clinical environment, contact areas are referred to, and often incorrectly, as entrance and exit sites[20]. The exit wound corresponds to the site where the current left the victim. Clinically, this often represents the worse area of tissue destruction. In high-voltage electrical burns, this contact site often appears as a 'blowout' type of wound because it appears as if the electric current 'exploded' from skin. Skin and subcutaneous tissue may be destroyed exposing thrombosed vessels, nerves, fascia, bones or joints (Fig. 4.5).

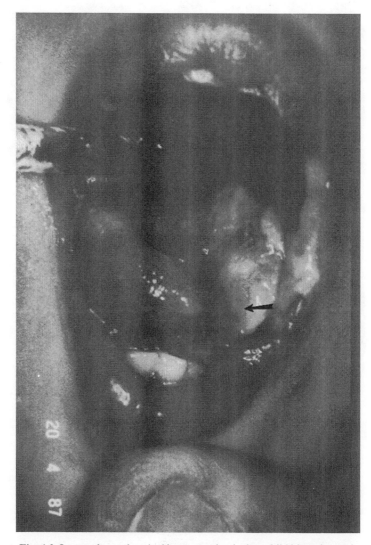

Fig. 4.3. Low-voltage electrical burn sustained when child bit on bare wire of electrical cord. Lip, gum and tongue burned. Tip of tongue was cut in half (see black arrow). Massive intra-oral oedema necessitated airway intubation in first 24 hours of injury.

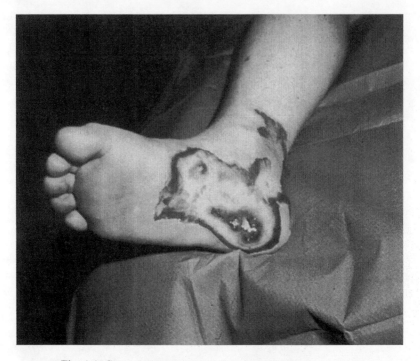

Fig. 4.4. Contact site on sole of foot from high-voltage electrical burn. There was no surrounding second-degree burn.

Gross inspection of the cutaneous injury does not give the examiner any indication as to the extent of involved underlying tissue. Electrical burns have been compared to icebergs. Deep or 'hidden' tissue damage may be present with a minor cutaneous burn. For practical purposes, the most common tissue injured is muscle. The 'hidden' tissue damage accounts for the greatest morbidity, functional impairment and cosmetic disfigurement associated with electric burns.

Oedema occurs in the skin, subcutaneous tissue and muscle when electrical current travels through the tissue. While the oedema is usually greatest around the contact sites, it extends for a considerable distance proximally and distantly and is worst in the first 24 hours after the burn. If compartmental pressure exceeds about 30 mm of mercury, muscle perfusion pressure is exceeded and ischaemia occurs, initially lymphatic, then venous, and finally arterial flow ceases. Oedema formation is accelerated by the rate and volume of resuscitation fluid administered. The presence of oedema does not imply that nonviable muscle is present, but the possibility certainly exists. The most common muscle compartments

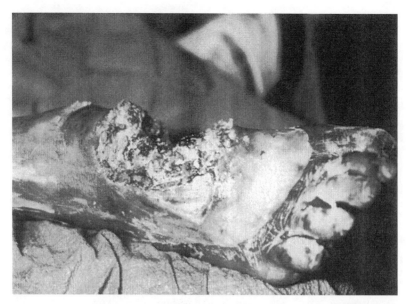

Fig. 4.5. A typical contact site referred to as 'blow out' injury. Often identified incorrectly as an exit wound.

affected are in the forearm and calf, where each has muscle compartments separated by two bones with tight, investing fasciae and intermuscular septa. The forearm and calf have two and four compartments respectively; all must be decompressed. The anterior and lateral compartments of the leg are most susceptible to increased pressure and manifest signs of ischaemia earliest. The physician treating an electrical burn must maintain a high index of suspicion because failure to recognize and decompress the compartments will result in additional muscle, often of the entire compartment, requiring extensive debridement and even amputation. In the PMH series, 90% of the fasciotomies were performed within 4 to 6 hours of injury; the rest were later because patients were transferred major distances to the unit.

The presence of any of the following physical signs or symptoms mandates immediate re-examination and appropriate therapeutic intervention: poor capillary refill, absent or diminished pulses, tight muscle compartment to palpation, paraesthesias, numbness, tingling, a cold extremity, and pigment in the urine. Although pigment indicates either haemoglobin or myoglobin, the latter is the common haemochromogen in electrical burns. It is noteworthy that nonviable muscle can be present in an extremity with palpable pulses and haemochromogens absent from the urine.

Myoglobinuria is characterized by pink to port wine coloured urine. The colour of the urine is directly proportional to the pigment load which is related to the volume of muscle damaged: the darker the colour of the urine and the greater the pigment load. Anyone either suspected of having muscle necrosis or involved in an accident with sufficient voltage to injure muscle must have the urine examined. The first urine sample obtained may be clear because it represents the volume in the bladder prior to the injury. Once fluid resuscitation commences, the urine may quickly change colour. Low-voltage household accidents are rarely accompanied by myoglobinuria. Regardless of the type of electrical accident, if myoglobin is present, both the rate and volume of the resuscitation fluid must be increased, and the need for fasciotomy determined.

A fasciotomy is both diagnostic and therapeutic[21]. While nonviable muscle may be identified through the fasciotomy sites, muscle may be ischaemic from hypoperfusion and hypovolaemia, or as a result of vascular compression from oedema in a tight muscle compartment. Once the intravascular volume and peripheral perfusion are restored, muscle perfusion improves, and clinical assessment of muscle viability is easier and more accurate (Fig. 4.6(a), (b)).

X-rays of the soft tissue surrounding the entrance and exit sites on rare occasions reveal free air. The air entered through the wound at the time of electric shock, and does not indicate the presence of an anaerobic infection. Soft tissue X-rays should be obtained if there is any reason to suspect skeletal injuries such as fractures and dislocations.

If the victim is thrown against something, or falls from a height, associated trauma is possible. Common injuries include: cerebral concussion/contusions, fractures, dislocations, especially vertebral, and bleeding from solid organ trauma. In the PMH series, there was one each of a traumatic rupture of a spleen, and bladder associated with a fall, and each patient required emergency laparotomy on the day of injury. Careful evaluation of the patient for the presence of blunt trauma is an integral part of the acute management.

Clinical examination of an extremity with a high-voltage contact point often reveals no evidence of muscle damage. Even at the time of fasciotomy, an accurate identification of the proximal and distal extent of necrosis is not possible. There is usually no sharp demarcation between the viable and nonviable muscle. Necrotic muscle is most prevalent under, and adjacent to, the contact sites, and the more distant the muscle from the contacts, the less the muscle necrosis. This is explained partially by visualizing an extremity as a volume conductor[5]. The current, and thus the heat produced

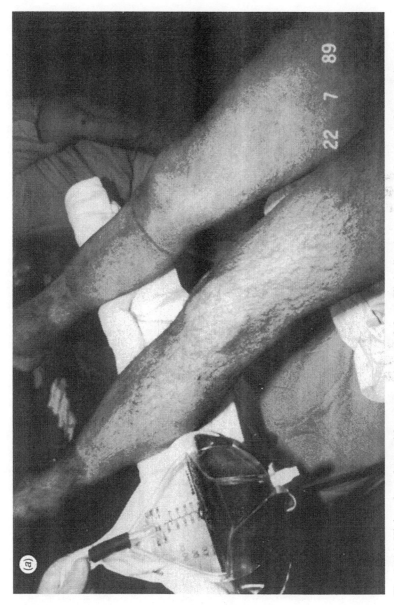

Fig. 4.6(a). High-voltage burn with a contact site on left foot. Clinically, there were no pulses in the foot and the anterior and lateral muscle compartments in the calf were swollen and tight to palpation. Note the dark urine indicative of myoglobin.

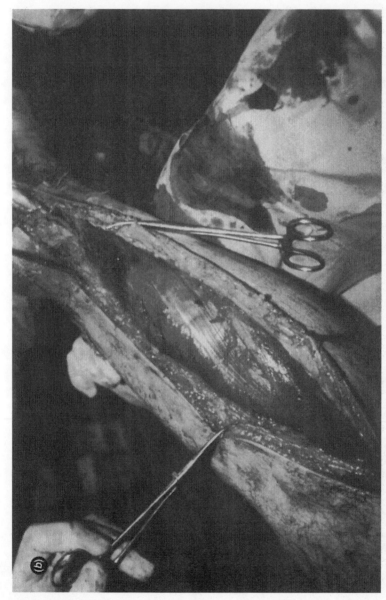

Fig. 4.6(b). Appearance of the leg after four-compartment fasciotomy. Note the massively swollen muscle bulging from the medial fasciotomy incision.

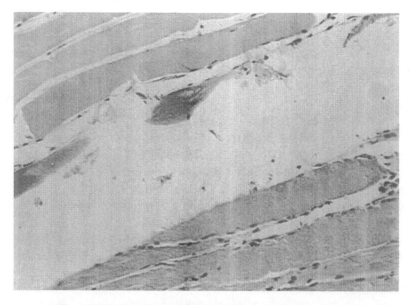

Fig. 4.7. This muscle was excised from an area with grossly viable muscle. Note, in the lower half of the section, the muscle has nuclei and there are muscle striations, indicating viable muscle. In the upper half, the muscle appears pale, and is without nuclei and striations, indicative of nonviable muscle.

at the time of injury, is concentrated at contact sites, the volume of the extremity increases proximally and decreases distally, explaining why tissue injury becomes less severe proximally and often worse distally. The classic clinical example of this is when a contact site is over the wrist. The hand and most of the upper forearm may be spared, but significant tissue damage exists at the wrist.

The phrase 'progressive muscle necrosis' is a term frequently used by surgeons when describing the phenomenon of having to subsequently debride muscle that had grossly appeared viable only several days before[22]. Whether this muscle was irreversibly injured at the time of the burn, yet grossly appeared normal at surgery, or was in fact initially uninjured and then subsequently died, still remains a mystery. This can be explained to a certain extent if muscle is biopsied and examined histologically (Fig. 4.7). In areas of grossly viable muscle, it is common to identify significant amounts of nonviable muscle. The clinician is simply not able to see microscopic areas of viable and nonviable muscle with the naked eye.

Because the clinical identification of nonviable muscle is difficult both acutely when the skin is intact, and even when the muscle is exposed, this may be a problem a number of days after the injury. Various tests have been proposed. The following three offer insight into the pathophysiology of the injury, but are not practical or useful in the clinical setting. Clayton *et al.* used $^{131}$Xe washout technique to identify muscle ischaemia[23]. A decrease in muscle blood flow was felt to represent nonviable muscle. Hunt *et al.* evaluated arteriography[24]. The findings substantiate what was apparent clinically, large calibre muscular vessels remain patent in areas with extensive muscle necrosis. Unfortunately, current arteriographic techniques do not provide sufficient resolution to allow visualization of the very small intramuscular branches, which are the sites of vascular thromboses. Typical vascular abnormalities noted in areas of injured muscle include spasm, narrowing, 'beading', and occlusion. Because of the potential nephrotoxicity of the dye when used in a hypovolaemic patient, as is often the case of a patient with a severe electrical burn, it is not recommended in the acute resuscitation period. Quinby *et al.* recommended using both frozen and permanent histological evaluation of tissue debrided to determine muscle viability[25]. The authors felt this technique minimized tissue loss and aided in the early closure of the burn wound. Unfortunately, the technique is both time-consuming and expensive. It may be possibly a valuable technique to guide debridement when cosmetic or functional considerations are of highest concern, such as on the face or hand. It is impractical when debriding large volumes of tissue in multiple locations.

Technetium-99m stannous pyrophosphate (Tc-PYP) scintigraphy was first proposed as a noninvasive diagnostic study to identify infarcted myocardial muscle[26]. It has also proved useful to identify nonviable skeletal muscle in electrical burns[27]. The agent is injected 24 hours after injury, and the suspected areas of muscle damage are scanned 2 hours later. Increased uptake of Tc-PYP indicates binding with intracellular calcium in irreversibly injured muscle. Blood flow must be intact to muscle for the binding to take place. An additional diagnostic benefit is also provided. The radioactive agent concentrates in viable bone after intravenous administration[28]. Lack of uptake in bone, under or adjacent to, contact sites indicates poor perfusion and possibly damaged bone (Fig. 4.8(a), (b)). Unfortunately, there is often overlying injured muscle which obscures the uptake in the bone. Absence of blood flow is indicative of irreversibly injured muscle and a 'cold' area is seen on scan (Fig. 4.9(a), (b)). Blood flow to areas of nonviable muscle enables the Tc-PYP to bind with the calcium that was released from the injured cells. These areas are identified on scan by increased uptake of the Tc-PYP or 'hot spots' (Fig. 4.7). Because the

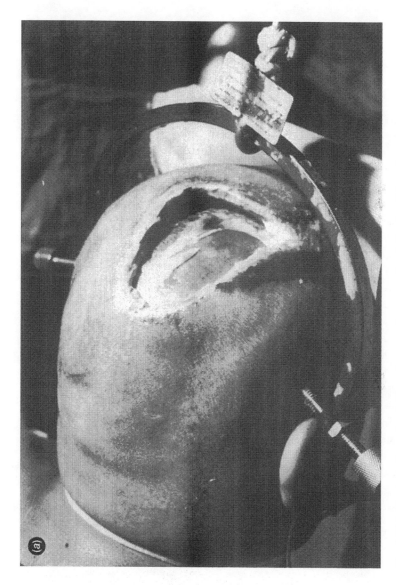

Fig. 4.8(*a*). Contact site on head. Bone is exposed, an associated C-spine dislocation present.

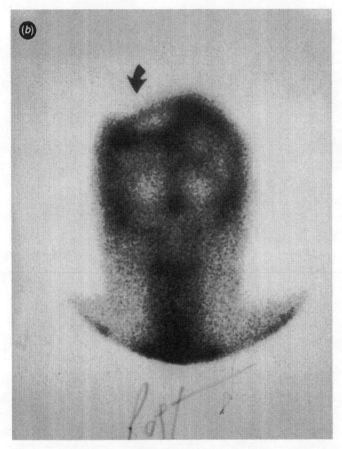

Fig. 4.8(*b*). A Tc-PYP scan of the calvarium. The 'halo' represents absent perfusion of the bone. A local scalp graft was rotated over the area on the seventh postburn day.

sensitivity of the scan is high, and the resolution of the X-rays so limited, care must be exercised when correlating scan-positive areas with the corresponding area view grossly. The scan graphically demonstrates the 'patchy necrosis' of muscle that so characterizes electrical burns. Muscle identified on scan as irreversibly injured may appear grossly normal, but, when a biopsy of the muscle is viewed histologically, varying proportions of viable and nonviable muscle are identified, the proportions depending on the location of the biopsy from the contact site. Clinical assessment of viability must always be the ultimate determinate as to whether muscle needs to be debrided.

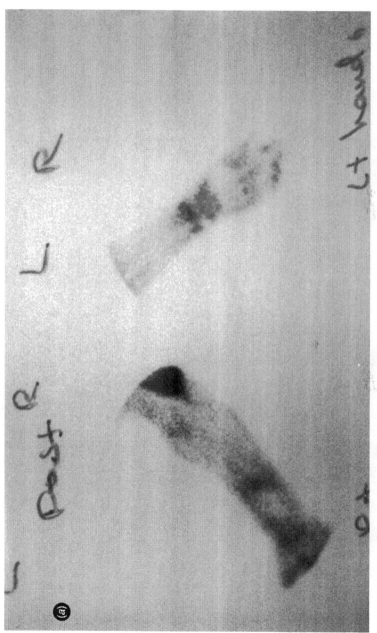

Fig. 4.9(a). A Tc-PYP scan of the right wrist demonstrating an area of nonviable muscle which has no blood flow and therefore a 'cold' spot surrounded by increased uptake 'hyperaemia' also indicative of nonviable muscle. The left hand is normal on scan.

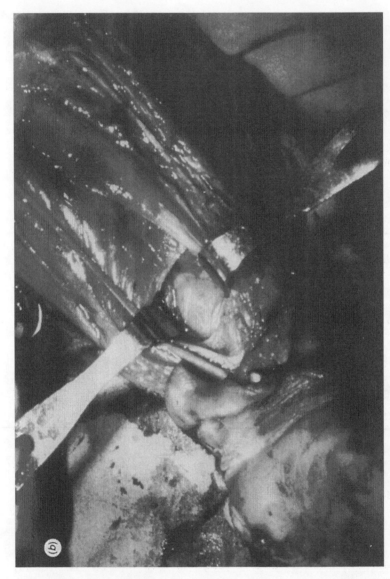

Fig. 4.9(b). At exploration of wrist, the superficial flexor muscles were grossly viable, but the pronator was nonviable (corresponding to the 'cold' spot on scan).

| Location | Number of patients |
|---|---|
| Upper extremity | |
| Above elbow | 12 |
| Below elbow | 12 |
| Hand | 1 |
| >1 digit | 20 |
| Lower extremity | |
| Above knee | 3 |
| Below knee | 11 |

Fig. 4.10. An analysis of amputation locations (49 patients).

The most serious soft tissue complication of an electrical injury is the loss of part, or all, of a limb. Rarely, a traumatic amputation occurs at the time of a high-voltage accident. In the PMH series, 49 patients required one amputation and 25 of them had multiple amputations (Fig. 4.10). Their mean TBSA was 20% and the number of operations ranged from 1 to 10 with a mean of 4. The mean postburn day for a major extremity amputation was 5. The mean length of stay was 40 days with a range of 9 to 196. An amputation was never performed unless the extremity was completely insensate, or was deemed to be functionally useless after all necrotic soft tissue was debrided. Surgical debridement was begun within 48 to 72 hours of injury and continued every 2 to 3 days until the majority of the soft tissue was debrided. Wound closure was usually accomplished within 10 days to 2 weeks. This virtually eliminated local and systemic sepsis originating from the wound.

Although abnormalities in cardiac rate and rhythm are not uncommon in the first 24 hours after an acute electrical burn, myocardial infarction is very rare. In the PMH series, less than 1% of the patients sustained myocardial damage[29]. Telemetry monitoring is only recommended for patients who received CPR after the accident, or had an abnormal 12 lead electrocardiogram. Several studies investigated whether elevated creatine kinase and specifically myocardial creatine kinase (MB-CK) were helpful in diagnosing myocardial injury. Housinger *et al.* showed a poor correlation between an increase in MB-CK, electrocardiographic abnormalities, and myocardial damage[30]. Most authors are of the opinion that elevation of cardiac enzymes is nonspecific, and positive isoenzymes in the absence of electrocardiographic findings should be interpreted with caution as to whether myocardial damage has occurred[31]. McBride *et al.* reviewed 36 patients with a high-voltage burn and concluded that cardiac injury is unusual and skeletal muscle can be the origin of elevated CK-MB[32]. The highest levels were found in normal skeletal muscle adjacent to the injury site[33]. However, Kahn *et al.* believed that an elevated CK-MB was indicative of myocardial injury and the magnitude of the elevation bore a strong relationship to the extent and number of extremity amputations[34]. Realistically, it may take 7 to 10 days for the surgeon to locate and debride all nonviable muscle. Unfortunately, this is not true for bone, cartilage, nerves, and tendons. It is often very difficult to assess the viability of these structures weeks after the burn. This visual inexactitude, coupled with a reluctance to debride tissue of such functional importance, leads to a very conservative surgical approach. As a result, the wound frequently becomes desiccated, bacterial colonization and local wound sepsis occurs, tissue necrosis ensues and debridement of previously viable tissue is the end result. Once all clinically obvious nonviable tissue is debrided, prompt wound closure with a local or distant soft tissue flap is recommended[35]. Even if the underlying tissue requires further surgery, the flap is elevated and local debridement continued. By following this management, all potentially viable tissue is salvagable[36].

Areas of the body with large cross-sectional diameters such as the thoracic and abdominal cavities are frequently traversed by electric current, but internal organ damage is very rare. Direct damage to the lungs or heart is always associated with an overlying contact site and necrosis of superficial tissue[37].

The overall incidence of nonspecific gastrointestinal symptoms and complications varies between 6 and 25%[38]. Nonspecific paralytic ileus associated with nausea and vomiting is the most common complication. Isolated cases of necrosis of the intestine, gall bladder, bladder and pancreas have been reported[39]. Even rarer are reports of intestinal perforation without an overlying abdominal burn[40,41].

While virtually any organ system may be affected acutely, others only manifest complications weeks or months after the injury. Miscellaneous delayed complications that have been reported include bone marrow aplasia[42], and abdominal aortic occlusion[43].

An interesting and, as yet, unexplained delayed complication is the appearance of cataracts[44]. Contact sites around the head, neck, and upper thorax are often present in patients who later develop cataracts. The earliest cataracts have been reported postburn is 3 weeks and the latest up to several years.

Immediate and delayed neurological complications are frequently encountered with electrical injuries. These may be temporary or permanent and are reported to occur in up to 58% of patients suffering from an electric burn[45]. Neurological disorders can involve the central nervous system,

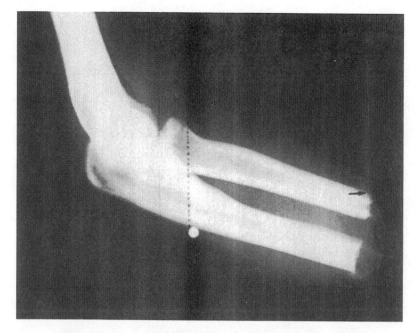

Fig. 4.11. Heterotopic calcification at distal margin of below-elbow amputation. Stump revision was necessary.

spinal cord, peripheral and sympathetic nerves[46-9]. When a patient presents with a neurological defect on admission and the contact site is over or adjacent to the involved nerve, there is a strong likelihood that the deficit will be permanent. Of course, local oedema may be responsible for acute neurologic deficits. A common example is a median or ulnar carpal tunnel syndrome caused by oedema from a contact site on the forearm. Surgical decompression of the carpal fascia must also include forearm fasciotomies.

An interesting delayed soft tissue complication, seen in some patients after an amputation, is formation of heterotopic new bone at the distal end of the stump[50] (Fig. 4.11). While it is impossible to predict which patient and what limb(s) will develop calcification, extremities requiring a major amputation (above or below knee and elbow) are most likely to develop it. Heterotopic calcification was not seen after minor amputations (finger or hand). The average time from amputation to diagnosis of new bone was 38 weeks with a maximum of 110 weeks. Surgical removal of the new bone was necessary because of skin breakdown at the stump, local pain or prosthetic-related problems.

**References**

1 Hiestand, D. & Colice, G.L. (1988). Lightning-strike injury. *Journal of Intensive Care Medicine*, **3**, 303–14.
2 Tribble, C.G., Persing, J.A. & Morgan, R.F. *et al.* (1984). Lightning injury. *Current Concepts in Trauma Care*, 5–10.
3 Hunt, J.L, Sato, R. & Baxter, C.R. (1980). Acute electric burns. *Archives of Surgery*, **115**, 434–8.
4 Rosenberg, D.B. & Nelson, M. (1988). Rehabilitation concerns in electrical burn patients: a review of the literature. *Journal of Trauma*, **28**, 808–12.
5 Hunt, J.L., Mason, A.D. Jr., & Masterson, T.S. *et al.* (1976). The pathophysiology of acute electric injuries. *Journal of Trauma*, **16**, 335–40.
6 Laberge, L.C., Ballard, P.A. & Daniel, R.K. (1984). Experimental electrical burns: low voltage. *Annals of Plastic Surgery*, **13**, 185–90.
7 Skoog, T. (1970). Electrical injuries. *Journal of Trauma*, **10**, 816–30.
8 Sances, A. Jr., Myklebust, J.B., Larson S. J. *et al.* (1981). Experimental electrical injury studies. *Journal of Trauma*, **21**, 589–97.
9 Robson, M., Murphy, R.C. & Heggers, J.P. (1984). A new explanation for the progressive tissue loss in electrical injuries. *Plastic and Reconstructive Surgery*, **73**, 431–7.
10 Lee, R.C., Gaylor, D.C., Bhatt, D. & Israel, D. (1988). Role of cell membrane rupture in the pathogenesis of electrical trauma. *Journal of Surgical Research*, **44**, 709–19.
11 Lee, R.C. & Kolodney, M.S. (1987). Electrical injury mechanisms: electrical breakdown of cell membranes. *Plastic and Reconstructive Surgery*, **80**, 672–9.
12 Ugland, O.M. (1967). Electrical burns. *Scandinavian Journal of Plastic and Reconstructive Surgery*, 2–74.
13 Moncrief, J.A. & Pruitt, B.A. (1979). Electric injury. *Postgraduate Medicine*, **48**, 189–94.
14 Sances, A. Jr., Larson, S.J. & Myklebust, J. *et al.* (1979). Electrical injuries. *Surgery, Gynecology and Obstetrics*, **149**, 97–108.
15 Hiebert, J.M., Thacker, J.G. & Edlich, R.F. (1979). Early management of commercial electrical current injuries. *Current Concepts in Trauma Care*, 8–14.
16 Burke, J.F., Quinby, W.C. Jr. & Bondoc, C. *et al.* (1977). Patterns of high tension electrical injury in children and adolescents and their management. *American Journal of Surgery*, **133**, 492–7.
17 Orgel, M.G., Brown, H.C., & Woolhouse, F.M. (1975). Electrical burns of the mouth in children: a method for assessing results. *Journal of Trauma*, **15**, 285–9.
18 Sadove, A.M., Jones, J.E. & Lynch, T.R. (1988). Appliance therapy for perioral electrical burns: a conservative approach. *Journal of Burn Care and Rehabilitation*, **9**, 391–5.
19 Baxter, C. (1970). Present concepts in the management of major electrical injury. *Surgery Clinics of North America*, **50**, 1402–18.
20 Solem, L., Fischer, R.P. & Strate, R.G. (1977). The natural history of electrical injury. *Journal of Trauma*, **17**, 487–91.
21 Holliman, C.J., Saffle, J.R., Kravitz, M. & Warden, G.D. (1982). Early surgical decompression in the management of electrical injuries. *American Journal of Surgery*, **144**, 733–40.

22 Zelt, R.G., Daniel, R.K., Ballard, P.A. & Brissette, Y. (1988). High-voltage electrical injury: chronic wound evolution. *Plastic and Reconstructive Surgery*, **82**, 1027–39.

23 Clayton, J.M., Hayes, A.C. & Hammel, J. *et al.* (1977). Xenon-133 determination of muscle blood flow in electrical injury. *Journal of Trauma*, **17**, 293–7.

24 Hunt, J.L., McManus, W.F., Haney, W.P. & Pruitt, B. A. (1974). Vascular lesions in acute electric injuries. *Journal of Trauma*, **14**, 461–70.

25 Quinby, Jr, W.C., Burke, J.F., Trelstad, R.L. & Caulfield, J. (1978). The use of microscopy as a guide to primary excision of high-tension electrical burns. *Journal of Trauma*, **18**, 423–9.

26 Buja, L.M., Tofe, A.J. & Kulkarni, P. V. *et al.* (1977). Sites and mechanisms of localization of technetium-99m phosphorus radiopharmaceuticals in acute myocardial infarcts and other tissues. *Journal of Clinical Investigation*, **60**, 724–40.

27 Hunt, J.L., Lewis, S., Parkey, R. & Baxter, C. (1979). The use of technetium-$^{99m}$ stannous pyrophosphate scintigraphy to identify muscle damage in acute electric burns. *Journal of Trauma*, **19**, 409–13.

28 Hartford, C.E. (1989). Preservation of devitalized calvarium following high-voltage electrical injury: case reports. *Journal of Trauma*, **29**, 391–4.

29 Purdue, G.F. & Hunt, J.L. (1986). Electrocardiographic monitoring after electrical injury: necessity or luxury. *Journal of Trauma*, **26**, 166–7.

30 Housinger, T.A., Green, L. & Shahangian, S. *et al.* (1985). A prospective study of myocardial damage in electrical injuries. *Journal of Trauma*, **25**, 122–5.

31 Harwood, S.J., Catrou, P.G. & Cole, G.W. (1978). Creatine phosphokinase isoenzyme fractions in the serum of a patient struck by lightning. *Archive of Internal Medicine*, **138**, 645–6.

32 McBride, J.W., Labrosse, K.R. & McCoy, H.G. *et al.* (1986). Is serum creatine kinase-MB in electrically injured patients predictive of myocardial injury? *Journal of the American Medical Association*, **255**, 764–8.

33 Nanji, A.A. & Filipenko, J.D. (1984). Non-myocardial source of CK-MB in a patient with electrical burn injury. *Burns*, **10**, 372–3.

34 Kahn, A.M. & Hoffman, R. (1985). Electric burn assessment: use of creatine kinase fractionation. *Journal of Burn Care and Rehabilitation*, **6**, 236–8.

35 Hunt, J., Purdue, G. & Spicer, T. (1983). Management of full-thickness burns of the scalp and skull. *Archives of Surgery*, **118**, 621–5.

36 Worthen, E.F. (1971). Regeneration of the skull following a deep electrical burn. *Plastic and Reconstructive Surgery*, **48**, 1–4.

37 Kirchmer, J.T., Larson, D.L. & Tyson, K.R.T. (1977). Cardiac rupture following electrical injury. *Journal of Trauma*, **17**, 389–90.

38 Miller, F.E., Peterson, D. & Miller, J. (1986). Abdominal visceral perforation secondary to electrical injury: case report and review of the literature. *Burns*, **12**, 505–7.

39 Newsome, T.W., Curreri, P.W. & Eurenius, C. (1972). Visceral injuries. *Archives of Surgery*, **105**, 494–7.

40 Xue-Wei W. (1980). Successful treatment of a case of electrical burn of the abdomen complicated with intestinal perforation. *Burns*, **8**, 128–30.

41  Williams, D.B. & Karl R.C. (1981). Intestinal injury associated with low-voltage electrocution. *Journal of Trauma*, **21**, 246–50.

42  Szabo, K. & Ver, P. (1983). Bone marrow aplasia after high voltage electrical injury. *Burns*, **10**, 184–7.

43  Reilley, A.F., Rees, R. & Kelton, P. *et al.* (1985). Abdominal aortic occlusion following electric injury. *Journal of Burn Care and Rehabilitation*, **6**, 226–9.

44  Saffle, J., Crandall, A. & Warden, G.D. (1985). Cataracts: a long-term complication of electrical injury. *Journal of Trauma*, **25**, 17–21.

45  Farrell, D.F. & Starr, A. (1968). Delayed neurological sequelae of electrical injuries. *Neurology*, **18**, 601–9.

46  Levine, N.S., Atkins, A. & McKeel, D.W. *et al.* (1975). Spinal cord injury following electrical accidents: case reports. *Journal of Trauma*, **15**, 459–63.

47  Jackson, F.E., Martin, R. & Davis, R. (1965). Delayed quadriplegia following electrical burn. *Military Medicine*, 601–5.

48  Silversides, J. (1964). The neurological sequelae of electrical injury. *Canadian Medical Association Journal*, **91**, 195–204.

49  White, J.W., Deitch, E.A. & Gillespie, T.E. *et al.* (1983). Cerebellar ataxia after an electrical injury: report of a case review of the literature. *Journal of Burn Care and Rehabilitation*, **4**, 191–3.

50  Helm, P.A. & Walker, S.C. (1987). New bone formation at amputation sites in electrically burn-injured patients. *Archives of Physical Medicine and Rehabilitation*, **68**, 284–6.

# 5

# The spectrum of electrical injuries

E.A. LUCE

## History

The commercial development of electrical energy began almost 150 years ago and was followed closely by the occurrence of serious injuries and fatalities. The first death may have been in 1879 in Lyon, France[1].

At present, over 1000 deaths occur each year in the United States, and electrical burns account for about 4% of the admissions to burn units.

The spectrum of clinical problems that occur from injuries secondary to electrical current span the household current injury of the oral commissure in a child to superficial palmar burns from a higher-tension source to that of a lethal high tension injury. Anatomically, high-tension electrical injury is devastating regardless of the area involved, whether skull, abdomen, or extremity.

Classifications of the type of electrical burns usually list three: thermal, arc, and direct electrical injury. A division of high-tension electrical injury into two subgroups, flash and 'true' has been found, by the author, to be useful. This division is based on the observation that some patients, although in contact with a high-tension source, actually sustained a flash pattern of burns and have a clinical course substantially distinct from that of the 'true' group. A 'true' high-tension electrical injury has the classic clinical features of a well-demarcated leathery full thickness site of current entrance and exit, although the distinction between entrance and exit wounds is not always obvious[2].

## Initial assessment and resuscitation

The initial assessment of the electrically injured patient should consider associated injuries sustained in a fall or other circumstances at the time of the accident. Careful questioning about the circumstances at the time of injury is essential. The patient, for example, may have fallen a distance, yet the historical fact may be lost in the concern with management of electrical burns.

Prompt fluid resuscitation of the electrical burn patient is the cornerstone for restoration of blood volume and prevention of acute tubular necrosis and failure. The volume of fluids necessary to adequately restore the intravascular volume and resuscitate the patient is much higher than in thermal burns. In addition, the combination of inadequate blood volume and the potential pigment load of myoglobin and haemoglobin pose a threat to renal function if such pigments should precipitate in the renal tubules. In the past, the use of agents such as mannitol, to increase renal perfusion, and sodium bicarbonate, to avoid pigment precipitation in an acid medium, have been a component of the resuscitation for electrical burns. The use of high-volume crystalloid such as Ringer's lactate without the addition of either bicarbonate or mannitol is preferred by the author. If the patient is adequately resuscitated, urine pH is either neutral or alkaline, particularly if Ringer's lactate is utilized.

In particular, the group of 'true' high-tension electrical burns required substantially more fluids than those high-tension burns that were judged to be more of a flash nature. Our experience, based on a retrospective review of patients, indicated that approximately 9 ml/kg/%BSA burned is necessary to adequately resuscitate a 'true' high-tension electrical burn.

Elderly patients, and those patients that have sustained both electrical and thermal burns with a substantial body surface area involvement, may require pulmonary artery catheterization to monitor cardiac function more accurately during resuscitation.

### Specific areas

Each anatomical region discussed: the skull, the trunk, and the extremities pose some particular problems for the clinician. Some of these problems have been successfully addressed with a distinct management plan. For others, the solution is less clear and some questions remain unanswered.

The appropriate management of the electrical burn wound has engendered considerable discussion and controversy. A dichotomy of opinion is evident in early reports and investigative work between those who adhered to a theory that high-tension electricity inflicts an injury with unique characteristics, intrinsic and separate from that of thermal burns[3]. Others attributed the injury to the heat of resistance generated by the passage of current[4]. The former concept gave rise to the conclusion that progressive or *de novo* necrosis occurred after the injury, possibly secondary to a delayed vascular phenomenon or occlusion from the current. Actually, experimental laboratory studies have not demonstrated evidence of the phenomenon of delayed or progressive necrosis[5]. Yet, the concept of progressive myonecrosis persists in many clinical discussions of the management of electrical burns. These arguments do not rest on theoretical grounds alone since, from this dichotomy, two different philosophies of the management of the electrical burn wound have emerged. One approach is to perform conservative, cautious debridement and delayed, even late, wound closure because of the fear that premature coverage will risk infection due to the incomplete removal of soft tissue that has become progressively necrotic. The other approach is early debridement and definitive repair. The point of difference is crucial because the final functional outcome may be compromised considerably by fibrosis and stiff joints. The potential for such complications is enhanced by prolonged closure of wounds, particularly in the extremity. In addition, rapid wound closure is advantageous in reducing pain, reversing the catabolic state, and hastening rehabilitation[6].

### The scalp and skull

The scalp and skull are frequently a contact or entry point in high-tension electrical burns, and the method of management is dependent on the depth of injury. The anatomical lesion has been described as saucer-like in configuration[7] when viewed in cross section. The deepest point of burn at the centre may expose cranium. With loss of the pericranium and exposure involvement of the underlying skull, coverage becomes problematic. The most conservative approach, now of historical interest only, was to leave the calverium exposed for an indeterminate time, usually months, and eventually the skull sloughed or was removed as a sequestrum. The subsequent defect was closed either with split-thickness skin grafts or flaps. The clinical course was often complicated by the occurrence of infectious complications of meningitis and epidural abscess[8]. An alternative approach, if performed sufficiently early in the postinjury period before the exposed bone has developed secondary osteomyelitis, is to excise the outer table and perform split-thickness skin grafts on the underlying diploic cavity. Clearly, the diploic cavity must be viable and the injury to the bone partial thickness only to obtain a vascularization of the split-thickness skin grafts. Often, the long-term durability of these skin grafts is not good, and the sequelae of recurrent ulceration and fibrosis may eventually dictate a more durable coverage.

If the injury is full thickness and the diploic cavity is destroyed, then the third option is early excision of the eschar and definitive flap coverage of the

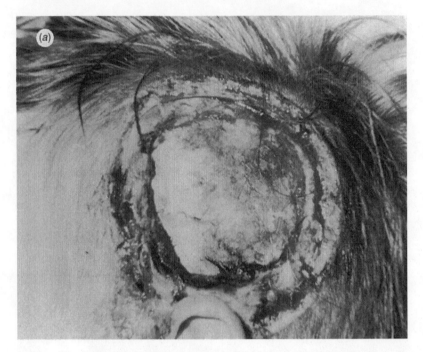

Fig. 5.1(*a*). High-tension contact point of the scalp with exposure and devitalization of underlying skull bone.

underlying exposed bone. Such an approach regards the devitalized bone as an *in situ* bone graft that will prosper beneath well-vascularized tissue[9]. If debridement and definitive coverage can be obtained before the bone becomes osteomyelitic, this approach is uniformly successful (Fig. 5.1 (*a–d*)). If the coverage defect is sufficiently large that the remaining uninjured scalp is inadequate to cover the exposed bone, free microvascular transfer of muscle or perhaps omentum is indicated.

Electrical burns of the scalp and skull raise several interesting questions:
1. *What is the effect of high-tension electrical current on bone?*
The occurrence of rarefaction, demineralization, and microfractures has been described in the past, but most available evidence is anecdotal in nature.
2. *What is the physiological basis for the development of central nervous system complications of paraplegia or quadraplegia on a delayed basis? What is the physiological basis for the development of nonfocal neurological signs and symptoms with problems with gait and balance, speech, memory, personality changes, or seizures?*

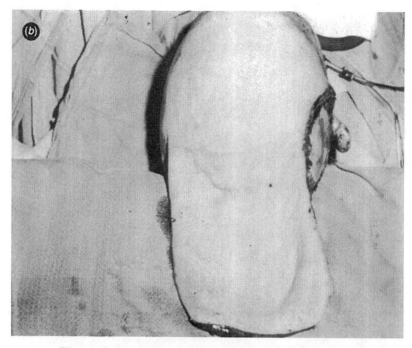

Fig. 5.1(*b*). A large occipital–parietal scalp flap. The nose is at the top of the figure.

Our experience with these complications has been limited to those patients who have sustained an entrance or exit wound of the scalp and skull, and this group seems at most risk. We have managed two patients with contact injury of the neck who developed a delayed onset of difficulty with gait and balance. Both of these patients had nonspecific neurological findings in the lower extremities and did not improve with follow-up.

3. *Why are the victims of high-tension electrical injury, particularly those with a contact point on the skull, at risk for the development of premature cataracts?*

The first presentation is a complaint of decreased visual acuity of delayed basis, usually 1 to 12 months postinjury, although the onset can be as late as $2\frac{1}{2}$ years postinjury[10]. The occurrence is usually bilateral and the incidence appears to be directly proportional to the magnitude of voltage exposure at the time of injury.

### Trunk, perineum

The primary concern in truncal electrical burns is injury to the intrathoracic or intra-abdominal contents. Entry and/or exit wounds may be contact

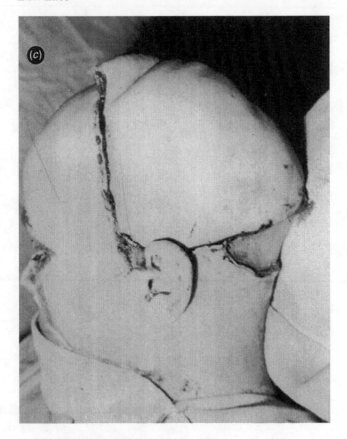

Fig. 5.1(c). The flap rotated into the defect.

points that conceal underlying damage to the thoracic or abdominal viscera. Two patients who had sustained a broad contact point of the anterior chest wall developed respiratory insufficiency in the early postinjury period and a radiographic picture, not unlike that seen in ARDS (adult respiratory distress syndrome), but the remaining lung paranchyma was radiologically normal. Both patients recovered with ventilatory support and positive end-expiratory pressure (PEEP). Injury to abdominal viscera from high-tension electrical burns is attended by a significant mortality[11,12]. A valuable clinical finding is a contact point on the anterior abdominal wall. The hypothesis is that a full-thickness injury of the abdominal wall has occurred and the adjacent intestine is damaged as well (Fig. 5.2). Perforation of the damaged intestine may occur on a delayed basis, and this delay may be the factor responsible for the significant mortality rate. The appropriate management of a high-tension contact

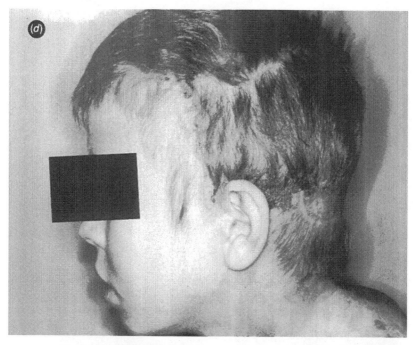

Fig. 5.1(*d*). Patient four months post-operatively. Wound has healed and no evidence of osteomyelitis is present.

burn of the anterior abdominal wall is immediate wound exploration and debridement. Sequential debridement of eschar, subcutaneous fat, and fascia and muscle, if indicated, is performed until viable tissue is encountered. Obviously, if the level of debridement is to the peritoneum, then an exploratory laparotomy is necessary to ascertain the status of the abdominal contents. The loop of injured intestine may lie anywhere within the abdominal cavity.

Full-thickness perineal injuries are managed optimally by early debridement and excision and definitive coverage.

Electrical injury to the abdomen poses additional questions:

1. *How do we explain the occasional case report of a patient who has sustained gangrene of an intra-abdominal viscus in the absence of a contact point on the abdominal wall?*

Such injuries appear extremely uncommon, but their occurrence is well documented[13].

2. *What is the pathophysiology that underlies the high incidence of late complaints of gastro-intestinal problems and dysfunction?*

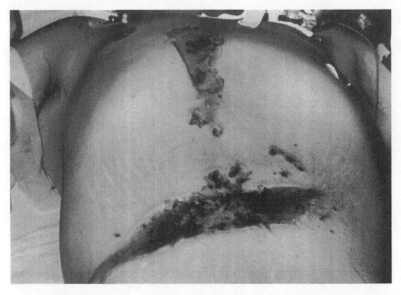

Fig. 5.2. High-tension linear contact point of the anterior abdominal wall as well as the mid-portion of the lower sternum.

### *Extremities*

The extremities are the most frequent site of high-tension electrical burns to injury, and have been the source of the most controversy in management. When the injury involves the upper extremity, the extremity or a portion is often lost. The eventual outcome in a group of such patients was dictated in a large part by the status of the extremity on acute presentation[14]. If the extremity was ischaemic without pulse, anaesthetic and held in a flexed and contracted position, amputation or salvage of a functionless part was a distressingly frequent result, despite aggressive decompression and debridement.

Virtually all such patients have been injured by grasping the line source or the ground. They sustain a significant cutaneous burn of the wrist in association with a palmar burn. The mechanism may be a tetanic contraction of the digits, wrist, and possibly elbow and shoulder. Arc burns occur at the flexion creases of the wrist, elbow, and axilla (Fig. 5.3). Exploration of the wrist burn will reveal a coagulative necrosis of the underlying structures, including muscle bellies, tendons, nerves, and most significantly the radial and ulnar arteries. Pulsatile flow can be traced to the level of the severe wrist burn and at that point the vessels are severely charred and nearly indistinguishable as discrete structures.

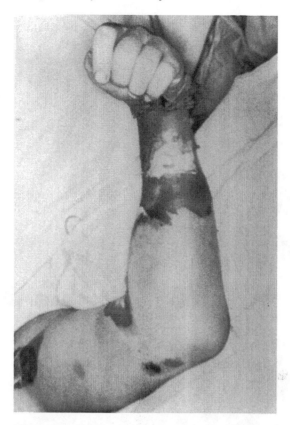

Fig. 5.3. Mummification of the distal one-half of the forearm and hand with arc burns at the elbow and axilla flexion creases.

The arc burns of flexion creases at the elbow and axilla often conceal a considerable amount of deep tissue necrosis. Additional areas of concealed necrosis may occur in the periosseous muscle groups even proximal to the level of the cutaneous burn (Fig. 5.4). Since bone is a poor conductor, perhaps the increased heat of resistance is responsible for the peri-osseous myonecrosis. These areas of myonecrosis also may be occult and unsuspected (Fig. 5.5(a)–(c)). Lastly, necrosis is not uniform or predictable. Patchy areas of necrosis of muscle can occur at the periphery of the central zone and may not be readily evident at the time of injury. Questionable muscle retained at early debridement provides the nidus for additional tissue loss. The resultant contamination and desiccation can perpetuate a cycle of compromised viability and diminished resistance followed by further infection, hypoxia, and further compromise of the circulatory

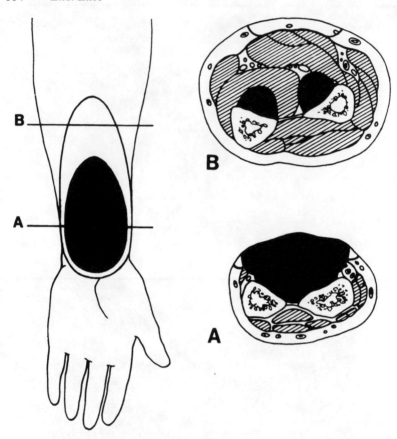

Fig. 5.4. Diagrammatic representation of the saucer-like configuration of the soft tissue component of electrical burns, yet peri-osseous muscle necrosis may be present proximal to the level of the most severe cutaneous injury.

status. Adjacent muscle, although viable yet compromised, may be adversely affected by the process and perpetuate the cycle.

Only early, aggressive, and complete debridement of devitalized skin and muscle can prevent this cycle and provide the setting for definitive coverage.

Electrical injuries should be considered appropriately a burn. Patients with high-tension injuries should have fasciotomy, usually in combination with escharotomy, wound exploration, and debridement accomplished in the first few hours postinjury. Debridement consists of the aggressive excision of devitalized muscle as judged by colour and lack of contractility to stimulation. Bleeding is often from larger vessels and does not represent

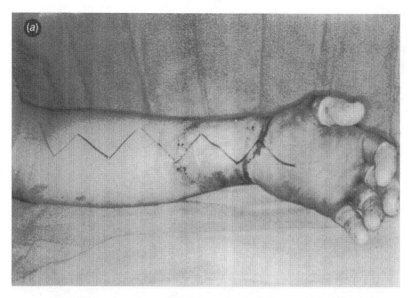

Fig. 5.5(*a*). A high-tension injury of the base of palm and wrist and forearm. The incisions for a forearm and hand fasciotomy are outlined.

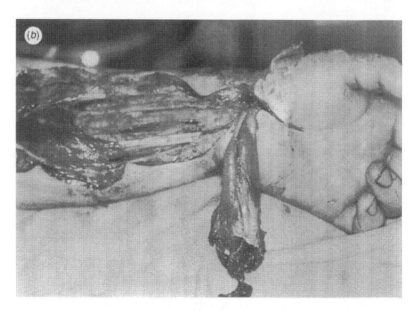

Fig. 5.5(*b*). Following debridement of the sublimus muscle groups, the underlying profundus tendons and muscle bellies were clearly viable.

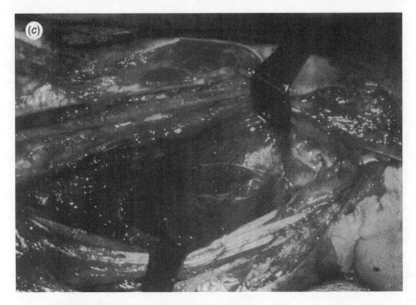

Fig. 5.5(*c*). After retraction of the volar structures, exposure of a clearly necrotic pronator quadratus is evident. Presumably, the muscle was damaged because of the peri-osseous location.

true nutrient flow to the muscle. Adequate debridement and exploration of the skip burns at the flexion creases should be performed acutely and particular attention directed to the deep and peri-osseous muscle groups (Fig. 5.6(*a*), (*b*)). The use of ancillary measures such as technitium scans or frozen-section microscopy has not gained widespread acceptance and application because of the considerable logistical problems these techniques present. Obviously, mummified extremities should be amputated at this acute setting (Fig. 5.7). Debrided wounds are covered with biological dressings of porcine skin or homografts.

The patients are returned to the operating room 24 to 48 hours later for a second wound exploration and debridement. At this juncture, the periphery of the zone of injury should be inspected carefully for areas of patchy necrosis. Skin wounds may need to be extended for proper exposure. Nerves and tendons are notable exceptions to this conceptual approach and should be preserved even if they appear devitalised. Definitive coverage is provided as rapidly as feasible. The systemic goals of pain relief, enhancement of nutrition, and deterrence of sepsis as well as the extremity rehabilitative goals of early motion and salvage of nerve and tendons are enhanced by early coverage. Early coverage can only be obtained by

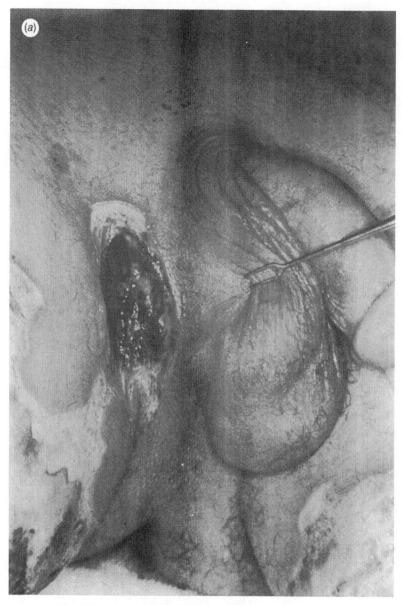

Fig. 5.6(*a*). An inguinal crease arc burn.

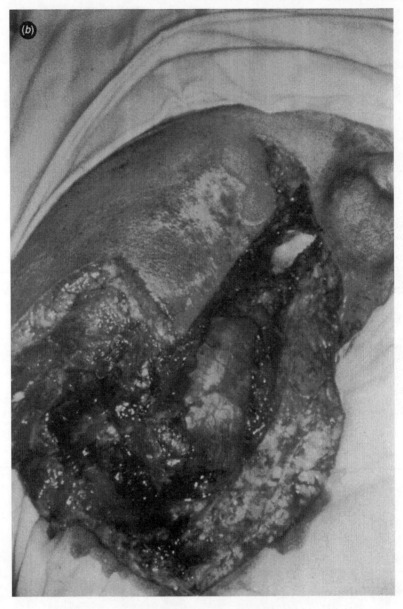

Fig. 5.6(*b*). After debridement and extension of incisions to ensure complete debridement, extensive defect is evident. In addition, the patient required a mid-thigh amputation of the extremity.

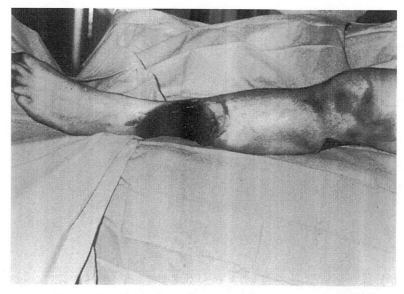

Fig. 5.7. Mummification of the lower extremity. Adequate debridement will require an above-the-knee amputation.

aggressive and complete debridement. Coverage has been provided by split-thickness skin grafts in the lower extremity and abdominal flaps or groin flaps in the upper extremity. Split-thickness skin grafts have been used on occasion on the upper extremity, but do not provide the stability of coverage often required. The use of free flaps for definitive coverage of upper extremity electrical injury wounds has been performed with some success[15,16]. Microvascular free tissue transfer is an attractive option for coverage of bone, tendon, and nerve, without the restrictive limitations of more conventional pedicle flaps. The concern that recipient vessels have sustained an occult injury that would contra-indicate free tissue transfer is not justified, and this technique deserves much wider application in the management of patients with electrical burns.

Therapeutic questions raised in management of high-tension injury of the extremities include:

1. *Can a better functional result be obtained in severe injuries by acute debridement and immediate coverage of damaged muscle with well-vascularized tissue? Could such muscle 'regenerate' or at least retain some functional capacity? Do we inflict additional injury by devascularization and the inevitable contamination of exposure with debridement?*

*2. What is the pathophysiological explanation for the late development of the skeletal complications of heterotopic bone formation and bone cysts?*

Although rarely reported in the past[17], the occurrence has been frequent in the group of patients who have required amputation secondary to high-tension electrical injury. Bone cysts have become inflamed secondarily and have culminated in sinus tracts that required curretement, packing, and secondary closure to obtain healing. Heterotopic bone formation has produced areas of skin erosion, difficulty with the prosthesis, and limitation of motion. The heterotopic bone formation is usually in the configuration of bone spicules, some of substantial length and not necessarily peri-articular in location. Does the passage of high-voltage current induce a change at a cellular level that stimulates osteogenesis?

### Summary

The traditional classification of high-tension injury is exposure to 1000 volts or greater. A further classification is possible based on the circumstances and the type and distribution of injury. Flash burns behave as thermal burns with a mixture of full- and partial-thickness injury without characteristic entry or exit wounds. The voltage in 'true' high-tension injury is usually considerably greater than 1000 volts. The subclassification of patients along such lines is important clinically since virtually all severe complications, including difficulty in resuscitation, amputations, and reconstructive procedures are limited to the 'true' subgroup.

Since adoption of an aggressive approach to electrical burns that includes acute exploration, early debridement, and definitive coverage, the duration of hospitalization in the 'true' subgroup has been reduced nearly by half (45.7 days vs. 23.1 days). Yet many questions still exist in the management of these patients with such a devastating injury.

### References

1 Luce, E.A. (1990). Electrical injuries. In *Reconstructive Plastic Surgery*, 3rd edn., McCarty, J.G. ed., W.B. Saunders.
2 Luce, E.A. & Gottleib, S.E. (1981). 'True' high tension electrical injuries. *Annals of Plastic Surgery*, **12**, 321–6.
3 Jellineck, S. (1936). Causation, pathology, and therapeutics of electrical injuries. *Edinburgh Medical Journal*, **43**, 587.
4 Jaffe, R.H. (1928). Electropathology, *Archives of Pathology*, **5**, 837.
5 Hunt, J.L., Sato, R.M. & Baxter, C.R. (1980). Acute electrical burns: current diagnostic and therapeutic approaches to management. *Archives of Surgery*, **115**, 434.
6 Luce, E.A. (1982). Discussion: rehabilitation following electrical injury. *Annals of Plastic and Surgery*, **8**, 442.

7 Stuckey, J.G. (1963). Surgical management of massive electrical burns of the scalp. *Plastic and Reconstructive Surgery*, **32**, 538.

8 Kragh, L.B. & Erich, J.B. (1961). Treatment of severe electrical injuries. *American Journal of Surgery*, **101**, 419.

9 Luce, E.A. & Hoopes, J.E. (1974). Electrical burn of the scalp and skull. *Plastic and Reconstructive Surgery*, **54**, 359.

10 Jaffe, J.R., Crandall, A. & Warden, G.D. (1985). Cataracts: a long-term complication of electrical injury. *Journal of Trauma*, **25**, 7.

11 Almgard, L., Liljedahl, S. & Nylen, B. (1965). Electrical burns of the abdomen. *Acta Chirurgica Scandinavica*, **130**, 550.

12 Yang, J.Y., Tsai, Y.G. & Noordhoff, M.S. (1985). Electrical burn with visceral injury. *Burns*, **11**, 207.

13 Williams, D.B. & Karl, R.C. (1981). Intestinal injury associated with low-voltage electrocution. *Journal of Trauma*, **21**, 246.

14 Luce, E.A., Dowden, W.L., Su, C.T. & Hoopes, J.E. (1978). High-tension electrical injury of the upper extremity. *Surgery, Gynecology and Obstetrics*, **147**, 38.

15 Grotting, J. & Walkinshaw, M. (1985). The early use of free flaps in burns. *Annals of Plastic Surgery*, **15**, 127.

16 Silverberg, B., Banis, J.E., Verdi, G.D. & Acland, R.D. (1986). Microvascular reconstruction after electrical and deep thermal injury. *Journal of Trauma*, **26**, 128.

17 Clark, G.S., Naso, F. & Ditunno, J.F. (1980). Marked bone spur formation in a burn amputee patient. *Archives of Physical Medicine Rehabilitation*, **61**, 189.

# 6

# Electrical trauma: pathophysiology and clinical management

ROBERT H. DEMLING

Electrical burn injuries account for less than 5% of admissions to major burn centres. However, the injury is much more complex than a skin burn and the morbidity and mortality rate is considerably higher. The mortality rate ranges from 3–15% with about 1000 deaths attributed to electrical current in the US each year. More than 90% of injuries occur in males, most between ages 20 and 34.

## Electrical current tissue damage

### *Pathophysiology*

The severity of injury to tissues is dependent on the amperage, i.e. the actual amount of current, passing through the tissues. It is impossible to know the amperage because of the variability of resistance and exposure time at the accident, but one can infer amperage from the voltage of the source at least as to high or low. A low-voltage source is capable of producing major cardiopulmonary complications and death if a sufficient current passes through the body (Table 6.1).

A high-tension source is usually required to produce the severe tissue necrosis characteristically seen along the path of the current. The damage is caused by both heat production and direct current damage. The initial resistance to flow of current, namely, skin or clothing, is overcome by the heat generated from the high voltage, and subsequent tissue necrosis occurs with continued contact. A dry hand may have sufficient resistance to avoid passage of current from a low-voltage source over a short time period. However, the generation of several thousand degrees at the contact site with a high-tension source will lead to an immediate local coagulation and

Table 6.1.

| Current in milliamps | Effect |
|---|---|
| High-tension source | Severe tissue destruction |
| 5000 or more | from heat and coagulation |
| | Cardiopulmonary failure |
| Household source | |
| 60 | Cardiac fibrillation |
| 30 | Respiratory muscle |
| | tetany: suffocation |
| 5 | Pain |
| 15 | Muscle tetany |

disruption of the electrical barrier. The current can now pass more readily through the tissues with a high water content, as water is an excellent conductor.

The mechanism of tissue damage itself is complex and not completely defined. There is clearly an injury to nerves, blood vessels, and muscle from the current itself, damaging the cells. Endothelial cell injury due either to heat or current will result in loss of protection against local clotting and microvascular thrombosis and tissue devascularization will result.

The resistance of tissues to passage of current is, in large part, dependent on water content, water being a good conductor. Tissue resistance in decreasing order from high to low is bone, fat, tendon, skin, muscle, vessels, nerve. With high-voltage injuries, the current passes through tissues indiscriminately.

The pathway of current can be somewhat unpredictable but, in general, current passes from a point of entry through the body to a grounded site; i.e. to a site of lower resistance to flow compared to air which is a poor conductor. Extremely high-voltage sources usually exit in multiple areas in an explosive fashion.

The severity of injury is also directly proportional to the duration of current flow. However, even extremely brief exposures to high amperage will produce massive tissue damage.

A vast array of injuries result from the electrical damage (Table 6.2).

### Cutaneous injury

The determination that a current injury to underlying tissue may be present is the finding of contact sites where the current enters and exits. Their

Table 6.2.

| Common complications | |
| --- | --- |
| Ventricular fibrillation | Muscle necrosis |
| Other rhythm abnormalities | Fractures |
| Respiratory arrest | Haemolysis |
| Seizures/coma | Renal failure |
| Mental changes | Haemorrhage |
| Hypertension | Limb loss |
| Retinal detachment | Anaemia |
| Cataract (delayed) | Paresis/paralysis and other neurological (delayed) |

presence is pathognomonic of an electrical injury beneath the skin.

The heat generated at the skin surface is dependent on the local resistance which, in the dry hand, can be sufficient to generate heat in excess of 1000 °C with high-voltage sources. This will lead to local mummification at the entrance. The skin appearance at the site of contact is often that of a well-defined charred wound which is depressed due to loss of tissue bulk. The latter is due to evaporation of local water content by the high temperature. The wound may sometimes appear like a typical deep flame burn, except that, in this case, the injury extends well below the dermis. The arc burn is basically a very deep thermal burn caused by the intense heat generated from the high-tension current.

Tissue appearance, at the site of current exit, varies considerably in magnitude. The appearance is often that which would be expected from an explosion, as pieces of cutaneous tissue are often absent, having been blown out by the immense energy of the exiting current.

### Muscle necrosis

Electrical burns more closely resemble a crush injury than a thermal burn. The damage below the skin where the current passes is usually far greater than the appearance of overlying skin would indicate. The immediate damage to these tissues is caused by the heat destruction of cells which is usually patchy in distribution along the course of the current. A massive release of intracellular contents with cell lysis may in part be responsible for the systemic toxicity evident early after injury. Fluid requirements are often massive, suggesting a generalized alteration in vascular permeability in injured tissues due to circulating inflammatory mediators. The second process is that of an apparent devascularization caused by injured blood vessels which thrombose over a several-day period. The third process is that of compartment syndrome with pressure necrosis especially prominent in nervous tissue and muscle enveloped by a nonyielding fascial covering. The fourth process is that of tissue infection.

There will be some immediate tissue death from heat coagulation. Dead muscle has a pale red to white appearance due to release of myoglobin content. The dead muscle is noncontractile and is often found near the entrance and exit areas as well as along the bone. Local blood vessels in the area are thrombosed. The immediate necrosis does not follow the anatomic division of muscles but is very uneven, reflecting the uneven nature of the current passage. Within minutes to hours of injury, the damaged, but still perfused, muscles begin to swell as vascular permeability appears to be altered. The release of intracellular osmotically active peptides may also accentuate the tissue oedema. The finite boundaries of the fascial envelope cause a rapid rise in tissue pressure which, when exceeding the 20–25 mm Hg microvascular hydrostatic pressure, produces further local tissue ischaemia as well as local compression nerve injury. A tissue pressure exceeding 30 mm Hg is clearly abnormal and must be decreased to avoid further damage. Oedema increases over the ensuing 24–48 hours.

Vascular thrombosis can occur immediately and over the ensuing 3–4 days due to initial current-induced vessel damage. The progressive devascularization results in a further loss of muscle tissue. The combination of endothelial cell damage and weakening of the vessel wall can lead not only to local thrombosis but also to local tissue haemorrhage.

The combination of these processes, the uneven nature of the necrosis and, in particular, the damage to muscles and nerves closest to bone, results in severe functional impairment and a high rate of amputation (30–40%). Eventual muscle atrophy, and replacement of injured muscle by fibrous tissue, is another cause of subsequent dysfunction.

### Cardiovascular

Immediate cardiac arrest is the most common cause of death after electrical injury. The process is due to both the direct alteration of rhythm by the current, leading to fibrillation, and to the depression of respiration, and subsequent hypoxia. Both brain and chest wall muscle changes will occur, leading to impaired ventilation. Hand-to-hand passage of a high-voltage current has a reported immediate mortality of 60%. The initial cardiac arrhythmia is often reversible, and cardiac resuscitation should be initiated at the scene. Current-induced myocardial necrosis is rare, although myocardial infarction can occur. The most common ECG changes seen other than fibrillation are sinus tachycardia and nonspecific ST-T wave changes. Systemic hypertension is quite common with high voltage, possibly due to a massive and sustained release of catecholamines.

A low flow state as a result of fluid protein and blood loss into the tissues is characteristic and must be aggressively treated to avoid additional shock-induced tissue damage. A crush-type injury invariably results in a massive fluid loss into the injured tissue.

Major vessel thrombosis is well described as is delayed rupture of large vessels with massive haemorrhage, even in the absence of surrounding tissue damage indicating the low resistance to flow within vessels. Aneurysms occurring weeks to months after injury, although uncommon, must be anticipated with good follow-up measures. Treatment is specific to the disease process.

### Renal

Renal failure is reported in 10% or more of injuries. Renal damage is caused by a multitude of processes. Myoglobin and haemoglobin released from damaged muscle and RBCs can precipitate in the renal tubules producing an acute tubular necrosis, ATN, picture. Myoglobin is colourless in circulating plasma while free haemoglobin is, of course, pink to red. Both, however, will produce pink to red urine. Myoglobin precipitation is accentuated by an acid urine and decreased by an alkaline urine. The muscle necrosis also produces a tissue injury very similar to a crush injury with evidence of distant organ dysfunction. The kidney, i.e. glomerulus, is a well-known target organ with this type of process. The low flow state caused by hypovolaemia simply will aggravate the injury. Direct renal vascular damage from the current also can result.

### Pulmonary

The immediate pulmonary abnormalities are the result of a CNS-induced hypoventilation or of chest wall neuromuscular dysfunction. Impairment of respiratory center activity and severe CNS damage will lead to hypoventilation which is frequently the cause of immediate death. Impairment of muscle activity in the chest wall caused by a chest burn, muscle damage, or second degree blunt traumatic injuries can impair compliance markedly. Injuries to the diaphragm are uncommon. Later pulmonary complications are comparable to those seen after thermal burn.

### Neurological

Both immediate and delayed neurological abnormalities are common. Acute CNS dysfunction with coma, seizures, motor and, to a lesser extent, sensory deficits are well described. Many of these abnormalities are permanent. In addition, a number of delayed injuries occur including both peripheral neuropathies and cord damage with paralysis.

### Abdominal viscera

Hollow viscus damage is not common but certainly can occur. Many of the injuries appear to be vascular in origin, although local heat-induced damage to the intestine has been described. Peptic ulcers, cholecystitis and gastro-intestinal bleeding can be seen. It is difficult, however, to sort out whether these latter types of processes are due to a specific current injury or simply a manifestation of severe trauma or the resulting shock.

### Orthopaedic

The most common orthopaedic injury occurs as a result of the severe immediate muscle spasm which is capable of producing long bone fractures and dislocation at major joints. Heat necrosis of local peri-osteum with subsequent production of nonviable bone and sequestrum formation is the next most common process. Devascularization of bone due to the same vascular injury affecting other tissues is less common.

### Ocular–otic

Again, both immediate and delayed injuries are noted. Conjunctival and corneal burns as well as ruptured eardrums are well described early changes. Late changes (up to 1 year) include cataract formation, tinnitus and decreased hearing.

### Hematological

Acute anaemia due to haemolysis and blood loss in damaged muscle is a characteristic finding. Clotting abnormalities, in particular, an initial consumptive coagulopathy, are also common.

### Infection

Infection in the areas of tissue necrosis and ischaemia is a major problem beginning several days after injury, particularly if a skin burn is also present which will potentiate cross-contamination from wound to wound. Control of the wound is much more difficult than with the skin burn, as topical antibiotics will not be able to reach subsurface pockets of infection.

### Hypermetabolism

A hyperdynamic, hypermetabolic state is seen characteristically beginning hours to several days postinjury. The process, initiated and perpetuated by inflamed injured tissue, leads to a marked increase in oxygen consumption and carbon dioxide production as well as to muscle catabolism and increased caloric demands.

## General treatment principles

### Monitoring

The first principle of treatment is making the diagnosis of an electrical injury. Since there is absolutely no way of ruling out deep injury on initial assessment, admission and observation are necessary. Cardiopulmonary monitoring and supportive care are clearly necessary, given the high incidence of cardiac arrhythmias and pulmonary dysfunction. An initial urinalysis is essential not only to verify adequate renal perfusion but also to check for myoglobinuria which if present will require special management. Blood gases and acid–base balance are of particular importance in avoiding an acidosis which will accentuate pigment deposition in the kidney.

Monitoring of peripheral perfusion and palpation of muscle compartments is of particular importance because of the concern of the development of compartment syndromes due to underlying muscle oedema. Compartment pressure can be monitored using several types of available systems. Determination of the need for fasciotomy are based either on the absolute value of tissue pressure or on the relationship of tissue pressure to blood pressure. Indications for an immediate fasciotomy include a tissue pressure greater than 40 mm Hg or a tissue pressure within 30 mm Hg of diastolic pressure. Usually the number itself is not used as an absolute indication but is compared with any clinical evidence of nerve compression, i.e. tingling, increased pain, or decreased sensation, or vessel compression. Motor nerve dysfunction is more difficult to assess, given the fact that muscle damage may be impossible to distinguish from nerve damage. Excessive tissue turgor is the single most useful sign of underlying muscle damage and the need for fasciotomy.

### Fluid management

The same basic principles apply as with a thermal burn alone. The primary resuscitation fluid is Ringer's lactate (or hypertonic lactated saline). There is no formula, however, to assist in management due to the unpredictable nature of the underlying tissue damage. In general, the fluid requirements per percentage of burn are 1.5 to 2 times that of a skin burn alone, given the nature of the added soft tissue injury. Colloid and blood are used more frequently during the early resuscitation period than after thermal burn alone due to haemolysis and to the increased whole blood losses into the damaged muscle and other deep tissues. Excessive crystalloid may accentuate muscle oedema and potentiate pressure necrosis even after fasciotomy, as this procedure does not totally eliminate the problem.

The rate of fluid administration is based on the amount necessary to maintain adequate perfusion using the same guidelines for burn shock management. The exception is the presence of urine myoglobin or other evidence of early renal impairment. If the urine is red or reddish–black, a massive myoglobin release from muscle has occurred and an increased washout of the tubular pigment is needed. A urine flow of 1 ml/kg/h or more is needed until pigment load has decreased. Mannitol (12.5 g for 2–4 h) is often required to maintain this level of output. In addition, sodium bicarbonate is often needed to maintain urine pH equal to or greater than 7 so as to minimize pigment precipitation. Loop diuretics may be needed, beginning the next day, to maintain a high urine flow, if pigment persists.

Furosemide increases tubular fluid flow and lowers renal vascular resistance. A similar approach at maintaining tubular patency is also initiated if evidence of nonpigment load renal dysfunction is noted from direct renal injury or that from disseminated intravascular coagulation (DIC) or low flow state.

Fluid and osmotic agents are temporizing agents, however, and the injured muscle, if a large amount is present, must be removed very early to prevent renal shutdown. Subsequent fluid, electrolyte, nutritional support and stress management follow the principles described for thermal burns.

### Infection control

In general, infection control is obtained by wound debridement. Tetanus prophylaxis is required in view of the risks of deep tissue necrosis in a relatively anaerobic environment. Broad spectrum antibiotics are not indicated as a prophylactic measure. However, perioperative antibiotics are indicated as with management of skin burns. The principal organism of concern in the initial 2–3 days is *Staphylococcus aureus*. Coverage with a cephalosporin or methicillin is appropriate. Later, organisms, such as *Pseudomonas aeruginosa* which thrives in a low-oxygen environment, will be the predominant organism. Topical antibiotics such as Silvidene and Sulfamylon can be used on the skin burns where an eschar is present.

### Escharotomy–fasciotomy

In general, if there is a circumferential deep burn and any evidence of impaired distal perfusion, i.e. decreased pulses, an escharotomy is necessary. If there is also a concomitant electrical injury to underlying tissue and increasing compartment pressure, evidenced by increased myoglobin, rigid muscle compartments, or of nerve or vessel compression, fasciotomy is indicated. The underlying muscle can then be inspected to determine viability. An electrocautery is often necessary with fasciotomy, as opposed to escharotomy, as fascial and muscle vessels may well be patent. The fasciotomy defect exposing the viable but injured muscle must be covered preferably with a biological or synthetic skin substitute to avoid desiccation. The escharotomy site and incisions through burn or nonviable tissue can be managed with topical antibiotics. It is not necessary, and is actually disadvantageous, to expose muscle groups which are not clearly involved in a compartment syndrome. The exposure of muscle increases the risk of colonization and infection.

### Wound management

The spectrum of injuries which can occur makes definitive comments on wound management difficult. In general, high-voltage burns with large amounts of necrotic muscle must be treated aggressively with surgical debridement, including early amputation of nonviable extremities, to minimize subsequent organ dysfunction, infection, and eventual mortality. An early aggressive surgical approach also maximizes the salvage of marginal tissue which is very susceptible to infection. If gross myoglobinuria is present for several hours or if there are large exit sites or mummification of a large entrance wound, one can nearly guarantee that a large amount of dead muscle is present.

Early excision of obviously dead muscle is performed as soon as hemodynamic stability is obtained, preferably in the first 1–2 days. Also the risks of renal failure increase as long as a large amount of dead and dying muscle is present.

The goal of subsequent surgical procedures is to conserve remaining viable tissue while removing neighbouring dead tissue. The uneven nature of the injury makes this approach difficult and very time consuming. Small, scattered areas of injured muscle will be reabsorbed and replaced by fibrous tissue. Physiological evidence of remaining infected dead tissue is often manifested by a high fever and tachycardia. The tissue along the bone is often the site of the necrosis.

### *Nutritional support*

Early nutrition of adequate calorie and protein intake is essential to minimize morbidity. The caloric requirements will be reflected in the degree of increase in oxygen consumption, which usually means 1.5–2 times normal calorie intake. Protein requirements with a major electrical burn are about 1.5 g per kg body weight per day.

### *Managing contact sites*

Entrance and exit sites of electrical injuries are more complex than a standard skin burn. The problem is that devitalized tissue exists below the burn especially at the exit site. Initial debridement to viable tissue should follow the same principles as with a thermal burn. However, it is best to use biological or synthetic temporary skin substitutes initially. Further necrosis of tissues is expected. After 3–5 days, the temporary skin substitutes (or moist dressings) can be removed, any residual necrotic tissue debrided and wound closure begun either with skin grafts or skin flaps. Tissue defects at entrance and exit may require tissue transfer. Initial closure with skin grafts is often preferred with the larger procedures to be performed later in a more stable patient.

### Thermal burns to the skin

The heat generated by arcing (jumping) of a high-voltage current from a high-tension wire toward the victim, will reach several thousand degrees as air has a high resistance. The heat will produce a fresh skin burn comparable to that of any explosion of volatile substances. In addition, the intense heat frequently causes clothes to catch fire, leading to deep burns. It is easy to overlook an electrical burn in the presence of a large skin burn. The subsequent soft tissue oedema and pain can be misinterpreted as due to the thermal injury rather than underlying damage.

The treatment is essentially identical to that for any cutaneous burn alone except that a higher urine output will be necessary if myoglobinuria is present. More fluid will be necessary and more initial cardiopulmonary support if an electrical burn is also present.

### Blunt trauma (free falls)

Well over half of high-voltage injuries occur to workers on towers and poles more than 20 feet above the ground. Free-fall injuries, therefore, are the result. The nature and magnitude of the injury depend on:

1 height of the fall
2 the impact surface (stopping distance)
3 body mass
4 body orientation on impact
5 distribution of impact forces
6 patient age, which affects tissue tolerance.

Some of the kinetic energy (KE) generated during the fall is converted to potential energy which is defined as $PE = mgs$ where $s$ is stopping distance. The greater the stopping distance, the more KE is dissipated as PE. Fortunately, the surface near power poles is frequently dirt rather than concrete. The majority of KE is converted to mechanical energy which is dissipated through the tissues, generating fractures and rupture of visceral organs.

Treatment is essentially the same as that for similar trauma in the absence of an electrical injury. Differences are primarily in the manner of treating fractures beneath burned skin or muscle damage where early fixation with hardware may not be as feasible. The major treatment problem, however, is failure to recognize the existence of the blunt injury in the electrical burn patient.

# 7

# Acute and delayed neurological sequelae of electrical injury

BAIBA J. GRUBE

DAVID M. HEIMBACH

## Introduction

Modern society has experienced a tremendous proliferation in the use of electricity. Like a bird perched on a high-tension wire, the human body is immune to shock so long as it is not part of the electric circuit[1], but current out of the constraints of its wire poses a dramatic hazard to life and limb. Despite safeguards, electrical injuries still account for 3% of all burn centre admissions and cause approximately 1000 deaths per year[1,2].

Electricity is a particularly temperamental and unpredictable maimer of young, working males injured on the job or while participating in recreational activities. In the United States, about one-third of the injuries occur in construction workers and another third in electricians[3].

Electrical injury can be likened to the 'Grand Masquerader' of thermal injuries, manifesting a variety of unpredictable immediate and delayed sequelae that even the most astute physician cannot anticipate always, yet ever must be prepared to recognize and treat. Any organ system may be involved, and damage may only become evident at some time distant from the injury.

Permanent neurological damage following major electrical burns has long been feared as a dreaded complication[4-12]. Immediate as well as subsequent complications can develop. Neurological complications involving either cerebral complaints (loss of consciousness, seizures, decreased memory, emotional lability, learning impairment or headaches) or peripheral complaints (sensorimotor loss, paraesthesias, paralysis, paresis, dysaesthesias, causalgia, or reflex sympathetic dystrophy) have been described.

### Review of literature

Neurological disorders from electric shock can be classified as cerebral syndromes, spinal syndromes and peripheral nerve syndromes[6]. In addition, the effects can be manifested immediately or can present after a long time delay[13]. The majority of neurological findings present in patients sustaining high-voltage injuries. The distinction between high voltage and low voltage depends on the source of information. Low voltage has been set at 380 V for safety[14], but the clinical data in the literature defines high voltage at variable levels, beginning somewhere between 380 V to 1000 V[15].

### Low voltage

There is a paucity of information regarding neurological sequelae with low voltage, since these injuries are usually relatively minor, rarely hospitalized and only mentioned incidentally in reviews of major electrical injuries. The morbidity may be greater than predicted[16]. The major complications from voltages between 120–240 volts include cardiac arrhythmias, respiratory compromise and death[17]. But, low-voltage electrical injuries have also been associated with some neurological changes, including loss of consciousness, paralysis and sensory deficits[13,18,19]. The resolution and/or evolution of symptoms as a function of time after injury was followed prospectively by Blom and Ugland[18]. Two patients with immediate symptoms from low voltage had neurological findings. One had loss of consciousness and another had loss of sensation of the right thumb. Both patients recovered completely. In this same series, 11 patients sustaining injury from 220–380 volts were given initial normal neurological exams and were followed for at least 1 year. One patient developed loss of sensation around the mouth, and another developed loss of the right fifth digit extensor function with loss of motor units in the *opponens pollicis* muscle. Panse[19] has described two patients with delayed onset of peripheral atrophy after sustaining low-voltage injury.

Panse[19] and Alexander[20] have described the delayed onset of spinal cord symptoms in several patients with low voltage, including amyotrophic lateral sclerosis, progressive atrophy of muscles associated with fasciculations and hyperaesthesia.

### High voltage

High-voltage injuries account for the largest fraction of major neurological complications. The incidence of immediate findings ranges from as low as

29%[9] to as great as 45% to 55%[5,12]. Although there are many cumulative reviews of neurological findings from high-voltage electrical injury, little is known in these reports about the evolution of symptoms as a function of time after injury.

### Cerebral syndromes

The most frequently reported neurological lesion is loss of consciousness, occurring in between 21% to 67% of the patients[5,12,21]. In Burke's series, all patients recovered and there were no permanent sequelae[21]. Burke postulates that most patients do not develop clinical permanent brain damage despite unconsciousness or deep burns to the calvarium because compensatory mechanisms render the changes undetectable. In another series, there were no memory deficits, impaired mental function or seizures, but several had amnesia for the event[12]. In a series of 14 case reports of patients with neurological sequelae, nine patients had loss of consciousness and eight developed delayed neuropsychiatric effects[13]. Symptoms resembled those of a concussion or confusion and included headaches, dizziness, vertigo, and occasional seizure activity. In addition, others exhibited psychoneurotic behaviour including impotence, headache, and personality changes. Persistent coma has a very bad prognosis, leading to death[5,12].

### *Peripheral nerve syndromes*

Peripheral nerve injuries may present as permanent deficits or as transient neuropathies. The incidence of acute peripheral nerve injuries is difficult to extrapolate from the published series. These injuries range between 5% to 23% of all neurological sequelae[2,4,5,9,21,22]. Peripheral injuries located at the site of devastated limbs are included in some publications and it is unknown which of these finite lesions were involved in early amputation. The most frequent peripheral injuries in most series occurred to the median nerve followed by the ulnar, radial and peroneal nerves[5,9,12,23]. Although infrequent, if the nerve sheath is intact, partial sensorimotor deficits can improve[2,24]. Early volar carpal tunnel release has been advocated by Butler and Gant[4] and Parshley *et al.*[25] in the oedematous arm and hand. Early surgical decompression of the median and ulnar nerves may improve the functional outcome if radial and ulnar arteries remain patent[26-28].

The effect of electricity on peripheral nerves has been examined in a rabbit model[29,30]. Animal experiments with graded potentials in the absence of possible heat effects have revealed a discrepancy in latency and duration of action potential between dorsal and ventral roots[14,29]. There were a longer latency and duration from dorsal roots. In addition, there was an increase in the threshold, resulting in inexcitability for 15 to 20 minutes. The greatest decrease in action potentials occurred in the fast fibres. The greatest decrease in conduction velocity occurred in the motor fibres. Both efferent and afferent limbs were affected similarly. Blom and Ugland[29] conclude that electric shock sufficient to injure man can produce dysfunction of peripheral nerves. In the absence of heat generation, the changes are produced by the current itself and are largely reversible.

Experimental data in the human ulnar nerve confirmed a prolonged latency, decrease in amplitude and conduction velocity[31]. These changes only affected the motor neurons and were completely reversible[32]. The conclusions from these studies implied that, in the absence of thermal destruction, the acute peripheral nerve dysfunction produced by electric current is transient and that complete recovery should occur.

### Delayed peripheral lesions

Delayed peripheral neuropathies including causalgia, motor weakness, paraesthesias, and hypaesthesia have been reported in several cumulative series[5,7], as well as in individual case studies[6,13,18,22]. Baxter[2] reports a very high incidence of delayed causalgia ultimately relieved either by sympathetic block or sympathectomy.

### Spinal cord syndromes

Transient spinal cord complaints have been described[4,7,9,12,13,33,34]. These transient lesions appear early, and rapid recovery within hours to days is the rule. Clinical manifestations include sensory and motor deficits, which can be partial or complete.

The more severe form of spinal injury is delayed, progressive and permanent[35,36]. In those cases where *post mortem* specimens were available, there was gross histopathological disruption consistent with a transverse myelitis. There is oedema of the cord and intravascular thrombosis, without evidence of infection.

### Histopathology

Although central, spinal, peripheral, and hysterical disorders of the nervous system occur with some frequency in nonfatal injuries, the sequelae are documented rarely histopathologically. With the aid of *post mortem* examinations, Critchley[37] describes histopathological changes including: focal petechial haemorrhages throughout the brain and medulla, chromatolysis of medullary cells, dilatation of the perivascular space, fragmentation of peripheral nerves, and ballooning of myelin sheaths. Unfortunately, the changes due to current often could not be differentiated from those that may have been caused by necrosis from heat, sepsis, or associated mechanical trauma.

The most interesting observation is that the changes are inconsistent and variable. Examination of some specimens after fatal high-voltage execution reveals no nerve cell changes. Langworthy[38] has shown that in rapid electrocution, nerve cell changes occur only at the sites directly transversed by current, but large, prolonged currents produce heat and cause neuronal changes similar to current alone. Transient changes can be observed in nerve cells[39]. The neuronal changes can be patchy in distribution, with normal cells lying adjacent to injured cells. Schwann sheath breakdown and cellular fusion have been noted.

### Thesis: What are the neurologic sequelae after electrical injury?

From the review of the literature, perhaps the most striking feature of neurological sequelae from electric current is the paucity of information on what the true incidence, severity and sequelae are. 'One person, electrocuted from an electric light main, is profoundly shocked; another makes contact with a considerably greater current and is little the worse'[37]. The authors have long been interested in the natural course of neurological symptoms at the University of Washington Burn Center and have followed these patients prospectively in conjunction with the Department of Neurology[40,41]. This compendium presents a 7-year experience of electrical injury at the University of Washington, with a particular focus on the neurological outcome. There were several specific questions addressed. Do low-voltage injuries have serious neurologic sequelae? What is the outlook for patients rendered unconscious by the current? Are peripheral neuropathies present on admission likely to be permanent? Are delayed neuropathies likely to develop and, if so, are they likely to be permanent?

### *Material and methods*

A review of 90 patients admitted to the University of Washington Burn Center who had sustained electrical current injuries during the period from 1980 to 1986 was undertaken to determine the extent and consequences of

Table 7.1. *Demographics*

| Patients | Age | TBSA | Lived | Died | ICU | Total stay |
|----------|-----|------|-------|------|-----|------------|
| Overall (90) | $31 \pm 13$ | $6 \pm 11$ | 86 | 4 | $5 \pm 10$ | $13 \pm 20$ |
| High voltage (64) | $31 \pm 12$ | $8 \pm 13$ | 60 | 4 | $6 \pm 12$ | $17 \pm 22$ |
| Low voltage (22) | $31 \pm 17$ | $1 \pm 1$ | 22 | 0 | $1 \pm 1$ | $4 \pm 5$ |
| Unknown (4) | $32 \pm 15$ | $4 \pm 4$ | 4 | 0 | $1 \pm 1$ | $8 \pm 11$ |

acute and delayed central and peripheral neurologic sequelae. Only patients with true electrical contact were included in the series. Patients who had sustained only flash or flame burns were excluded if there was no history of current passage or clear evidence of entrance or exit wounds. All injuries from current greater than 380 V[14] were considered to be high-voltage injuries. Neurology consultants examined patients with high-voltage injuries at the time of admission. Patients who developed neurological symptoms after discharge from the hospital were referred for neurological evaluation, electromyographic studies and/or neuropsychiatric assessment as indicated by the complaints.

### Results

The demographics of this patient population are shown in Table 7.1. There were 2305 admissions to the University of Washington Burn Center between 1980 and 1986; electrical injuries accounted for 4% of these admissions. The voltage was known in 86 patients. There were no lightning strikes. The mean age was similar for both high- and low-voltage groups. The length of stay in the intensive care unit and the total hospital stay were shorter for low-voltage injuries. There were four deaths (4%), all in the high-voltage group. Two of the deaths occurred in patients who had suffered severe anoxia at the time of initial injury. The third death occurred in a patient who sustained multiple severe injuries, including a basilar skull fracture, pelvic fracture, cervical spine (C2/3) fracture dislocation and a severe liver disruption. The fourth death occurred in a 35 year-old patient who sustained an 84% total body surface area flame burn in addition to the electrical burn. There were 82 male and 8 female victims.

The actual electrical potential could be determined in 76 patients. There were 22 patients in the low-voltage group, 10 struck with 110 V and 12 with 220 V. The tissue injury and neurologic consequences in this group are skewed from all low-voltage injuries, since asymptomatic patients without tissue destruction are not generally admitted to the hospital. The actual voltage was known in 54 of the 64 patients in the high-voltage group and the median voltage was 7200 V with a range from 440 V to 150 000 V. Entrance wounds were identified in 78 patients and exit wounds in 68 patients. One or both upper extremities account for 82% of the entrance wounds. Twenty-one per cent of the exit wounds could be identified in the upper extremities, 30% in the lower extremities, 28% on the trunk or on multiple sites, and 21% were unidentified. The majority of high-voltage injuries occurred at work (72%) compared to only 38% of those in the low-voltage group. Most low-voltage injuries (57%) occurred at home. Fourteen patients underwent 18 amputations, seven of upper extremities, eight lower extremities, two patients required toe amputations, and one underwent finger amputation. The extremities that underwent amputation secondary to massive thermal tissue destruction were considered to have a permanent sensorimotor deficit in the isolated limb and were not considered in the symptomatic group of patients unless they developed neurological sequelae in the stump or elsewhere.

### Low voltage

Twenty-two patients sustained low-voltage injuries. Eleven patients had no presenting neurological complaints and none developed subsequent problems. The remaining 11 had one or more neurological symptoms including: seizures (1), motor weakness (4), decreased sensation (5), left hemiparesis (1), and loss of consciousness (4). In the final outcome, the symptoms had completely resolved in nine of these patients, and, in the other two, the symptoms were resolving. The high incidence of symptoms in this low-voltage group is due undoubtedly to a skewed patient population, since it is policy to discharge from the emergency room patients who sustained 110 V and 220 V injuries unless they had some associated indication for admission.

### High voltage

Sixty-four patients sustained high-voltage injuries. There were 21 patients in the high-voltage group who had no neurologic deficits at the time of admission. Four of these patients developed dysaesthesias and shooting pains in amputated extremities, and one of them underwent excision of a painful neuroma without resolution of symptoms. A fourth patient developed bilateral hip weakness and pain 1 month after injury, but did not follow through with neurological consultation.

### Loss of consciousness

Loss of consciousness occurred in 29 of the 64 patients in the high-voltage group (45%). Eight patients (28%) in this group required CPR prior to admission. Six patients remained comatose at admission. Three of these patients never regained consciousness and died (9%). The other three comatose patients regained consciousness in the hospital, but all of them had persistent central neurological deficits. Three patients with momentary loss of consciousness developed new central neurological symptoms. Over all, 20 patients who transiently lost consciousness became completely asymptomatic, while six had evidence of persistent or delayed central neuropathy. The final central symptoms ranged from the slight symptom of amnesia for the accident (one patient) to global hyperreflexia with aphasia and bilateral clonus (one patient). Other deficits included: a slight deficit in memory and learning by neuropsychiatric evaluation (one patient), poor short- and long-term memory with hypoxic encephalopathy and violent behaviour (one patient), an isolated Babinski with normal neuropsychiatric evaluation and a hand sensorimotor deficit by EMG (one patient), and a post-traumatic stress disorder with cortical visual field deficit by visually evoked responses (one patient).

Forty-five per cent of our patients suffered transient loss of consciousness. Eighty-seven per cent of those who had transient loss of consciousness had no sequelae. Half of the patients who remained comatose died, and the other 50% developed persistent central deficits including: decreased memory, aphasia, and violent behaviour. Three patients with transient loss of consciousness had some permanent impairment including decreased memory and a post-traumatic stress disorder.

Other initial central nervous system problems in the high-voltage group included seizures and paralysis. Seizures were present in three patients and all resolved. Two patients developed new seizures at some point during their hospitalization. Five patients had initial paralysis that resolved promptly. One patient had transient paresis that resolved.

### Acute peripheral neuropathy

Twenty-two patients with high-voltage injuries presented with one or more peripheral neuropathies including: motor loss (16), decreased sensation

(16), paraesthesias (1), paralysis (1), and pain (2). Of the 16 motor lesions: eight resolved, two improved, four persisted, and two progressed. The motor lesions which resolved included: generalized upper and/or lower extremity weakness (5), and dysfunction of the median (2), ulnar (2), or radial (1) nerves. Two patients presented with four claw hands. Immediate carpal tunnel release brought partial improvement to three hands and no improvement to the fourth. The motor lesions which progressed included deterioration of a peroneal nerve, a tibial nerve and ulnar and median nerves. The four motor deficits that have not resolved include one patient with a complete median, ulnar and radial nerve motor deficit with sensory sparing who underwent eventual amputation, one weak left hand (2 years after injury), one complete median and ulnar sensorimotor deficit (6 years) and complete sensorimotor loss from an associated C5/6 fracture dislocation. The sensory lesions resolved in seven, improved in three, progressed in two, and persisted in five. The paraesthesias resolved in one. Initial pain symptoms resolved in both. One or more peripheral neuropathies occurred in 34% of our high-voltage injuries. The immediate peripheral neuropathies resolved or improved in 64% and persisted or progressed in 36%. The median, ulnar and radial nerves were most often implicated. Three out of four decompressed hands that presented in tight finger flexion recovered some sensory and motor function.

### Delayed peripheral neuropathy

Eleven patients developed relatively minor additional or new delayed symptoms which included; muscle weakness (5), sensory deficit (3), paraesthesias (4), and new pain symptoms (4). In only one of the patients was the combined sensorimotor deficit significant – a young man sustained injuries to both wrists, but had complete hand function except decreased light touch in one hand. This rapidly recovered by EMG, but he developed delayed radial sensorimotor nerve deficits and bilateral carpal tunnel symptoms 5 months postinjury. He remains unemployed. Of the four patients who developed new motor symptoms, one resolved, two improved and two persisted. Of the three sensory deficits, one improved and two persisted. Delayed paraesthesias occurred in four patients and resolved in two, but persisted in two. Delayed chronic pain symptoms occurred in four patients and remained in three. Delayed dysaesthesias developed in two patients and resolved in one. No patients developed delayed spinal cord symptoms. Eleven patients developed 18 peripheral neuropathies, most of relatively minor consequence. However, 50% of them persisted. In the most significant case, a patient developed bilateral carpal tunnel symptoms which could fall into Blom's[42] classification of perineural scarring, since the entrance wounds were located at both wrists.

### Summary

Low-voltage injuries generally do not have any major sequelae. Approximately half of the patients with high-voltage injuries had loss of consciousness at the scene, but recovery was good unless associated with anoxia. About one-third of the patients with high-voltage injury experienced acute peripheral neuropathies. About two-thirds of these resolved. Delayed peripheral neuropathies occurred in about one-fifth of the patients injured by electric current. The symptoms are less likely to resolve, but are generally mild. Delayed central or spinal cord lesions are recognized sequelae, but are uncommon.

### Pathophysiology of electrical injury

A knowledge of the basic laws of physics is critical in order to understand the extent and severity of electrical injury. A multitude of factors contribute to the manifestations of electrical injury including current and type of current, length of time of contact, electrical density, voltage and the electric field produced, tissue and environmental resistance, and current pathway.

Despite an understanding of the laws of physics, there still exists substantial controversy in the mechanism of conversion of electrical energy into tissue destruction[43]. This is particularly evidenced in the diverse manifestations of neurological symptoms in response to electrical current. Although there remain many unanswered questions regarding the specific electrophysiological cellular interactions causing alterations in function, there are some known data about the nerve cell, the anatomic configuration of the nervous system which may elucidate the reasons for the diversity in presentation.

Researchers are investigating the flow of electricity in the body and proposing new theories about the effects of electrical current on cells and cell membranes that may supply answers to the perplexing problems encountered from electrical current. Although a treatise on the pathophysiology of electricity is beyond the scope of this chapter, several relevant facts about electrical current, the nervous system and new concepts about electrobiology may account for the clinical symptoms detected in patients in response to electrical injury.

### The laws of physics

If the body becomes a part of the electric circuit, the extent of injury is defined by the current and the duration of the shock[43]. The current is defined by Ohm's Law which states that current ($I$) is directly proportional to the voltage ($V$) and inversely proportional to the resistance ($R$), $I = V/R$. The voltage is the driving force that forces the ions to move in one direction[3]. The resistance is a measure of how difficult it is for electrons or ions to flow through the conducting medium. Although the determinants of Ohm's Law can be defined experimentally in mammalian models, in the accidental injury situation, the only known quantity is the voltage. Resistance of the interface is unmeasurable and, therefore, current is undefinable in absolute terms.

### *Resistance*

The impedance to the flow of current is important to evaluate in determining whether a particular voltage will be associated with a physiological response. The resistance to current flow is a combination of intrinsic tissue properties and extrinsic factors.

Ever since the discovery of bioelectrical events, investigators have been interested in the alterations of current produced by the intervening tissues[44]. The body has a very high external resistance in intact skin and a low ionic internal resistance. Internal tissues have their own complex intrinsic resistances and may contribute to the alterations observed in voltage measurements[45]. A few broad generalizations can be made about the conductivity of biological materials. Cell-free fluids: urine, amniotic fluid, bile, cerebrospinal fluid and plasma have the lowest resistance[45]. The addition of cells to plasma decreases its conductance 2.5 fold[46]. Flowing blood exhibits a lower resistance than stationary blood[47]. Skeletal muscle and nervous tissue have a considerable degree of electrical anisotropy (unequal conductance dependent upon direction of flow), that precludes generalizations about their conducting properties. Nerve fibres are long, thin tubes filled with electrolytes that have a higher resistance when measured transversely than along the fibre length[48]. Grey matter, consisting largely of cell bodies, conducts better than white matter, which is composed of anisotropic fibre tracts. This discrepancy in resistance between transverse and longitudinal flow may therefore contribute to the disparate sequelae from electrical injury.

### Current path

An investigation of current distribution and density requires the isolation of representative portions of the current path and the determination of the percentage of total current carried by each of the segments of the circuit[49]. The passage of 60-cycle current in various anatomical configurations has been evaluated for currents ranging from 10 to 50 mA in a cat model[49]. Electric current passed through the animal as though it were passing through a structureless gel, always chooses the shortest path from contact to contact without deflection by anatomical landmarks. The amount of current carried by the aorta, vena cava, spinal cord and long muscles of the back was the same when current passed from forefoot to hindfoot. However, when current passed from forefoot to forefoot, a significant amount of current passed through the spinal cord at the level of the seventh cervical segment. The course of the current within the body is difficult to determine in the accidental situation, but some of the variable and/or delayed symptoms may arise from the localization of current in specific peripheral nerves or spinal segments.

## Biophysical mechanisms for neurological sequelae from electricity

The mechanism(s) of tissue injury still remain somewhat controversial. Some attribute tissue destruction to thermal injury; others, to a specific action of the current. Neither explanation alone seems to answer the question completely. Studies with isolated nerve preparations show significant membrane injury that is reversible[29,30]. The extent of thermal destruction can depend on the degree of associated tissue perfusion[2]. Animal models have also shown progressive tissue necrosis which can be diminished with nonsteroidal anti-inflammatory agents implicating arachidonic acid metabolites[50]. Only through an elaboration of both thermal and nonthermal electrical effects can we gain a better understanding of a very complex neurological injury pattern.

### Thermal destruction – joule heat

Tissue destruction by electricity occurs at least in part by the conversion of electricity into heat. There is some controversy as to which tissues are the largest 'heat sink' generating the greatest temperatures. The controversy stems around the question of whether a material of extremely high resistance, such as bone, produces the greatest amount of heat, or whether a low resistance, but high-volume tissue, such as muscle, develops the greatest heat capacity. Patterns of current distribution and temperature generation have been examined in experimental animal models[51,52] and proposed on the basis of theoretical calculations[43]. Each will be discussed below separately. An understanding of the current repartition and heat generation are critical in order to understand the patterns of injury to the tissues encountered along the course of the current.

Joule's Law describes the conversion of electrical energy into heat in a solid conductor. Heat production in joules is proportional to the power dissipated and the duration of contact. Joule heat $(J)$ is the heat production and is described by the following equation: $J = I^2RT$.

### Uniform resistance volume conductor model

Experimental studies in rats suggest that an electrical burn is simply a thermal injury[52]. Although it has been suggested that the severity of tissue injury may be related to differences in absolute resistances, Hunt[52] suggests that the clinical significance of this may be immaterial once the external resistance of the skin has been overcome. The extent of tissue necrosis in the rat model is related to the volume of tissue, rather than to specific individual tissue resistances. Once the high resistance of the skin has been overcome, the internal tissue, except bone, acts as a low-resistance volume conductor in this small animal model. Although the initial temperature of muscle rises more rapidly than in bone, both tissues attain the same temperature by the time the current arcs. It is a self-limited, nonprogressive injury that terminates when the current arcs. Muscle injury occurs at the time of initial insult and does not progress.

The concept of finite, irreversible, complete tissue damage is disputed by some on the basis of clinical observations[14,53,54]. High-tension electrical injuries produce nonuniform tissue destruction[28,54].

### Inhomogeneous resistance composite tissue model

The disparate clinical findings have stimulated scientists to search for a more thorough explanation for tissue destruction from electrical injury by joulean heat. Recent investigations on the flow of current and heat generation have generated both theoretical models and sophisticated large animal experiments. These suggest that the magnitude of heat production during an electrical injury is complex and depends on the current density, the conductivity of the tissues, and the spatial arrangement of the tissues in relation to the entry and exit points of the current. The clinical applicability to human victims, however, remains to be confirmed. The discrepancy in current flow and heat production along a given path in these animal models must affect all adjacent tissues, including the nerves.

A mathematical explanation for tissue loss from electricity has been proposed by Lee and Kolodney[43] in a one-dimensional arm model consisting of composite tissues. They theorize that, when tissues are electrically in parallel, the greatest heating occurs in the most conductive tissue, the muscle, which then proceeds to transfer heat to adjacent tissues, like bone. If the tissues are in series, the heat generation is inversely proportional to the tissue conductivity. The skin can be viewed as being in series with the other tissues since all the current must pass through the skin from the power line. This may account for the extensive thermal destruction seen at the skin contact point with the power source. The skin has the lowest conductivity and therefore the highest heat generation capacity when it is modelled in series.

Support for this theoretical model has been generated by using a reproducible high-voltage model in primates[51,55]. When a computer-activated system delivers a preselected energy level in kilojoules to a primate upper extremity, the predominant current load is carried in the muscle, the tissue occupying the largest cross-sectional area in the arm. Chilbert *et al.*[55], also, observed that most of the current will flow through the largest conducting volume of the lowest resistivity in concentration directly related to the cross-sectional diameter. Although it appears that muscle is the greatest tissue conductor, there is a nonuniformity in maximal flow of current within muscle groups. The flexor muscles of the forearm carry approximately 64% of the current, confirming that most of the current flow is through the largest conducting volume of the lowest resistance[51].

The highest recorded temperature values occur in the muscles of smallest cross-sectional diameter and in tissues of highest inherent resistance. Long, thin muscles, such as the brachioradialis, or the flexors along the radial aspect of the forearm, and the origins and insertions of major muscle groups register more current per cross-sectional area and thus greater heat generation and more tissue necrosis.

Approximately 20% of the current passes through the bone. Bone temperatures are sufficiently elevated to result in prolonged dissipation of heat to the surrounding tissues, the peri-osseum and deep muscle groups. An interesting phenomenon was observed in the primate model. As the path of current courses along the longitudinal axis of the forearm, the cross-sectional composition of the limb changes from low resistance muscle to high resistance bone and tendon at the antecubital fossa and axilla. The current is rerouted at these anatomical levels. Traditionally, the deep lesions in the antecubital fossa have been ascribed to arcing[56], but this phenomenon was not observed in the primate model of Daniel *et al.*[51] They attribute the destruction in these areas to a redirection of current from deep muscle towards the surface tissues because the current encounters high resistance bone and tendon and a significantly reduced cross-sectional area of muscle.

After the termination of current flow and heat generation, the dynamics of temperature flux depend on blood perfusion, heat conduction and air convection at the skin surface. In the theoretical model where muscle reaches the highest temperature, the cooler bone and the hotter muscle equilibrate in 10 minutes, whereas skin may never reach the temperatures of the underlying muscle because it loses heat from the surface by convection[57]. In addition, blood flow has a profound effect on the rate of cooling[58]. If perfusion is impaired, re-equilibration of temperature may require many hours.

The experimental data above recognize the variability of current flow and heat generation within a given segment of the animal body depending on the complex configuration of the tissues. Although only the current and heat in the muscle and bone compartments are investigated, the anatomical course of the nerves in relationship to the volume, shape and location of the muscles and bone may play a significant role in the determination of specific early and late nerve lesions.

### Nonthermal tissue destruction by electricity

Exposure to intense electric fields can produce a wide spectrum of tissue injury ranging from charring to the gradual development of neurologic deficits[6]. As noted above, joule heating has been incriminated as the mediator of tissue damage. However, the nonuniform distribution of cellular injury[54] and the delayed cellular alterations[29] are not well explained by the immediate effects of thermal destruction.

### Electric field hypothesis

Electrical fields are capable of damaging cells by nonthermal means as well as thermal mechanisms[57]. Blom and Ugland[29] examined the effects of electric shocks of 250 to 1700 mA on the cell membrane and noted there to be transient changes in resting membrane threshold, which rapidly reversed. Similarly, Dalziel[59] demonstrated that subthreshold electric fields applied to bilayer lipid membranes developed increased permeability which was reversible. Rupture of cells by strong electric fields is well documented, and is a commonly used tool for membrane research and for encapsulation of pharmacological agents normally impermeable to the biological lipid membrane[42]. The local electric field is of sufficient magnitude to cause electrical breakdown of cell membranes and cell lysis[60].

There are two possible mechanisms for electrical breakdown of cell membranes: direct compression of the cell membrane[61] and the stretching of transient aqueous pores in the lipid bilayer[62]. Current evidence supports the pore theory[42,57]. The expansion of pores beyond a critical radius can create a mechanically unstable membrane which will rupture.[62]

Cell size and orientation may also be important in the electric field strength model[57]. Lee[57] proposes that large elongated cells, such as muscle and nerve cells, are more vulnerable to electrical breakdown. In a simple geometric model for nonspherical cells, the maximum voltage drop depends on the cell orientation with respect to the electric field[57,63]. The greatest voltage drop is observed when the long axis of the cell is parallel to the electric field. Lee *et al.*[57] postulate that a 1-cm long muscle cell aligned in the direction of the electric field of 200 V/m is sufficient to rupture the cell without producing joulean heat[58]. They have recently shown in an *in vitro* rat skeletal muscle model that electric field strengths of 10–300 V/cm, comparable to those sustained by man in electrical accidents (1 to 100 kV/m), are capable of rupturing skeletal muscle cells without any evidence of joule heating[64]. This appears to be cell-type dependent, since there were no changes in the fibroblasts. The susceptibility of muscle and nerve cells to electric field effects may account for the clinical observations noted by Ponten[53] that muscle under normal skin 25 cm from the entrance site can be necrotic, but the blood vessels are still patent.

### Inflammatory mediator model

The evidence for immediate irreversible tissue necrosis versus progressive tissue destruction remains controversial[2,14,52–55]. Progressive tissue loss in electrical injuries has been proposed in a rat model to be due to metabolites of arachidonic acid[65]. Sequential histochemical analysis of tissue at the entrance wound and along the proximal peri-osseum revealed progressive accumulation of thromboxane. Treatment with antithromboxane agents halted the evolution of tissue necrosis and preserved limb length.

## Conclusions

The neurological sequelae from electrical injury are diverse. A review of the literature presents a summary of the central, peripheral and spinal symptoms encountered from electric shock. A large series of patients treated at The University of Washington is presented to elucidate the outcome of acute and delayed neurological symptoms. The basic laws of electricity and how they affect nervous tissue are reviewed. Possible mechanisms for the disparate neurological symptoms and their evolution are presented.

### References

1 Dalziel, C.F. (1972) Electric shock hazard, *IEEE Spectrum*, **9**, 41.
2 Baxter, C. (1970). Present concepts in the management of major electrical injury, *Surgery Clinics of North America*, **50**, 1401.
3 *Accident Facts*, (1987). National Safety Council.
4 Butler, E.D. & Gant, T.D. (1977). Electrical injuries with special reference to the upper extremities. *American Journal of Surgeons*, **134**, 95.
5 DiVincenti, F.C., Moncrief, J.A. & Pruitt, B.A. (1969). Electrical injuries: a review of 65 cases. *Journal of Trauma*, **9**, 497.
6 Farrell, D.F. & Starr, A. (1968). Delayed neurological sequelae of electrical injuries, *Neurology*, **18**, 601.
7 Hunt, J.L., Sato, R.M. & Baxter, C.R. (1980). Acute electrical burns. *Archives of Surgery*, **115**, 434.
8 Rouse, R.G. & Dimick, R.G. (1978). The treatment of electrical injury compared to burn injury: a review of pathophysiology and comparison of patient management protocols, *Journal of Trauma*, **18**, 43.
9 Solem, L., Fischer, R.P. & Strate, R.G. (1977). The natural history of electrical injury. *Journal of Trauma*, **17**, 487.
10 Sturim, H.S. (1971) Management of major electrical injuries, *Journal of Trauma*, **11**, 959.
11 Varghese, G. Mani, M.M. & Redford, J.B. (1986). Spinal cord injuries following electrical accidents. *Paraplegia*, **24**, 159.
12 Wilkinson, C. & Wood, M. (1978). High voltage electric injury. *American Journal of Surgery*, **136**, 693.
13 Silversides, J. (1964). The neurological sequelae of electrical injury. *Journal of the Canadian Medical Association*, **91**, 195.
14 Skoog, T. (1970). Electrical injuries. *Journal of Trauma*, **10**, 816.
15 Jaffe, R.H. (1928). Electropathology: a review of the pathologic changes produced by electric currents. *Archives in Pathology*, **5**, 837.
16 Moran, K.T. & Munster, A.M. (1986). Low voltage electrical injuries: the hidden morbidity. *Journal of the Royal College of Surgeons of Edinburgh*, **31**, 227.
17 Robinson, D.W., Masters, F.W. & Forrest, W.J. (1969). Electrical burns: a review and analysis of 33 cases. *Journal of Surgery*, **57**, 385.
18 Blom, S. & Ugland, O.M. (1967). Peripheral nerve injuries in electrical

burns. *Scandinavian Journal of Plastic and Reconstructive Surgery* (suppl) **2**, 45.

19  Panse, F. (1931). Die Schadignungen des Nervensystems durch technische Electrizitat. *Mschr Psychiatric Neurology*, **78**, 193.

20  Alexander, L. (1936). Clinical and neuropathological aspects of electrical injuries. *Journal of Industrial Hygiene*, **20**, 191.

21  Burke, J.F., Quinby, W.C., Bondoc, C. *et al.* (1977). Patterns of high tension electrical injury in children and adolescents and their management. *American Journal of Surgery*, **133**, 492.

22  Hartford, C.E., Ziffren, S.E. (1971). Electrical injury. *Journal of Trauma*, **11**, 331.

23  Brokenshire, B., Cairns, F.J., Koelmeyer, T.D. *et al* (1984). Deaths from electricity. *New Zealand Medical Journal*, **97**, 139.

24  Sachatello, C.R. & Stephenson, S.E. (1965). Management of high voltage electrical burns: a review of 16 cases. *American Journal of Surgery*, **31**, 807.

25  Parshley, P.F., Kilgore, J. & Pulito, J.F. (1985). Aggressive approach to the extremity damaged by electric current. *American Journal of Surgery*, **150**, 78.

26  Engrav, L.H., Gottlieb, J.R., Walkinshaw, M.D., Heimbach, D.M., Trumble, T.E. & Grube, B.J. (1989). Electrical injury with immediate median and ulnar nerve palsy at the wrist. Presented at Northwest Society of Plastic Surgeons, Seattle, Wa.

27  Holliman, C.J., Saffle, J.R. & Karvitz, M. (1982). Early surgical decompression in the management of electrical injuries. *American Journal of Surgery*, **144**, 733.

28  Mann, R.J. & Wallquist, J.M. (1975). Early decompression fasciotomy in the treatment of high voltage electrical burns of the extremities. *Southern Medical Journal*, **68**, 1103.

29  Blom, S. & Ugland, O.M. (1967). II. Experimental study. Electrical injury to peripheral nerves: AE experiment in cats and rabbits. *Scandinavian Journal of Plastic and Reconstructive Surgery*, (suppl), **2**, 53.

30  Uruquhart, I.R.W. & Noble, E.C. (1929). Experimental electric shock II. *Journal of Industrial Hygiene*, **11**, 154.

31  Blom, S. & Ugland, O.M. (1967). B. Experiments in Man, *Scandinavian Journal of Plastic and Reconstructive Surgery*, (suppl), **2**, 68.

32  Blom, S., Hagbarth, K.E. & Skoglund, S.E. (1964). Post tetanic potentiation of H-reflexes in human infants. *Experimental Neurology*, **9**, 198.

33  Christensen, A., Sherman, R.T., Balis, G.A. *et al* (1980). Delayed neurologic injury secondary to high voltage current with recovery. *Journal of Trauma*, **20**, 166.

34  Petty, P.G. & Parkin, G. (1986). Electrical injury to the central nervous system. *Neurosurgery*, **19**, 282.

35  Jackson, F.E., Martin, R. & Davis, R. (1965). Delayed quadriplegia following electrical burn. *Military Medicine*, **130**, 601.

36  Levine, N.S., Atkins, A., McKeel, D.W. *et al.* (1975). Spinal cord injury following electrical accidents: case reports. *Journal of Trauma*, **15**, 459.

37  Critchley, M. (1934). Neurological effects of lightning and of electricity. *Lancet*, **4**, 68.

38 Langworthy, O.R. (1930). *Bulletin Johns Hopkins Hospital*, **47**, 11.
39 Langworthy, O.R. (1932). *Journal of Industrial Hygiene*, **14**, 87.
40 Grube, B.J., Heimbach, D.M. & Copass, M.K. (1988). Neurologic consequences of electrical burns. *Pacific Coast Surgical Annual Meeting*, San Francisco.
41 Grube, B.J., Heimback, D.M., Engrav, L. & Copass, M.K. (1989). Neurological consequences of electrical burns, submitted to the *Journal of Trauma*.
42 Benz, R., Beckers, F. & Zimmermann, U. (1979). Reversible electrical breakdown of lipid bilayer membranes: A charge–pulse relaxation study. *Journal of Membrane Biology*, **48**, 181.
43 Lee, R.C. & Kolodney, M.S. (1987). Electrical injury mechanisms: Dynamics of the thermal response. *Plastic and Reconstructive Surgery*, **80**, 663.
44 Nichter, L., Bryant, C.A. & Kenney, J.G. (1984). Injuries due to commercial electric current. *Journal of Burn Care and Rehabilitation*, **5**, 124.
45 Geddes, L.A. & Baker, L.E. (1967). The specific resistance of biological material – a compendium of data for the biomedical engineer and physiologist, *Medical and Biological Engineering*, **5**, 271.
46 Rosenberg, D.B. & Nelson, M. (1988). Rehabilitation concerns in electrical burn patients: a review of the literature. *Journal of Trauma*, **28**, 808.
47 Sigman, E., Kolin, A., Katz, L.N. & Jochim, K. (1937). Effect of motion on the electrical conductivity of the blood. *American Journal of Physiology*, **118**, 708.
48 Burger, H.C. & van Dongen, R. (1960–61). Specific electric resistance of body tissues. *Physics in Medical Biology*, **5**, 431.
49 Weeks, A.W. & Alexander, L. (1939). The distribution of electric shock in the animal body: an experimental investigation of sixty cycle alternating current. *Journal of Industrial Hygiene*, **21**, 324.
50 Robson, M.C., Del Beccaro, E.J. & Heggers, J.P. (1979). The effect of prostaglandins on the dermal microcirculation after burning, and the inhibition of the effect by specific pharmacological agents. *Plastic and Reconstructive Surgery*, **63**, 781.
51 Daniel, R.K., Ballard, P.A. & Heroux, P. *et al.* (1988). High-voltage electrical injury: acute pathophysiology. *Journal of Hand Surgery*, **13A**, 44.
52 Hunt, J.L., Mason, A.D. & Masterson, T.S. *et al.* (1976). The pathophysiology of acute electrical injuries. *Journal of Trauma*, **16**, 335.
53 Ponten, B., Erickson, U. & Johansson, S.H. *et al.* (1970). New observations on tissue changes along the pathway of current in an electrical injury. *Scandinavian Journal of Plastic and Reconstructive Surgery*, **4**, 75.
54 Quinby, W.C., Burke, J.F. & Trelstad, R.L. *et al.* (1978). The use of microscopy as a guide to primary excision of high-tension electrical burns. *Journal of Trauma*, **18**, 423.
55 Chilbert, M., Moretti, D.J. & Swiontek, T. *et al.* (1988). Instrumentation design for high-voltage electrical injury studies, *IEEE Transactions in Biomedical Engineering*, **35**, 565.
56 Luce, E.A. & Gottlieb, S.E. (1984). 'True' high-tension electrical injuries. *Annals of Plastic Surgery*, **12**, 321.

57  Lee, R.C. & Kolodney, M.S. (1987). Electrical injury mechanisms: electrical breakdown of cell membranes. *Plastic and Reconstructive Surgery*, **80**, 672.
58  Eberhart, R.C. (1985). Thermal models of single organs. In *Heat Transfer in Medicine and Biology*, A. Shitzer and R.C. Eberhart, eds, Chap. 12, New York: Plenum Press.
59  Dalziel, C.F., Ogden, E. & Abbott, C.E. (1943). Effect of frequency on let-go currents. *Transactions AIEE*, **62**, 745.
60  Teissie, J. Knutson, V.P., Tsong, T.Y. *et al.* (1982). Electric pulse-induced fusion of 3T3 cells in monolayer culture. *Science*, **216**, 537.
61  Crowley, J.M. (1973). Electrical breakdown of bimolecular lipid membranes as an electromechanical instability. *Biophysical Journal*, **13**, 711.
62  Weaver, J.C., Powell, K.T.R. & Mintzer, R.A. *et al.* (1984). The electrical capacitance of bilayer membranes: The contribution of transient aqueous pores. *Bioelectrochemistry and Bioenergetics*, **12**, 393.
63  Klee, M. & Plonsey, R. (1976). Stimulation of spheroidal cell: the role of cell shape. *IEEE Transactions in Biomedical Engineering*, **23**, 347.
64  Lee, R.C., Gaylor, K. & Prakah-Asante, B. *et al.* (1987). Skeletal muscle cell rupture by pulsed electric fields. *IEEE/Ninth Annual Conference of the Engineering in Medicine and Biology Society*, Boston, Nov. 13, 0712.
65  Robson, M.C., Murphy, R.C. & Heggers, J.P. (1984). A new explanation for the progressive tissue loss in electrical injuries. *Plastic and Reconstructive Surgery*, **73**, 431.

# 8

# Paediatric electrical burns

CRISTINA FREXES KEUSCH
GEORGE GIFFORD
ELOF ERIKSSON

### Introduction

The leading cause of accidental death in the home for children ages 1 to 14 years is burn-related injury[1]. Electrical burns compose a small percentage of paediatric burns, varying from an incidence of 1.6% in those less than 2 years of age to 3.8% in the adolescent. Although relatively less frequent, electrical burns are of prime importance in light of their potentially devastating local and systemic effects. The limb amputation rate is reported to occur in up to 40% of these cases with death occurring in up to 7%[2].

Electrical injury may be of two types: low tension or high tension. One thousand volts is the approximate minimum value for the high-tension category of injury.

### The injury

#### Low-tension injuries

The majority of electrical injuries in young children are of the low-voltage type. Low-tension injuries typically occur in the home and result from contact with relatively low-voltage alternating household current (110 V). The most common sites of injury are the mouth and the hand.

Oral injuries most commonly result from biting on an electrical cord or sucking on an electrical wall socket[3] (Fig. 8.1). The most commonly affected site is the upper and lower lip and the connecting commissure (43%), with tongue involvement in 26% and alveolar involvement in 10%. Typically, the centre of the wound is depressed and charred with an overlying exudate. Surrounding oedema increases over 2 hours and gradually resolves over a 2-week period. The eschar separates within 2 to 3

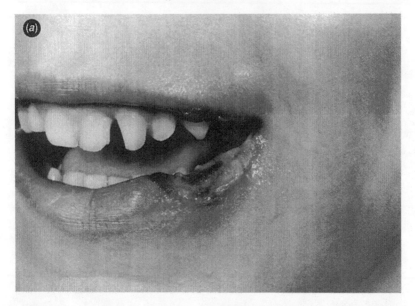
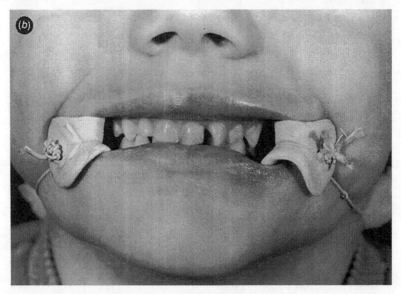

Fig. 8.1(*a*). Electrical burn of the lower lip (a typical 'cord bite'); (*b*) application of an oral commissure splint; (*c*) appearance 1 year later following 4 months of splinting; (*d*) normal position, shape and range of motion of the oral commissure are maintained.

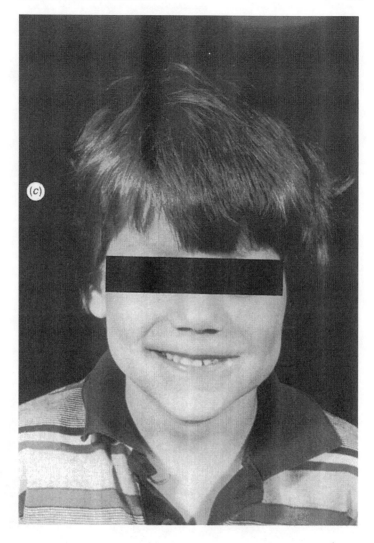

weeks, at which time bleeding from the labial artery may occur, with a reported incidence of 24%[3].

The hand is another frequent entry or contact site in paediatric low-tension (as well as high-tension) injuries (Fig. 8.2). Exit wounds are most commonly found at the grounding site, i.e. the lower extremities, with the current travelling along the path of least resistance. These injuries typically result from manual manipulation of live cords or sockets. Local injury consists of partial- or full-thickness thermal burns.

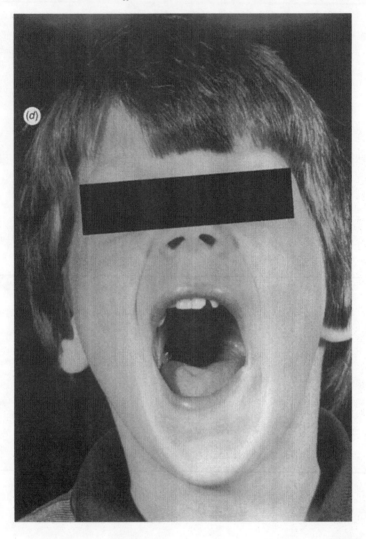

Systemic side-effects in low-voltage injuries are relatively rare. Cardiac arrhythmias, renal failure, and myonecrosis generally do not occur unless an alternating current source, as seen with incandescent lights and appliances, is present. These currents are more dangerous due to their tetanizing effects, such that the victim is unable to remove himself from the electrical source[4,5].

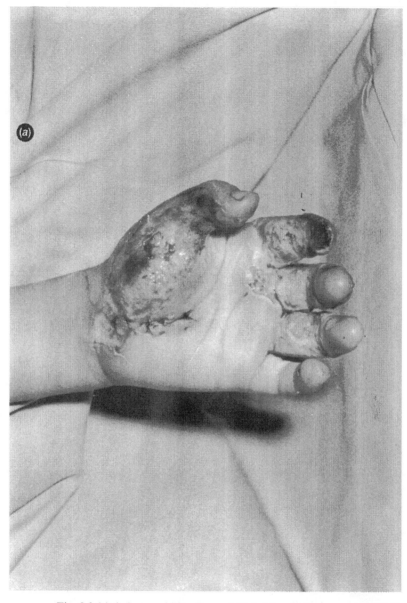

Fig. 8.2 (*a*) A 4 year-old boy burned his left hand on an exposed 110 V
wire. This figure shows appearance following initial debridement and
carpal tunnel release immediately after admission; (*b*) & (*c*) 48 hours later,
final debridement with groin flap coverage; (*d*) & (*e*) 1 year postburn there
is a flexion contracture at the thumb IP joint, with otherwise good range of
motion.

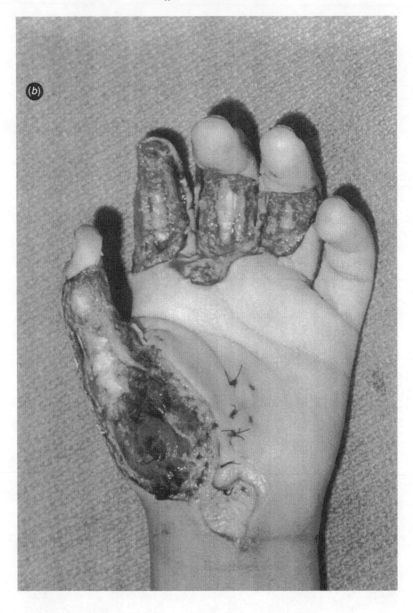

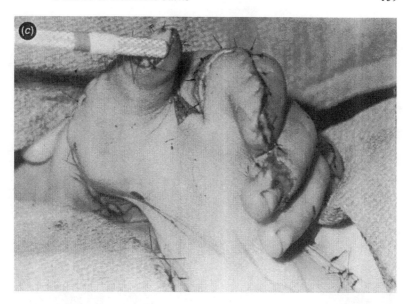

### High-tension injuries

A higher proportion of electrical injuries in older children or adolescents are of the high-tension type. These typically occur away from the home and are more often the result of occupational or recreational activity[1]. Electrical wires are a common source of these injuries and the extremities are the most frequently involved sites. The upper extremity, particularly the hand, is involved in 50–75% of these cases[2,6] (Fig. 8.3).

The cutaneous effects of high-tension electrical burns are typically devastating, with widespread tissue destruction. Thermal injury is mediated by different mechanisms.[4]

### Current effect

This is seen at skin entry and exit sites. A deep thermal burn results here due to the great resistance encountered at these sites which in turn produces large quantities of heat. These skin wounds are characteristically leathery or charred and full-thickness loss may be seen. The entry site is often dry and depressed, whereas the exit wound is raised and irregular[4]. The current travels along the path of least resistance (neurovascular bundles). Bone is the most resistant tissue to the electrical current and it therefore generates the greatest heat, accounting for the greater destruction of para-osseous muscle along the path of the current as compared to more superficial sites[6].

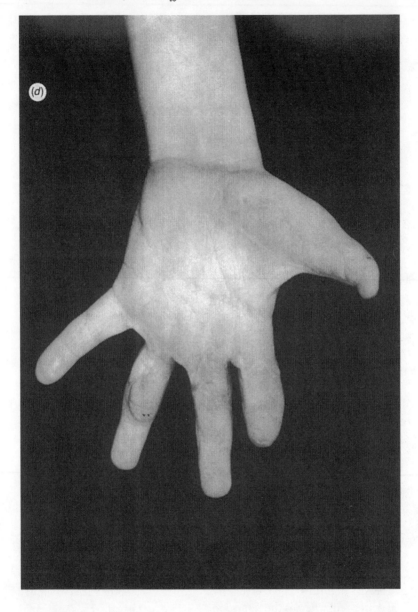

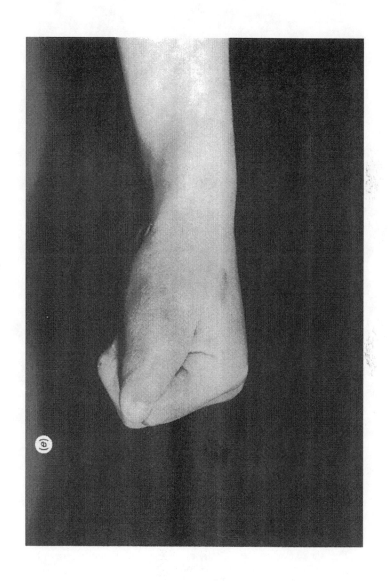

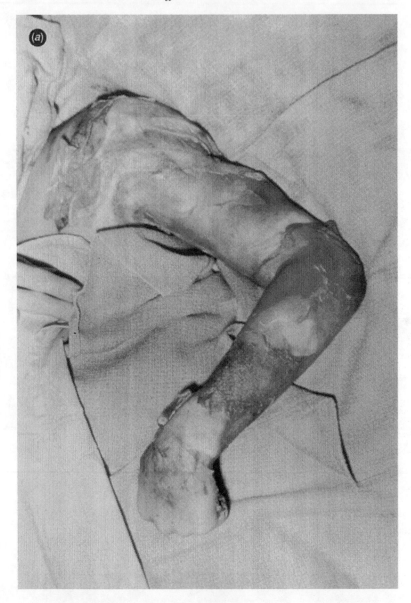

Fig. 8.3 (*a*) High-tension electrical injury to the left upper extremity in a 9 year-old boy who fell from a tree onto a power line; (*b*) amputation of this extremity was required; (*c*) rehabilitation was achieved with a myoelectric prosthesis.

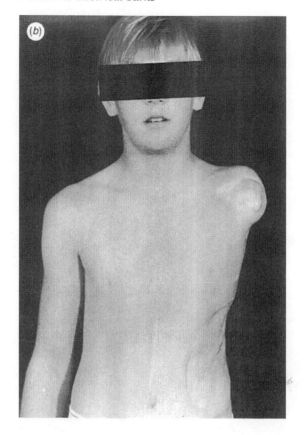

### Arc burn

This occurs when a current courses external to the body from contact to ground. Air particles are ionized by high-tension current and extremely high temperatures are generated. The hand and flexor surfaces of the arm are most commonly involved due to the tetanic spasms of the arm which bring these areas into close proximity. Deep burns result at the sites of entry and exit of the arc.

### Flame burn

This is a typical thermal burn resulting from an electrical injury which then secondarily ignites clothing. These are typically full thickness burns.

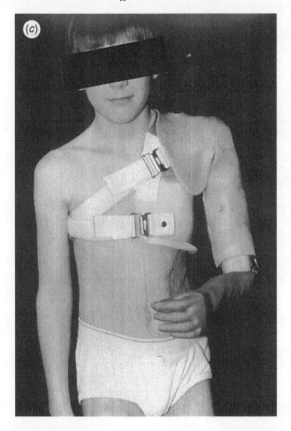

### Systemic effects

High-tension injuries are complicated potentially by cardiac, renal, neurologic or other associated injuries. Cardiac injury results from transmission block, coronary artery spasm, coronary endarteritis, or diffuse myocardial damage[7]. Cardiac dysrhythmia or infarction may occur.

Renal injury is mediated either through myoglobinuria and resultant acute tubular obstruction or, less commonly, through direct thermal injury to the renal parenchyma[4]. Neurological aberrations are felt to be the most frequent nonfatal sequelae of electrical injury[4]. Findings range from transient loss of consciousness, to epilepsy or spinal cord injury. Interestingly, unless there is loss of brain tissue, the brain seems to survive the injury without sequelae.

Other associated injuries include muscle and tendon disruption due to tetanic contractions, intra-abdominal organ injury due to direct electrical injury or through the effects of stress, cataracts, and bone injury including fractures (typically related to a fall), and peri-osteal necrosis.

### Treatment

#### General principles

In both low- and high-tension injuries, the victim must be safely disengaged from the power source. Cardiopulmonary resuscitation and monitoring, as needed, are begun. Vigorous intravenous hydration, particularly essential in high-voltage injury, is initiated. Complete examination with evaluation for possible associated injuries is performed, and baseline cardiac, renal and hepatic studies are obtained and followed.

#### The wound – low-tension injury

As mentioned previously, low-tension injuries usually result in limited local injuries with relatively few systemic effects.

Treatment of labial contact burns has changed over the years with management directed away from surgical treatment, as proposed by Gifford, *et al.* in 1971[3] to nonoperative management in the form of splints[8].

Wound contraction, as well as the sphincter-like action of the orbicularis oris muscle, are important factors contributing to scar contracture in these wounds. Custom-made splints, designed to maintain constant tension opposing the forces of the contracting scar, have shown excellent results with avoidance of operative therapy in most cases[8]. Hospitalization is generally not required, and treatment is continued for 6 to 12 months. The resultant effect is a soft and pliable, healed wound without contracting potential.

Delayed labial artery bleeding, typically occurring at 21 days, is readily controlled with pressure and an adrenalin-soaked sponge. Rarely, ligation of the labial vessel may be required.

Low-voltage injuries of the hand may be managed locally with saline-soaked gauze initially. Surgical excision is performed at the earliest possible date followed by immediate reconstruction with a skin graft or flap (local, regional, or distant)[9].

### The wound – high-tension injury

These injuries predominantly involve the hand as the entry site and the contralateral upper extremity, the lower extremity, the thoraco-abdominal region or the scalp as the exit site[6]. Entry and exit sites represent areas of full thickness necrosis which are sharply demarcated from normal skin. The greatest damage along the path of the current typically occurs in the extremities, due to the smaller cross-sectional areas of these parts. This follows from the 'volume conduction theory' which states that heat is directly proportional to current density, which is defined as flow per unit cross-sectional area[10].

Another important factor in planning debridement of these wounds is that para-osseous muscle is typically more extensively injured than other nearby tissues. Often, the external wound is only the tip of the iceberg in terms of tissue destruction by electrical injuries.

An aggressive approach is required for treatment of these injuries[6,9]. Tetanus prophylaxis is given. Following initial resuscitative efforts, the patient should be taken to the operating room for debridement of devitalized tissues and decompressing escharotomies and fasciotomies. This should be done generally within the first 3 hours following admission. The wound is packed with sterile saline gauze. Another debridement is then carried out 48 hours later and every 48 hours thereafter until the remaining tissue in the wound is viable. The technetium (Tc-99m) pyrophosphate muscle scan described by Hunt *et al.* was found to be helpful in guiding debridement procedures[11]. Here, injured muscle shows increased tracer uptake, whereas nonviable muscle shows no tracer uptake.

Vascular occlusion due to arterial thrombosis occurs at the time of the initial injury and requires urgent treatment. Amputation may be indicated if limb injury has been massive with total necrosis of the limb.

Wound closure is attempted as soon as complete debridement has been carried out. This minimizes bacterial colonization and allows cover of vital structures. If no important structures are exposed, the wound is simply skin-grafted. Exposure of bone, joint, nerve, blood vessel or tendon necessitates cover with a pedical flap or free flap. Attention must be directed to placement of the vascular anastomosis away from the zone of injury.

Active and passive range-of-motion exercises are started soon after admission and are interrupted only in the immediate postoperative period. At the same time, the patient is measured for a compression garment. If the patient is to be fitted for a prosthesis, this is done as early as possible.

### Outcome

Low-tension electrical injuries, if properly managed initially, in general carry a good prognosis. Oro-labial burns ultimately do well if the patient is compliant with nonoperative management for the prescribed time period. In contrast to the requirement for surgical revision in the majority of cases (83%) as reported in 1971[3], nonoperative management is successful in most cases today[8]. Only 3% of the patients followed by Silverglade and Ruberg at the Ohio State University College of Medicine required surgical intervention. These were full-thickness, circumoral burns in which surgery is uniformly required and splints here are used as an adjunct in therapy to maintain the normal commissure position and shape.

High-tension injuries, in general, are associated with limb amputation rates of up to 70%[12] and mortality rates of 2 to 15%.[6] Similar figures are given in the paediatric population, with a reported limb amputation rate of 41% and mortality rate of 7%[2].

### Conclusion

Paediatric electrical injuries are predominantly of the low-tension type until the adolescent years when high-tension injuries become more prevalent. The mouth and hands are the most frequently involved sites. Nonoperative management is stressed for low-tension injuries of the oral region.

Operative management of high-tension injuries to the hands is stressed with an emphasis on frequent debridement and early soft tissue coverage. With these guidelines, optimal results can be expected in treating these difficult injuries.

### References

1 East, M.K., Jones C.A. & Feller, I. *et al.* (1988). Epidemiology of burns in children. In *Burns in Children: Pediatric Burn Management*, Carvajal, H.F. & Parks, D.H. eds, vol. 1, 3–10, Chicago: Year Book Medical Publishers Inc.

2 Burice, A.F., Quinby, W.C. & Bondoc, C. *et al.* (1977). Patterns of high tension electrical injury, in children and adolescents and their management. *American Journal of Surgery*, **133**, 492–7.

3 Gifford, G.H., Marty, A.T. & MacCollum, D.W. (1971). The management of electrical mouth burns in children. *Pediatrics*, **47**, 113–19.

4 Monafo, W.W. & Freedman, B.M. (1987). Electrical and lightning injury. In *The Art and Science of Burn Care*, Boswick, J.A. ed. pp. 241–53, Rockville: Aspen Publishers Inc.

5 Edelman, P.A. (1986). Chemical and electrical burns. In *Management of the Burned Patient*, Achauer, B.M., ed., pp. 183–202, Norwalk: WB Saunders Co.

6 Zelt, R.G. & Daniel, R.K. (1989). Electrical injury. In *Current Therapy in Plastic and Reconstructive Surgery*, pp. 29–33, Marsh, J.L. Ed. Toronto: BC Decker Inc.

7 Bingham, H. (1986). Electrical burns. In *Clinics in Plastic Surgery*, Ruberg, R.L. ed., pp. 75–85, Philadelphia: WB Saunders Co.

8 Silverglade, D. & Ruberg, R.L. (1986). Nonsurgical management of burns to the lips and commissures. In *Clinics in Plastic Surgery*. Ruberg, R.L. ed., pp. 87–94, Philadelphia: WB Saunders Co.

9 Pribaz, J.J., Eriksson, E. & Smith, D.J. (1991). Acute management of the burned hand. In *Plastic Surgery Education Foundation Instructional Courses*, Russel, R.C. ed., vol II. St. Louis: CV Mosby Co, in press.

10 Nichter, L.S., Bryant, G.A. & Kenney, J.G. *et al.* (1984). Injuries due to commercial electric current. *Journal of Burn Care and Rehabilitation*, **5**, 124–37.

11 Hunt, J.L., Lewis, S., Parkey, R. *et al.* (1979). The use of technitium 99m stannous pyrophosphate scintigraphy to identify muscle damage in acute electrical burns. *Journal of Trauma*, **19**, 409–13.

12 Luce, E.A. & Gottlieb, S.E. (1984). 'True' high-tension electrical injuries. *Annals of Plastic Surgery*, **12**, 321–6.

# 9

# Surgical technique for salvage of electrically damaged tissue

LAWRENCE J. GOTTLIEB
JONATHAN SAUNDERS
THOMAS J. KRIZEK

The triad of cutaneous injury, occult soft tissue destruction and multiple organ damage secondary to high-voltage electrical injury may lead to a potentially devastating scenario. The management of the injured soft tissue can be particularly challenging because treatment decisions directly affect both the acute resuscitation of the patient and the long-term functional result. Opinions regarding the timing and extent of the initial debridement and subsequent wound closure in patients that have sustained significant soft tissue injury secondary to electrical trauma are far from uniform. These differences of opinion and consequent varied therapeutic approaches evolve from different understandings of the pathophysiologic mechanism of this injury.

Several mechanisms have been postulated to explain the particular form of tissue destruction caused by high-voltage electrical injury. Artz[1] and Rouse and Dimick[2] equate electrical trauma with the injury associated with a crush syndrome. Lee[3] believes that nonthermal electrical damage at the cellular level is an important component. Many others[4-6], however, ascribe the damage caused by electrical trauma to heat generated by the passage of current through the tissues, the joule effect.

Although any one of the above theories may account for acute cell death, none of them adequately addresses the concept of progressive tissue necrosis. This concept has a major influence on soft tissue management. Key questions about soft tissue management include:

1 Does all lethal tissue injury occur immediately? or
2 Does progressive tissue damage occur after electrical trauma?
3 If tissue damage is progressive, is it preventable?
4 Can nonviable tissue be reliably identified?
5 Is there an optimal time sequence for debridement and coverage?

6 How should one handle tissue of questionable viability at the initial debridement?

The concept of progressive necrosis in electrical trauma has been investigated by Robson and associates[7]. They demonstrated that cellular injury leads to an increase in thromboxane production with a consequent vasoconstriction and thrombosis in the microcirculation, followed by further necrosis. They also postulated that this process could be prevented through the use of prostaglandin inhibitors. Lee[3] also addressed progressive necrosis, demonstrating experimentally that the nonthermal electrical component perforates the cell membrane of nerve and muscular cells causing potentially reversible cell membrane changes and subsequent delayed cell death. On the other hand, Zelt[8] analysed electrical trauma in a primate model via gross observation, light microscopy, angiography and electrophysiologic nerve conduction. He concluded that progressive necrosis does not occur.

If one accepts the concept that the major damage from electrical trauma is the result of thermal injury, then perhaps the dynamic zone of stasis postulated by Jackson can be extended to include electrical injury. Janzekovic[9] has described preservation of this marginal, potentially reversible, zone of stasis in thermal burns by tangential debridement and immediate physiologic coverage.

To achieve maximal tissue salvage in patients with high-voltage electrical injury, a uniquely aggressive therapeutic regimen was instituted. This approach is based on the theory that the tissue injury by the thermal component of electrical trauma may indeed have a dynamic zone of stasis which can respond to immediate physiologic closure.

In addition to the direct tissue damage caused by the electrical and thermal components of electrical injury, muscle may be irreversibly damaged by the subsequent increased pressure within its fascial compartments. The initial step for tissue salvage is the early recognition and immediate treatment of compartment syndrome via escharotomy and fasciotomy. The critical importance of preventing progressive tissue loss secondary to pressure by complete early decompression cannot be overemphasized. Decompression is followed by radical operative debridement of *all* nonviable soft tissue. Viable muscle, which we define by colour and contractibility, is preserved, as are noncharred tendons and nerves. Marginal muscle when intermixed with healthy appearing muscle is also spared.

If, after initial debridement, the remaining tissue appears adequate for long-term function, then *immediate* wound closure is performed. If the magnitude of debridement required is such as to preclude expectation of reasonable long-term functional recovery, amputation is performed. In the situation where the viability of tissue which is potentially critical for function is indeterminate, a more traditional care plan is utilized and definitive debridement is postponed for 24 hours. Immediate coverage is not appropriate for all patients.

The treatment of the right upper extremity of a recent patient illustrates the philosophy. A 54 year-old right-hand dominant male was transferred to the University of Chicago Burn Center after sustaining a high-voltage electrical injury. He was working on a fire hydrant when a 7500 V line fell on the posterior aspect of his neck. His main contact points were his neck and right hand. Additional cutaneous injuries were noted on his left hand and left thigh. Initial exam of his right hand revealed deep burn to his wrist with severely charred thenar skin and flexed wrist and fingers. His right hand was swollen, cool and tense (Fig. 9.1). Neurological examination revealed a low median and ulnar neuropathy. Examination of the left hand was similar to the right, but clearly less extensive and without neuropathy. After stabilization of his airway and initiation of acute fluid resuscitation, the patient was taken to the operating room, within 2 hours of arrival to the Unit.

Both arms were decompressed simultaneously with extensive fasciotomies and decompression of the carpal tunnel and Guyon's canal, bilaterally. No devitalized tissue was encountered on the left side. On the right hand (Fig. 9.2), devitalized skin was overlying the thenar muscles, and the wrist was debrided as was the majority of the superficial head of the flexor pollicis brevis muscle and the abductor pollicis brevis muscle. All of the extrinsic flexor muscles of the distal one-third of the right wrist, and the pronator quadratus muscle, were all clearly nonviable and therefore acutely debrided. The remaining thenar muscles and proximal portion of the flexors revealed an admixture of pink and pale portions. The remaining flexors contracted when stimulated by the electrocautery, whereas the thenar muscle did not. The median nerve was firm to palpation and was decompressed with an internal neurolysis under microscopic control for a length of 16 cm. The exposed, devascularized tendons and nerves as well as the remaining marginal muscle were acutely closed with a rectus abdominus muscle free flap. Microvascular anastomosis was performed at the level of the brachial artery and vein just distal to the elbow, and a split-thickness skin graft was placed over this muscle (Fig. 9.3). A biopsy of the remaining thenar muscle was performed prior to closure and at 3 months postoperati-

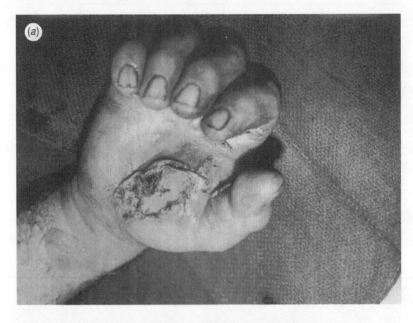

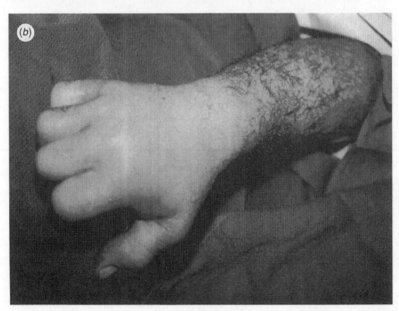

Fig. 9.1 (*a*) Right hand contact point over thenar eminence; (*b*) dorsum of right hand demonstrating acute swelling.

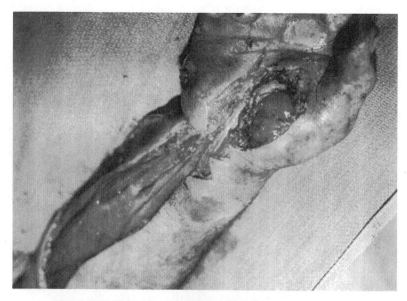

Fig. 9.2. Right hand and forearm volar fasciotomy – superficial portion of thenar muscles are dark and haemorrhagic.

vely (Fig. 9.4). Split-thickness skin allograft was placed on the decompressed left forearm. Forty-eight hours later this was exchanged for an autograft when the neck injury was addressed. Both upper extremities healed without drainage or infection. Examination 6 months postoperatively of the left upper extremity was normal while the right side had a persistent medial and ulnar neuropathy.

### Discussion

This aggressive approach to wound closure is unique. In other series, wounds are debrided two to four times prior to definitive coverage. The practice of delayed coverage stems from the fear of covering areas of dead muscle which may act as a depository for secondary bacterial seeding. It is thought that these risks are minimized if impending compartment syndromes are released prior to irreversible muscle damage and these decompressed wounds are closed early, before contamination, desiccation and autolysis occur. The advantage is potential salvage of more tissue. Successful grafting of bone, tendon, nerve and muscle all have been documented throughout the medical literature. If adequately decompressed residual muscle, devascularized tendon, nerve and bone are covered

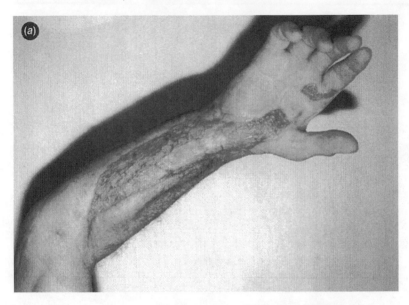

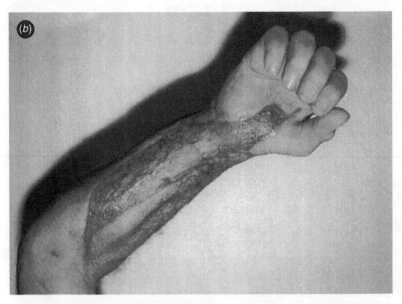

Fig. 9.3. Right hand and forearm 3 months after rectus abdominus free flap. (*a*) active extension of fingers; (*b*) active flexion of fingers.

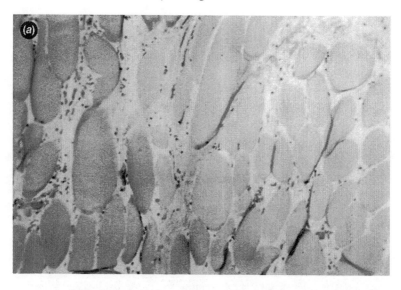

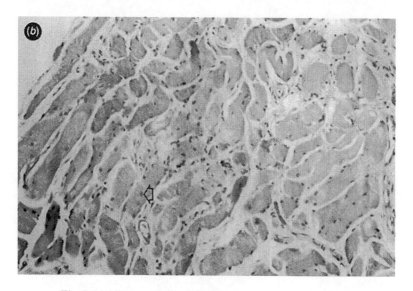

Fig. 9.4 (*a*) Biopsy of remaining thenar muscle prior to closure with free flap demonstrating varying degree of injury. (125x); (*b*) re-biopsy of thenar muscle 3 months post-operatively. Demonstrating myopathic changes consistent with fibre regeneration. Note variation of fibre size and centrally located nuclei (125x).

with well-vascularized tissue, prior to bacterial contamination and autolysis, this tissue should act like a composite graft. Although much of the salvaged muscle will atrophy, residual muscle cells can survive and subsequently hypertrophy[10].

Through early complete fasciotomies and the immediate utilization of well-vascularized healthy tissue, coverage of the marginally healthy regions of electrical injury may enable us to salvage potentially nonviable tissue. This method leads to a more expedient recovery with potentially improved long-term functional results.

### References

1 Artz, C.P. (1967). Electrical injury simulates crush injury. *Surgery Gynecology and Obstetrics*, **125**, 13116.

2 Rouge, R.G. & Dimick, A.R. (1978). The treatment of electrical injury compared to burn injury: a review of pathophysiology and comparison of patient management protocols. *Journal of Trauma*, **18**, 43–7.

3 Lee, R.C. & Kodney, M.S. (1987). Electrical injury mechanisms: electrical breakdown of cell membranes. *Plastic and Reconstructive Surgery*, **80**, 672.

4 Baxter, C.R. (1970). Present concepts in the management of major electrical injuries. *Surgery Clinics in North America*, **50**, 1401.

5 Hunt, J.L., Mason, A.D. Jr, Masterson, T.S. *et al.* (1976). The pathophysiology of acute electric injuries. *Journal of Trauma*, **16**, 335–50.

6 Lee, R.C. & Koldney, M.S. (1987). Clinical injury mechanisms: dynamics of the thermal response. *Plastic and Reconstructive Surgery*, **80**, 663.

7 Robson, M.C., Murphy, R.C. & Heggars, J.P. (1984). A new explanation for the progressive tissue loss in electrical injuries. *Plastic and Reconstructive Surgery*, **73**, 431.

8 Zelt, R.G., Daniel, R.K., Ballard, P.A. & Brissette, Y. (1988). High voltage electrical injury: chronic wound evolution. *Plastic and Reconstructive Surgery*, **82**, 1027–39.

9 Janzekovic, Z. (1970). A new concept in the early excision and immediate grafting of burns. *Journal of Trauma*, **10**, 1103.

10 Maxwell, L.C. & Moody, M.R. (1988). Muscle fiber regeneration in grafted skeletal muscles. *Journal of Reconstructive Microsurgery*, **4**, 161–6.

# Part III:

Tissue responses

# 10

# The role of arachidonic acid metabolism in the pathogenesis of electrical trauma

MARTIN C. ROBSON
PETER G. HAYWARD
JOHN P. HEGGERS

An electrical injury is a unique and thoroughly devastating form of trauma. The clinical pictures following cellular damage due to electrical current comprise more of a syndrome than a specific injury. The syndrome consists of varying degrees of cutaneous burn combined with 'hidden' destruction of deep tissue[1]. The electrical insult results in progressive tissue necrosis in excess of the originally apparent trauma, somewhat resembling the injury of crush trauma[2,3]. Controversy exists as to whether this is a slow manifestation of irreversible muscle damage secondary to the original current passage[4-6], or whether it is actively progressive ischaemic necrosis secondary to ongoing macrovascular or microvascular compromise[1,7,8,9].

The cause of the controversy is a poor understanding of the pathophysiology. Because the injuries comprise a syndrome, the inciting cellular mechanism(s) for the pathophysiology may be multiple. Historically, the mechanism was thought to be heat. Passage of electric current through a solid conductor results in conversion of electric energy into heat, the joule effect. The amount of heat can be determined by Ohm's Law and the joule effect. Ohm's Law states that the current travelling through tissue is determined by the voltage ($V$) divided by the resistance ($R$). Heat production in joules is proportional to the power dissipated multiplied by the duration of contact and is expressed by the equation $J = I^2 RT$ where $J$ is the heat production, $I$ is the current, $R$ is the tissue resistance, and $T$ is the time of contact[1]. The extent of injury depends on the type of current, the pathway of flow, the local tissue resistance, and the duration of contact[5,10-14].

Two theories attributing the pathological changes seen following electrical injury to generated heat have been postulated. The first emphasizes the differences in tissue resistance to current flow to explain the observed changes following electrical injury[15]. Tissue resistance progressively increases from nerve to blood vessels, muscle, skin, tendon, fat, and bone. Bone, having the greatest resistance, generates the most heat according to the joule effect. This would cause greater necrosis in the deep peri-osseous tissues, a situation frequently observed in this syndrome. However, the majority of current would preferentially travel along the lines of lesser resistance, particularly the blood vessels[12,16,17]. These vessels are injured, but not immediately thrombosed[18]. According to this theory, the progressive muscular necrosis is attributed to these vascular lesions leading to delayed arterial occlusion and progressive ischaemic necrosis[7-9].

Another theory questions the existence of progressive muscle necrosis. Hunt *et al.* found that the internal milieu of an experimental animal's body acts like a volume conductor of a single resistance and not as if it were composed of tissues of varying resistances[5]. With the onset of current flow, amperage and temperature rise in parallel throughout the limb. By the time of current arcing, both muscle and bone temperatures are equal. However, they observed that it takes bone longer to dissipate the heat and suggested it was this prolonged elevation in temperature that accounted for the peri-osseous 'core' of necrotic muscle seen clinically. They also thought that involved muscle and vessels sustain irreversible damage at the time of current passage with immediate microscopic muscular coagulation necrosis and small nutrient artery thrombosis. To support this concept are reports that progressive occlusion of major-sized vessels have not been documented arteriographically in the experimental situation or clinically[4,6,19].

Progressive microvascular deterioration beyond the resolution of radiographic evaluation is not ruled out by a failure to delineate progressive changes arteriographically. Quinby *et al.*, and Luce *et al.*, in describing the microscopic changes of questionably viable muscle emphasized the mixed 'patchy' nature of the electrical injury[20,21]. Normal muscle cells can be seen immediately adjacent to necrotic cells with pyknotic nuclei, and normal patent vessels can exist adjacent to thrombosed vessels, reminiscent of the 'zone of stasis' in the thermal burn[12]. Progressive small vessel thrombosis and deterioration of the microvasculature could convert these areas of 'patchy necrosis' into complete tissue loss.

There is a problem with attributing the entire pathophysiology responsible for the syndrome of electrical injury to heat. Lee and Kolodney have demonstrated through electrical and mathematical modelling that joule heating is often not sufficient to explain the tissue necrosis seen[22,23]. When the current passes transversely across a limb, the tissue would be arranged electrically in series. In this situation, the tissue with lower conductivity and higher resistance would generate the greatest amount of heat. This situation would mimic the theory suggested by Baxter[15]. However, as Lee and Kolodney suggest, most clinical situations probably place the tissues electrically in parallel[22]. When current enters an upper extremity and transverses the entire body to another contact point on the lower extremity, they have shown this to be the case. They have also shown the tissue with greatest conductivity to generate the most heat. They suggested that muscle would generate the greatest intensity of joule heating and the adjacent bone would be heated secondarily. This would corroborate the theory proposed by Hunt *et al.*[5] The bone heated secondarily would dissipate heat quite slowly. Lee and Kolodney showed this dissipation to be prolonged in a state of poor perfusion[22]. The cause of this poor perfusion in electrical injury will be discussed later.

Although the mathematical modelling appeared to explain the different theories for joule heating as a cause for cellular damage in electrical injuries, it also showed that often the amount of heat is not sufficient to explain tissue damage at sites distant from the current contact[22]. However, Lee and Kolodney demonstrated that an electric field can be of sufficient magnitude to cause electrical breakdown of cells and cell lysis[23]. They point out that rupture of cells by strong electric fields is well documented[24]. Electric fields stronger than a threshold magnitude and turned on faster than the mechanical response of a membrane can rupture bilaminate lipid membranes[25].

It appears that these various observations are all correct in select situations following electrical trauma. That is the reason for describing the clinical response as a syndrome. Perhaps a way of unifying these theories is to look at the cellular response to the initial electrical insult. To do this, one needs to look at the immediate and delayed cellular damage following contact with an electric field. This unifying concept is the same as for other causes of soft tissue trauma such as thermal burning, frostbite, or other injuries in which patients present to the emergency department with what appears to be relatively minor injuries and, after a period of days, lose large amounts of tissue[26]. Similar circumstances occur with crush injuries in which muscle damage appears to worsen under intact skin, and in avulsion injuries in which the flap looks healthy at the time of admission only to become necrotic over a few days.

The immediate damage is similar and fairly well delineated for all of these injuries. Similar mechanisms are postulated following electrical trauma. The traumatic insult results in a degree of cell shock. The intracellular energy system changes stored adenosine triphosphate (ATP) to cyclic adenosine monophosphate (AMP), and the sodium pump becomes ineffective as the cell membrane becomes permeable to sodium and calcium ions[27,28]. As part of the immediate cellular injury, proteases are released, and these can trigger both the coagulation cascade and complement degradation. Degradaton products such as $C_5A$ begin the immunologic cascade, and the soft tissue responds by increased vascular permeability and chemotaxis[26]. The mast cell, stimulated by these tissue proteases coming out of the injured cell, produces more cyclic AMP. Penneys has shown that injury also activates phospholipase A, which cleaves phospholipids that are bound to cholesterol and triglycerides in the cell membrane[29]. This results in the metabolism of arachidonic acid which, when released, helps to activate the platelet plug. The other activity from the proteases is the initiation of chemotaxis. The respiratory burst of the leukocyte occurs producing more arachidonic acid metabolites. This also produces free oxygen radicals necessary for the initial control of bacteria at the site of injury.

It appears that any traumatic soft tissue injury results in these immediate effects[26]. However, except in the most severe cases of soft tissue injuries, the immediate effects may not result in tissue necrosis. This is the case in clinical electrical injuries in which tissue proximal to the site of contact often appears uninjured.

The major causes of soft tissue loss in the various clinical presentations of the electrical syndrome are due to delayed effects. Robson et al. suggested the aetiology and a method to control these delayed effects in an experimental electrical injury[1]. Their laboratory had previously shown that progressive tissue loss in burns and frostbite was due to progressive dermal ischaemia mediated by various metabolites of arachidonic acid[30-33]. These substances, especially prostaglandin $F_{2a}$ and thromboxane $A_2$, are vasoconstrictors and platelet aggregators and theoretically detrimental to tissue following trauma. By blocking their production, they had been able to reverse the progressive ischaemia seen following burns and frostbite and to provide increased tissue survival. Heggers and Robson have postulated that cellular integrity depends on a homeostatic relationship between $PGE_2$ and $PGF_{2a}$[34]. Injury to the cells disrupts this, causing a shunt in arachidonic acid metabolism toward thromboxane production. Production of this vasoactive prostanoid in large amounts leads to vasoconstriction, thrombosis, progressive ischaemic necrosis, and further thromboxane production.

Because Arturson[35] suggested that various forms of trauma could activate phospholipase A to cleave the phospholipids from the cell membrane to begin the arachidonic cascades, and because heat and electrical disruption of the cell membrane were forms of trauma, the definitive experiment linking arachidonic acid metabolites to the pathophysiology of electrical trauma was reported in 1984[1]. A rat model, modified from that described by Buchanan *et al.*, was used to provide a reproducible electrical injury to the hind limb[19]. The modification was to deliver 250 volts AC for 10 seconds, since higher voltages were found to produce instant mummification and unacceptable mortality rates. Male Sprague–Dawley rats were anaesthetized with intraperitoneal sodium pentobarbital, and their left forelimbs and right hand limbs shaved. The rats were placed on an insulated platform and 5 mm wide wire mesh leads were applied with the positive lead around the ankle joint of the right hind limb and the negative lead around the left forelimb. Electrodes were attached to a transformer set to deliver 250 volts ac. Current was delivered to the animals for 10 seconds, sufficient to produce a visible burn at the electrode sites. This model appeared to mimic the progressive injury of a high-voltage injury in the human since the limb progressed from normal to autoamputation over a 72-hour period.

The experiment was divided into two parts with the first evaluating the production of arachidonic acid metabolites in different parts of the injured limbs serially over 72 hours, and the second part evaluating the efficacy of blocking arachidonic acid metabolism on tissue preservation. In part one, immediately after receiving the current and at 8, 24, 48, and 72 hours after injury, animals were sacrificed and their right hind limbs amputated. Cross-sections of the limb were taken at three levels: (1) distal, immediately above the electrode site; (2) midlevel, immediately above the knee joint; and (3) proximal, immediately distal to the inguinal ligament. These sections were fixed, coded, and stained for prostaglandin $E_2$ (PGE$_2$), prostaglandin $F_{2\alpha}$ (PGF$_{2\alpha}$), and thromboxane $B_2$ (TxB$_2$) using the peroxidase–antiperoxidase (PAP) method described by Heggers *et al.*[36]. The results showed that distally immediately beneath the electrode, there were high levels of thromboxane. However, far proximally in an area which looked grossly normal for the first 48 hours and eventually proceeded to autoamputation, the thromboxane was very high initially only in the deep peri-osseous tissue. Superficially, next to the skin which appeared to be totally normal, thromboxane was nonexistent at time zero but progressively rose until the point at which the skin was dead and the leg autoamputated.

In Part 2 of the experiment, animals were divided into groups after receiving the electrical insult: the groups which received no treatment and served as a control or were treated with a systemic antithromboxane agent, a topical antithromboxane agent, a nonspecific prostaglandin blocker, or the combination of systemic and topical antithromboxane drugs. Surviving limb length was the measure of success. All attempts were successful compared to the untreated controls, with the best results due to the combination of systemic and topical antithromboxane agents. In this group, surviving limb length was 79.8% compared to 37.2% in the control animals[1]. Total salvage of the limb occurred in some animals.

The demonstration of arachidonic acid metabolites in increasing amounts in tissue following electrical trauma allows a unifying concept for the various theories regarding the pathophysiology of these injuries. Both joule heating and cell membrane disruption can activate the arachidonic acid cascade. Once initiated, the various immediate effects of trauma produce more of these mediators[26].

This concept allows other clinical observations to be clarified. Many of the inflammatory mediators can cause marked vasoconstriction of the microcirculation. This would decrease perfusion of an anatomic part and markedly decrease the rate of cooling. Another concept difficult to explain by previous theories is that of 'patchy necrosis'. This has been reported in most clinical and experimental electrical injuries[1,20,21]. Since tissue perfusion can be both macroscopic and microscopic, local production of ischaemia-causing mediators due to cell rupture in an electric field could result in 'patchy necrosis'. Certainly, in the experiment reported by Robson *et al.*, when tissue was stained specifically for $TxA_2$, a patchy distribution was seen[1]. They postulated that the elevated thromboxane production by the injured cells could easily provide the impetus for converting areas of 'patchy' necrosis into areas of complete tissue loss.

The observed and reported increase in tissue necrosis in the peri-osseous tissue becomes quite clear when one combines all of these theories. In Baxter's scenario, the bone provides the greatest amount of joule heating[15]. In the theories by Hunt *et al.*, and Lee and Kolodney, the muscle produces the highest immediate heat, but the bone prolongs the time of heating[5,22]. If mediators are produced by the two mechanisms discussed above, perfusion next to the bone will be less because of vasoconstriction of the microvasculature, temperatures will rise, and more injurious mediators will be produced. Therefore, the increased death of tissue needs no further explanation.

It now seems quite straightforward to explain the presence of deep necrosis beneath unaffected skin. Skin temperature distant from the point of contact may never rise to the lethal range in an electrical injury.[22] The fact that this apparently uninjured skin may progressively necrose may be due to progressive ischaemia caused by inflammatory mediators and not the electrical event itself. This would be similar to other forms of trauma which activate the arachidonic acid cascade and would allow a unifying concept regarding progressive tissue loss.

There has been resistance to accepting this unifying concept for the pathophysiology of tissue injury following electrical trauma. Part of this has been due to semantics. Historically, there was the idea that there was delayed muscle necrosis and, therefore, early debridement and wound closure was contraindicated. This led to weeks of serial debridement, desiccation of the open wound, and infection. This vicious cycle indeed led to further tissue necrosis. Kuzon *et al.* and Zelt *et al.* designed a model in a primate which showed that this delayed muscle necrosis did not occur and suggested that debridement and definitive wound closure could occur much earlier[37,38]. Similarly, Silverberg *et al.* have advocated early debridement and closure[39]. The arachidonic acid metabolites are activated immediately after injury. Their effects begin at that time and most of the ischaemia produced by them would be expected to be complete by 72–96 hours. Any attempt to pharmacologically block their effects must be done in the immediate post-traumatic period. Therefore, Zelt and Daniel's recommendation to decompress and adequately explore the injury immediately and to provide definitive debridement and wound closure between the third and the fifth day is totally compatible with the concept of a progressive mediator-induced injury over a limited timespan[6]. To delay beyond that time has no physiological basis, and to allow the wound to remain open invites further loss of tissue. Desiccation alone actually stimulates the production of thromboxane.

Most clinicians who advocate early wound closure in electrical injuries suggest the definitive debridement and closure not be done in the first 48–72 hours. This makes sense to allow the progressive or 'nonimmediate' cellular effects to be manifest. If, as Lee and Kolodney suggest, those cells not coagulated by joule heating die because of membrane disruption, this will not be recognized grossly at the time of initial decompression and exploration[23]. It will be recognized several days later when the arachidonic acid metabolites have caused microvascular ischaemic cell death. It is, at that time, that the necrotic tissue can be excised and the wound closed.

Based on the results of the experiments discussed in this paper and the unifying concept of tissue injury, clinical treatment of patients with high-voltage electrical injuries has been changed. After admission and stabilization, the muscular compartments are immediately released, the nerves decompressed, a topical antithromboxane agent applied, and it is believed the progressive injury is limited. This appears to allow earlier definitive

186     *M.C. Robson, P.G. Hayward and J.P. Heggers*

reconstruction than was seen historically with delayed necrosis due to desiccation and infection that frequently would have ended up with an amputation.

### References

1 Robson, M.C., Murphy, R.C. & Heggers, J.P. (1984). A new explanation for the progressive tissue loss in electrical injuries. *Plastic and Reconstructive Surgery*, **73**, 431–7.
2 Rouse, R.G. & Dimick, A.R. (1978). Treatment of electrical injury compared to burn injury. *Journal of Trauma*, **18**, 43.
3 Artz, C.P. (1967). Electrical injury simulates crush injury. *Surgery, Gynecology and Obstetrics*, **125**, 1316.
4 Hunt, J.L., McManus, W.F., Haney, W.P. & Pruitt, B.A. (1974). Vascular lesions in acute electrical injuries. *Journal of Trauma*, **14**, 461.
5 Hunt, J.L., Mason, A.D., Masterson, T.S. & Pruitt, B.A. (1976). Pathophysiology of acute electrical injuries. *Journal of Trauma*, **16**, 335.
6 Zelt, R.G. & Daniel, R.K. (1989). Electrical injury. In *Current Therapy in Plastic and Reconstructive Surgery*, Marsh, J., ed., pp. 29–33.
7 Baxter, C.R. (1990). Present concepts in the management of major electrical injuries. *Surgery Clinics of North America*, **50**, 1401.
8 Ponten, B., Erickson, U. & Johansson, E.H. *et al.* (1970). New observations on tissue changes along the pathway of the current in an electrical injury. *Scandinavian Journal of Plastic and Reconstructive Surgery*, **4**, 75.
9 Skoog, T. (1970). Electrical injuries. *Journal of Trauma*, **10**, 816.
10 Sances, A., Larson, S.J., Mykelbust, J. & Cusick, J.F. (1979). Electrical injuries. *Surgery Gynecology and Obstetrics*, **149**, 97.
11 Esses, S.I. & Peters, W.J. (1981). Electrical burns: pathophysiology and complications. *Canadian Journal of Surgery*, **24**, 11.
12 Mann, R.J. & Wallquist, J.M. (1975). Early decompression fasciotomy in the treatment of high voltage electrical injury of the extremities. *Scandinavian Medical Journal*, **68**, 1103.
13 Jaffe, R.H. (1928). Electropathology: a review of the pathologic changes produced by electric currents. *Archive of Pathology*, **5**, 837.
14 Sances, A., Myklebust, J.B., Larson, S.J., Darin, J.L., Swiontek, T., Prieto, T., Chilbert, M. & Cusick, J.F. (1981). Experimental electrical injury studies. *Journal of Trauma*, **21**, 589.
15 Baxter, C.R. (1970). Present concepts in management of major electrical injury. *Surgery Clinics of North America*, **50**, 1401.
16 Solem, L., Fischer, R.P. & Strate, R.G. (1977). Natural history of electrical injury. *Journal of Trauma*, **17**, 487.
17 Sturim, H.S. (1971). The treatment of electrical injuries. *Journal of Trauma*, **11**, 959.
18 Jaffe, R.H., Willis, D. & Bachem, A. (1929). The effect of electrical current on arteries. *Archives of Pathology*, **7**, 244.
19 Buchanan, D.L., Erk, Y. & Spira, M. (1983). Electrical current arterial injury: a laboratory model. *Plastic and Reconstructive Surgery*, **72**, 199.
20 Quinby, W.C., Burke, J.F., Trelstad, R.L. & Caulfield, J. (1978). The use of microscopy as a guide to primary excision of electrical burns. *Journal of Trauma*, **18**, 423.

21  Luce, E.A., Dowden, W.L., Su, C.T. & Hoopes, J.E. (1978). High tension electrical injury of the upper extremity. *Surgery and Gynecology and Obstetrics*, **147**, 38.

22  Lee, R.C. & Kolodney, M.S. (1987). Electrical injury mechanisms: Dynamics of the thermal response. *Plastic and Reconstructive Surgery*, **80**, 663.

23  Lee, R.C. & Kolodney, M.S. (1987). Electrical injury mechanisms: Electrical breakdown of cell membranes. *Plastic and Reconstructive Surgery*, **80**, 672.

24  Teissie, J., Knutson, V.P., Tsang, T.Y. & Lane, M.C. (1982). Electric pulse-induced fusion of 3T3 cells in monolager culture. *Science*, **216**, 537.

25  Benz, R., Beckers, F. & Zimmermann, U. (1979). Reversible electrical breakdown of lipid bilayer membranes: A charge-pulse relaxation study. *Journal of Membrane Biology*, **48**, 181.

26  Robson, M.C. (1989). The immediate and delayed cellular damage following soft tissue trauma. In *Essays in Surgery*, Zarins, C. ed., pp. 153–8.

27  Teissie, J. & Tsang, T.Y. (1980). Evidence of voltage-induced channel opening in Na/K ATPase of human erythrocyte membrane. *Journal of Membrane Biology*, **55**, 133.

28  Lee, R.C., Gaylor, D.C., Bhatt, D. & Israel, D. (1988). Role of cell membrane rupture in the pathogenesis of electrical trauma. *Journal of Surgical Research*, **44**, 709.

29  Penneys, N.S. (1980). Prostaglandins and the skin. *Current Concepts*. Kalamazoo: The Upjohn Co.

30  Robson, M.C., DelBeccaro, E.J. & Heggers, J.P. (1974). The effect of prostaglandins on the dermal microcirculation after burning and the inhibition of the effect by specific pharmacological agents. *Plastic and Reconstructive Surgery*, **63**, 781.

31  DelBeccaro, E.J., Robson, M.C., Heggers, J.P. & Swaninathan, R. (1980). The use of specific thromboxane inhibitors to preserve the dermal microcirculation after burning. *Surgery*, **87**, 137.

32  Robson, M.C., DelBeccaro, E.J., Heggers, J.P. & Loy, G.L. (1980). Increasing dermal perfusion after burning by decreasing thromboxane production. *Journal of Trauma*, **20**, 722.

33  Raine, T.J., London, M.C., Goluch, L., Heggers, J.P. & Robson, M.C. (1980). Antiprostaglandins and antithromboxanes for treatment of frostbite. *Surgical Forum*, **31**, 556.

34  Heggers, J.P. & Robson, M.C. (1983). Prostaglandins and thromboxanes. In *Traumatic Injury – Infection and Other Immunologic Sequelae*, Ninneman, J., ed., Baltimore: University Park Press.

35  Arturson, G. (1984). How are prostaglandins and leukotrienes involved in immunological alterations? A discussion. *Journal of Trauma*, **24** (suppl), S128.

36  Heggers, J.P., Loy, G.L., Robson, M.C. & DelBeccaro, E.J. (1980). Histological determination of prostaglandins and thromboxanes in burned tissue. *Journal of Surgical Research*, **28**, 110.

37  Kuzon, W.M., Zelt, R.G., Green, H.J., Ballard, P.A., Pynn, B.R., Plyley, M.J., McKee, N.H. & Daniel, R.K. (1986). Skeletal muscle energy metabolism following high voltage electrical injury. *Surgical Forum*, **37**, 621.

38 Zelt, R.G., Ballard, P.A., Common, A.A., Heroux, P. & Daniel, R.K. (1986). Experimental high voltage electrical burns: role of progressive necrosis. *Surgical Forum*, **37**, 624.

39 Silverberg, B., Banis, J.C., Verdi, G.D. *et al.* (1985). Microsurgical reconstruction for the electrical and deep thermal injury. *Proceedings of the American Burn Association*, **17**, 129.

# 11

# Thermal damage: mechanisms, patterns and detection in electrical burns

PAUL HÉROUX

## Thermal damage in electrical burns

Even brief 50–60 Hz electric shocks at currents between approximately 100 mA and 4 A carry a significant risk of cardiac fibrillation. Beyond 4 A, that risk is reduced considerably because the myocardium is completely depolarized by current passage; on current interruption and after a few seconds at rest, the heart starts beating again spontaneously. At currents beyond 4 A, however, burns can occur through joule heating due to high voltage, long contact time or both.

In electrical burns, intolerable temperature rise in muscle is the prime cause of tissue necrosis (immediate or delayed) and consequently of limb amputation. Although there is evidence that, in some cases, electric lesions may be morphologically different from thermal lesions, specifically in the appearance of vesicular nuclei[1], it has not been demonstrated that the necrotic zone in electrical burns extends outside the thermally damaged volume. Perhaps the strongest evidence for the dominant role of thermal damage is that patterns of temperature rise coincide with tissue damage at the anatomical level.

## Mechanisms of hyperthermic cell death

### Topic factors: thermal stress

By contrast with death from other mechanisms, cell death specifically by hyperthermia is thought to occur rapidly[2]. Mortal heat stress first stops the movement of mitochondria which become pale, swollen and vesiculated. The loss of mitochondrion function is detectable by a vital dye technique monitoring the decrease of its phosphorylation potential. Further, all cellular and intracellular movements cease, cytoplasm and nucleoplasm develop a mottled appearance and both cell and nucleus shrink[3]. The identification of the mitochondrion as the early site of damage lends support to the view that thermal death results from a form of metabolic exhaustion due to increased expenditure with rising temperature and to simultaneous elimination of the ATP synthesis pathway. It is known that prethermal-shock nutritional deprivation enhances thermal killing[4]. It is understood that inhibition of ATP synthesis at the mitochondrion mechanically affects the membrane–cytoskeleton connection, as cytoskeleton maintenance depends heavily on ATP; membrane blebbing and hyperpermeability then result in a collapse of cell polarization[5]. Cellular events similarly dependent on cytoskeleton function, such as the operation of the spindle in mitotic cells, are also highly thermosensitive[6].

Histologically, rapid hyperthermic death has been reported for both tumour and normal tissues in the form of interphase nuclear pyknosis[7-10]. Various cells, including erythrocytes, which fragment to form spherocytes at 49 °C, die within a narrow range of temperatures, despite, in the case of erythrocytes, somewhat different metabolic pathways and the absence of mitochondria[11].

### Systemic factors: perfusion

Data on severe heat injury show that small vessel changes occur within as little as 5 to 10 minutes, resulting in damage to the endothelial cell membranes which ultimately triggers the coagulation system and leads to thrombosis[12,13]. More discrete challenges lead to changes in the pH of muscle from 7.1–7.4 to higher values when heated to 43.5–45 °C, but to decreases to values as low as 6.6 when raised above 46°C[14]. Survival-threatening rises may therefore occur in an acidic environment which is known to enhance cell killing[15]. Systemic acidosis also tends to develop over 6 hours if electrical burn victims are untreated[16]. Because greater cell killing occurs in tumours *in vivo* than *in vitro* by the same heat dose, the possibility cannot be excluded that cell death progresses over time[17], partly by either immunological or systemic mechanisms dependent on vascular damage[18]. Whether necrosis could be reduced by optimal management of perfusion to the wound is the subject of considerable controversy. Although more perfusion may stabilize pH, it may also under some circumstances favour the formation of higher concentrations of free radicals.

Anaesthetists have noticed that thermal injury results in dystropic skeletal muscle dysfunction and hypersensitivity to acetylcholine[19]

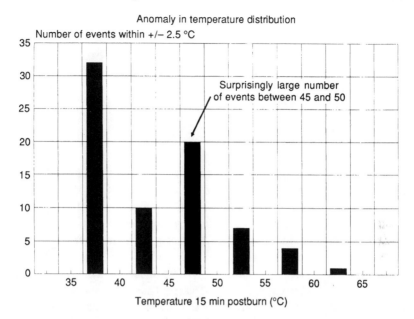

Fig. 11.1 Thermal decays observed in the forearms of primates reveal unanticipated action of vasoconstrictive mechanisms.

through a persistent release of catecholamines. Acetylcholine is related intimately to perfusion regulation in muscle by interactions with sympathetic nerve stimulation[20] and endothelium-derived vascular relaxant factor[21]. Perhaps electrical burns can destroy vasomotor control[22], favouring accumulation of intravascular water[23].

The group at the Royal Victoria Hospital[24] observed thermodynamic anomalies in a model of electrical burns in primates which may relate to vasomotor control. The tests monitored temperature decays following electrical burns using thermistors implanted in muscles of the forearm. The data showed that both the crest temperature and the temperature 15 minutes after shock were recorded at values between 45 and 50 °C more frequently than expected (Fig. 11.1). Some of the decays showed horizontal plateaux as long as 6 minutes (decay slope was normally 0.64 °C per minute), at a temperature always very near 48.2 °C, close to the thermal death limit of the tissue.

The interpretation was that a powerful vasoconstrictor was released at a specific temperature, leading to the apparently adiabatic intervals[25]. The enzyme acetylcholinesterase from muscle shows a 60% drop in activity from 42 to 48 °C (due to inactivation of the monomeric 4 S enzyme), followed by a plateau, the second stage of inactivation starting at 51 °C and ending at 57–60 °C[26]. A possible interpretation is that the observed stoppage in thermal decays in muscle would result from the thermal characteristics of acetylcholinesterase activity (enzymatic activity often shows partial recovery when a heat-denatured enzyme is returned to normal temperatures).

### Heat dose: thermal death equation

Calculations predicting damage to tissue from its temperature history use the Maxwell–Boltzmann equation and the threshold 'activation energy' as a base. The equation determines, from the mechanics of molecular collisions, the fraction of a group of molecules that possess a motion energy larger than the activation energy. The assumption is that thermal killing depends on a biochemical reaction which needs a minimum energy to occur. As more molecules possess that minimum energy (the fraction rises with temperature), the reaction rate increases. This simple theory has been used to explain the rate of both chemical (within a reasonable temperature range) and, more surprisingly, biochemical reactions (within a more restricted range). It is widely known in chemistry as the Arrhenius equation. More recently, the Arrhenius equation has been applied to *in vitro* and *in vivo* heat-killing. The theoretical framework is not extensive enough to describe cell death because heat-killing likely involves irreversible reactions beyond the mechanistic assumptions of the Maxwell–Boltzmann equation and because many reactions may be coupled or sequenced simultaneously. But, these theoretical difficulties do not stop experimentalists from fitting data to the mathematical expressions[27].

In practice, the Arrhenius equation, when suited with the activation energy known to occur in biological materials ($\sim 149$ kcal/mol; this corresponds to '75 000' in the equation below), states that, in the temperature range relevant to heat killing, an increase of 1° will increase the reaction rate by a factor very close to 2.

Temperature–survival data from various investigators is scattered among a variety of tissues and experimental animals. Temperature is applied for various durations, and is sometimes inconstant over the test period. Also, the histological techniques used in assessing the temperature-related damage are far from uniform, specifically in the weight given to acute (24 h) versus chronic damage. The virtue of the equation is that it yields $D$, the percentage of cells dying from exposure, from any number of $T$ values, the temperatures in Kelvin at the start of each second. The

Table 11.1. *Necrosis limits for a 2.75 min hyperthermic episode*

| Author | Temperature | Animal | Tissue |
|--------|-------------|--------|--------|
| 37,38 | 50.90 | Swine | Skin |
| 17 | 49.28 | Swine | Muscle |
| 2 | 49.01 | Mouse | Carcinoma and sarcoma |
| 39 | 48.63 | Monkey | Retina |
| 40,41 | 48.14 | Rat | Rhabdomyosarcoma |
| 42 | 48.11 | Human | Skin |
| 43 | 48.01 | Rat | Rhabdomyosarcoma |
| 43 | 47.64 | Rat | Rhabdomyosarcoma |

summation is carried out over the hyperthermic episode, and therefore takes complete temperature history into account.

$$D = \Sigma\exp(232.34 - 75\,000/T)$$

Analysis of experiments carried out in primates showed that the temperature decay over time in muscles was such that the hyperthermic period was approximately equivalent in inflicted damage to 2.75 minutes at the crest temperature (and no damage thereafter). The data of other investigators were brought to that common comparison point using the thermal death equation. This procedure generated Table 11.1.

As can be seen, with proper correction, a surprisingly tight grouping of the necrosis limit temperatures among a variety of test animals and tissues is displayed. It is thought that this coherence is in great part caused by the swiftness of the transition from living to dead (within 1°) which has been observed by many investigators and which is represented by the large coefficient (75 000) in the thermal death equation. As can be seen below in computations carried out from real temperature histories (primate experiments), theory predicts almost no damage at 47 °C and total death at 49 °C (Fig. 11.2).

This mixed theoretical–experimental system of tissue assessment allows an adjustment for tissue specificity which is represented in the equation by the value '232.34'. The equation was set so that a 2.75 min exposure to 48 °C results in 50% tissue death, while 48.95 °C results in 100% tissue death. In some locations, the temperature rises are such that the tissues rate much beyond the 100% dead limit (extremely large values of $D$). The numerical variations can be restricted to a more reasonable range by using a 'damage index' derived from the value of $D$ which allows all damage levels to be

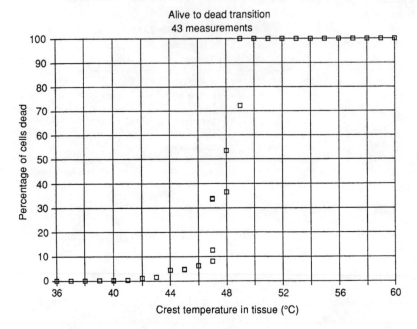

Fig. 11.2. Swift transition in thermal damage from 47 °C to 49 °C. Note
that values beyond 100% are equalled to 100%.

encompassed within a range of 10 arbitrary units. This 'damage index' is
computed as follows:

$$\text{Damage index} = 0.2556 \ln D = 0.2556 \ln \Sigma \exp (232.34 - 75000/T)$$

With this variable, the viability limit (50% dead) is equal to 1. All tissues
with a damage index beyond 1 are therefore potentially necrotic, death
being total at 1.18 (100% dead). When the damage index calculated from
experimental data is plotted against the crest temperature reached in the
tissue, a tight dependency is obtained (Fig. 11.3).

The decay of temperature in tissues is therefore sufficiently repeatable,
and the contribution of the high readings sufficiently dominant, that a good
assessment of damage can be obtained from a single value: the crest
temperature. A possible exception to this would be the tissues immediately
surrounding the large arteries, where the perfusion is so high that
temperature decays are considerably accelerated, resulting in reduced
damage. In fact, the large arteries are known to be largely immune to
temperature-induced damage in electrical accidents. This immunity would
not apply to smaller vascular structures, however, since it is known that the

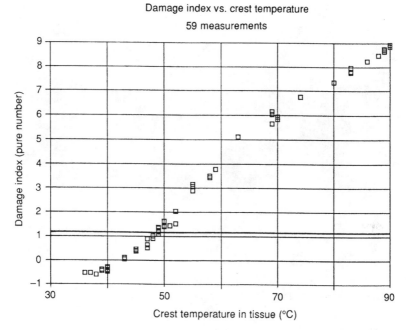

Fig. 11.3. The damage index computed and the crest temperature reached in the tissue rate tissue damage almost equally.

blood is thermally at equilibrium with tissues beyond the arteriole level[28].

From the previous considerations, it would be expected that electrical accidents result in a given pattern of temperature rise within a limb – due to local current circulation and specific tissue resistivities – which would label some tissues as viable and others as necrotic, and that little transition zone should exist[25]. This picture, while probably broadly correct, rests on considerations of topic thermal stress alone and on the applicability of Maxwell–Boltzmann statistics to situations as complicated as tissue survival in the human body. It would be incongruous to view it as more than a first approximation of thermal damage.

## Patterns of thermal damage in a primate model of electrical accidents

From 1982 to 1987, a project aimed at improving the treatment of severe electrical burns was conducted by Dr R.K. Daniel at the Royal Victoria Hospital in Montreal and funded by the Canadian Electrical Association. This first project conducted numerous tests using a hand-to-hand acute and

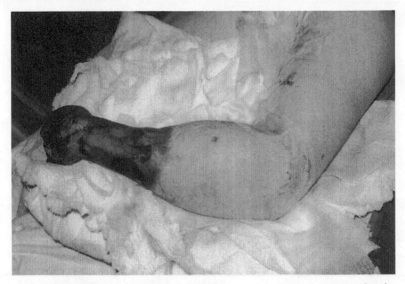

Fig. 11.4. Severe case of electrical burn in a human arm, showing coagulation limit (mid-arm) and skip wounds (elbow).

chronic electrical burn model in primates (injury to hands and arms occurs in 75% of clinical cases). The obvious similarities between selected clinical cases and primate experiments convinced the investigators of the adequacy of the model (see Figs 11.4 and 11.5). Three types of measurements were obtained by direct implantation of probes before shock administration in decorticated, anaesthetized primates: temperatures, currents and potentials (Fig. 11.6).

The final report[29] arrived at five practical conclusions.

1  In electrical burns, patterns of injury beyond the electrode contact area are anatomically determined. Hot spots can be repeatedly observed in specific locations such as the cubital fossa.
2  Tissue injury may extend more proximally deep within muscle than superficially.
3  Heat is the predominant mechanism of injury.
4  Progressive necrosis does not play an influential role in wound evolution.
5  Diagnostic aids are desirable for improving electrical burns treatment, as actual damage cannot be properly gauged by the surgeon in many cases.

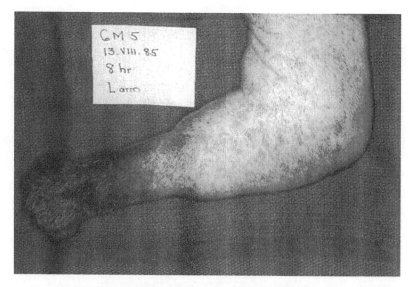

Fig. 11.5. Severe case of electrical burn in a primate arm, showing coagulation limit (mid-arm) and skip wounds (elbow).

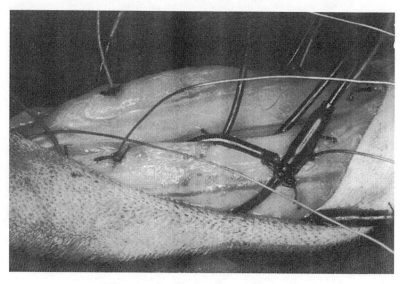

Fig. 11.6. Decorticated, anaesthetized primates were implanted with current, voltage and temperature probes before shock administration. Figure shows appearance immediately after burn.

### Macroscopic patterns

#### Peri-electrode damage

An appreciable part of the heat involved in an electrical burn is usually concentrated near the contact points because current there must flow through skin rather than below it (the skin is relatively resistive) and also across the longitudinal structures of the limb rather than along them. This peri-electrode damage is further increased when large energies are injected since the electrode contact will dry out and increase its resistance relative to the rest of the body. The wound at the contact site is therefore usually significant and visible.

Past work on electrical burns has often focused on peri-electrode damage sites, often differentiated as 'entry' and 'exit' wounds since damage at the 'exit' wound appears more extensive. Because alternating current produces the wound, these terms should be more properly labelled as 'first' and 'second' contact wounds. Destruction is more substantial at the second point of contact since in most scenarios arcing and higher contact resistance should concentrate heat there rather than at the first contact which is usually a good prehension or supporting (low resistance) location. Since the same current flows through the two contact sites in simple situations, differences in wound severity are due to different contact resistances.

#### Inter-electrode damage

In contrast to flame, electricity can generate within the body internal wounds along a current path extending from one contact point to another. In the case of a hand-to-hand burn in a human, for example, current passed through the chest usually leaves it intact, since its bulk allows a dispersion of the current to density values sufficiently low that no significant heating will occur. The limbs have small cross-sections, however, and current densities remain significant all along their length. It has been known for some time[30] that various tissues have different specific impedances and that a number of them, such as muscle, have conductivities that vary with the direction of measurement. Examination of current[31], potential and temperature readings shows that the current and injury patterns are relatively complex[24].

The experimental model in the primate has allowed us to observe that so-called inter-electrode damage is often determined by the anatomy of experimental animals in a region lying between, and distant from, the electrodes.

The inter-electrode wound is insidious because it may be enclosed by tissues of normal appearance, as explained below. It may have a dramatic effect on prognosis in the case of hand-to-hand burns since the whole arm can progressively be lost although the only superficial wounds visible initially were in the hands and in the distal part of the forearm.

### Peri-osseous damage

Measurements in the primate model showed that the predominant current load is carried in muscle, with some unexpectedly high current concentrations in the medullary portion of long bones. Probes circling various anatomical groups gave current readings which were surprisingly high for bones (Fig. 11.7), around which it is known clinically that damage concentrates (see specific locations in Figs 11.10 and 11.11). The specific resistance of the medullary canal and epiphysis is much lower than that of the cancellous bone matrix. Although no temperature readings were made in bones, a likely explanation for the observations is that the specific electrical power dissipated there is higher than in muscles (since the specific conductivity of the canal is higher than that of the muscles connected in parallel), leading to larger thermal rises. (Principles of electrical heat repartition state that among elements in parallel, the low resistance component receives a larger fraction of total power, while among elements in series, more power goes to the high resistance element. Also, matching the impedance of the source yields highest power transfer. 'Impedance of the source' includes all elements connecting power to the segment under consideration: wiring and connecting body parts.)

### Skip wounds

Small skin lesions were observed systematically, occasionally in pairs, at the elbow and shoulder levels in the absence of electrical arcing, which could not be detected by eye or on video in the 4000 V tests (arcing had been mentioned as the cause of the so-called skip wounds). This indicated a superficial deviation of high current densities to these locations, although little underlying damage was detected. The current deviation was presumably caused by the presence of electrically resistive structures within the joint. When thermal probes were preplaced in the lesions's locations, substantial temperature rises were measured. Arcing is an unlikely cause of skip wounds in the elbow or axilla because bridging tissues containing electrolytes ($\sim 30$ ohms impedance) by an electric arc would necessitate about 1 kA to obtain the $\sim 30$ kV necessary to break down the distance between skip wound pairs. This is much above the 3 A used in the tests. Also, no severe burns were observed on the skin, as would be expected from

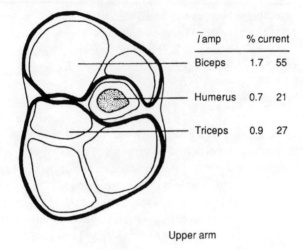

| $\bar{I}$ amp | % current |
|---|---|---|
| Biceps | 1.7 | 55 |
| Humerus | 0.7 | 21 |
| Triceps | 0.9 | 27 |

Upper arm

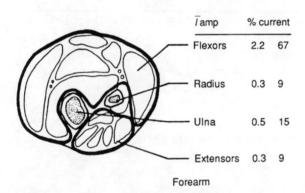

| $\bar{I}$ amp | % current |
|---|---|---|
| Flexors | 2.2 | 67 |
| Radius | 0.3 | 9 |
| Ulna | 0.5 | 15 |
| Extensors | 0.3 | 9 |

Forearm

Fig. 11.7. Forearm and upper arm currents measured in primate experiments: in bone, note the high current to area ratio.

electric arcs. Although contact within skin folds can produce the wounds, careful placement of the limbs during tests confirmed that the wounds occurred without it.

### *Concentration at origins and insertions*

The overall pattern of injury is illustrated in Fig. 11.8. The proximal rise in damage at the origin of the flexor carpi ulnaris can be explained by diminishing cross-section (Fig. 11.9) and corresponding increase in current density. Also, in the forearm, higher temperatures were observed along the radial aspect where the long flexors have a relatively smaller cross-sectional

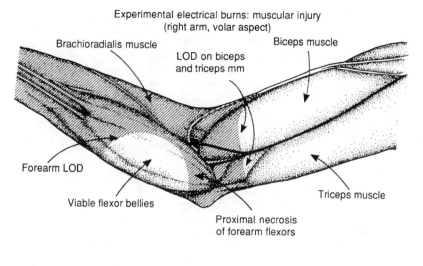

Experimental electrical burns: muscular injury
(right arm, volar aspect)

Brachioradialis muscle

LOD on biceps
and triceps mm

Biceps muscle

Forearm LOD

Viable flexor bellies

Triceps muscle

Proximal necrosis
of forearm flexors

Shaded area represents
grossly nonviable muscle.

LOD: Line of demarcation between grossly
viable and nonviable muscle.

Fig. 11.8. Muscle injury shows a concentration at the elbow level.

diameter than those on the ulnar border (Fig. 11.10). Major muscle groups therefore seemed subject to higher current densities towards their origins and insertions, which resulted in a discontinuous pattern of injury.

### Core damage

At the level of the single muscle, it is sometimes observed that damaged tissue is surrounded by muscle of normal appearance. Examination revealed more extensive damage to the deeper musculature which often extended proximally beneath or within viable-appearing muscle (Fig. 11.11).

### Pattern of damage and specific energy

As previously mentioned, the pattern of temperature rise is determined by anatomical particularities, which result in simultaneous occurrence of both sub-lethal and lethal damage in the left–middle portion of Fig. 11.12.

In general, the temperature rises observed were greater as the energy injected into the limb increased. This is particularly true in the forearm, but not in the upper arm (Fig. 11.13) where at higher energies, heat transfer seems limited by forearm impedance. Unfortunately, the slight decrease in

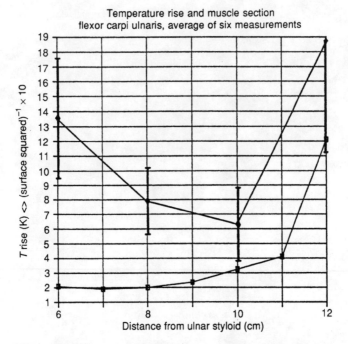

Fig. 11.9. The two curves show observed temperature rises (upper curve, with ± σ-error bars) in the proximal segment of flexor carpi ulnaris and the variation of the inverse cross-section of the muscle (proportional to current density) in the same region. Proximal rise in temperature is explained by diminishing cross-section and increased current density. Temperature rise to the left of the graph is due to proximity of electrode.

temperature with increasing energy seen in the upper arm (Fig. 11.13) is not enough to obtain tissue vitality, as depicted in Fig. 11.12.

### Progressive necrosis

From a medical therapist's point of view, severe electrical burns represent potentially difficult cases. After a treatment (of the electrode region) has been applied, necrosis sometimes occurs, even after several days, in structures that were previously thought to be healthy. This phenomenon, specific to electrical wounds, is designated 'progressive necrosis'. It usually necessitates repeated surgical interventions and amputations to excise necrotic tissues. It is believed, however, that 'progressive necrosis' may be the eruption of pre-existing inter-electrode damage. The scattered tissue damage may lie under normal skin or muscle, and therefore elude clinical and even intra-operative observation. Analysis of the recorded temperature

Cross-sectional template
(right arm, mid-forearm level)

Anterior

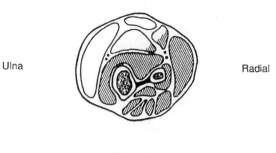

Ulna                    Radial

Posterior

Shaded area represents nonviable muscle.

Fig. 11.10. Cross-sectional damage in the forearm.

Experimental electrical injury:
injury to biceps muscle

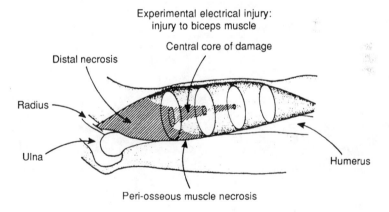

Shaded area represents grossly nonviable muscle.

Fig. 11.11. Core damage in the biceps.

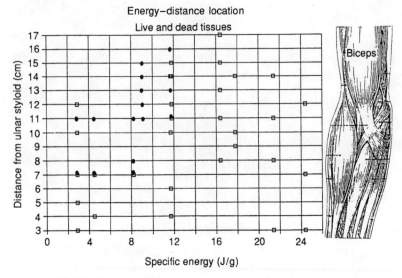

Fig. 11.12. Energy–distance determination of tissue vitality. Filled circles denote live tissues, open squares dead tissues.

Crest temperature vs. specific energy

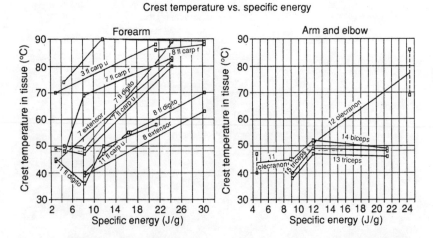

Fig. 11.13. Crest temperature vs specific energy. High power leads to a less severe burn in the upper arm as opposed to the forearm, past a critical energy. Numbers preceding muscle designations indicate distance in cm from ulnar styloid. Measurements obtained from flexor sublimis digitorum and flexor profundus digitorum were not distinguished in the analysis.

histories showed that according to thermal-kill parameters, only 8.7% of recorded sites would lie at a damage index between 10% and 90% (doubtful vitality) although the sites were consciously selected to assess the vitality of transitional tissues. This small percentage indicates that marginal heat stress is not a likely cause of progressive necrosis. Late recognition of decaying tissue may be the problem.

Angiographic findings included a sharp demarcation between patent and nonpatent vascular trunks: cubital fossa in the radial artery and at a more distal location in the ulnar artery[32]. Serial films revealed an increased number of nutrient vessels in viable regions adjacent to nonviable areas. Ulnar nerve conduction studies showed loss proximal to the cubital fossa with no recovery.

### *Microscopic patterns*

Electricity is relatively easily transported through the human body by extracellular electrolytes (40% of all body fluids), specifically the interstitial (30%) and vascular (10%) fluids. Intracellular electrolytes (60% of all body fluids), on the other hand, are contained within relatively insulating barriers, the cell membranes.

In practice, the useful conductivity of extracellular fluids can be severely limited by obstacles such as cell bodies, calcified material or fibrous sheets. Yet, under some conditions, intracellular fluids can contribute to electrical conductivity by passing electrical currents through punctured or partly permeable cell membranes.

Light microscopy of muscle in the transition zones revealed patchy cellular necrosis intermixed with viable cells[29]. Affected cells in proximity to normal cells were found generally towards the periphery of the muscle fascicle. This unevenness was also manifested in the penetration of macrophages. Therefore, although the damage occurs in the core of muscle at the macroscopic level, it tends to come superficially in the fascicles. This surprising pattern may be explained by an uneven distribution of current flow.

### Detection of thermal damage by electrical impedance spectroscopy

Thermal damage can be detected by various methods, in suspended cells or in tissues, *in vitro* or *in vivo*, in the laboratory or in the operating room. Each method has its advantages and problems. A common problem is that the results are difficult to interpret in the context of guiding surgical decisions. This results partly from specific defects of the burn assessment methods, but mostly from an incomplete understanding of burn pathophysiology. The inadequacy of simple techniques such as gross appearance, colour, bleeding from a scalpel cut, response to pinching, and contractility by a 2 mV nerve stimulator, have prevented the surgeon from assessing the wound accurately. The laboratory has tried to provide further help; unfortunately, the methods available do not, at the moment, provide determinations capable of reassuring the surgeon that he is making the best decision.

For example, cell viability is often evaluated using a dye (trypan blue and others) exclusion test. Such tests evaluate plasma membrane integrity. In many cases, however, the fraction of dye-excluding cells continues to decrease after dye exposure is discontinued. Thus, after a heat challenge, it is difficult to specify a time when the fraction of dye-excluding cells will correlate with truly viable cells, and this fraction often depends on the parameters of the treatment.

Other examples can be found in the systemic investigations performed in burn patients. These assessments often focus on the circulation because surgeons observe a close correlation between perfusion and viability of tissues. Arteriography can be used to document the patency of major blood vessels, and sodium fluorescein can be used to confirm perfusion to the microcirculation level. However, over time, fluorescein will permeate even unperfused tissue, and will penetrate in the cytoplasm even of viable cells.

Conventional histology[33], histochemistry and vital microscopy can be used to determine damage limits. However, each method presents problems either of practicality or interpretation – especially when viewed in a perspective of continuous wound evolution – which has prevented any of the methods from becoming widely accepted. This lack of diagnostic methods has prompted further work in the area of the assessment of thermal damage to muscle tissue.

The ideal technique would identify without ambiguity excision margins; more realistically, it would yield irreversible damage limits and a definition of regions within which tissue survival is imperiled but still possible. These limits would be defined using specific, physiologically relevant variables.

Another requirement is that the technique be quick and minimally invasive, so that chronological data can be obtained in the laboratory and from patients.

Until now, measurements of electrical impedance have had few medical applications. The classical techniques involve measurements on large regions of the body at a single frequency ($\sim 50$ kHz) with the goal of estimating the resistivity variations associated with the passage of blood. Applications include the determination of total body fat, total body electrolytes, heart stroke volume and respiratory activity[34].

The fact that the electrical conductivity of tissues is altered under pathological conditions has been known for some time[35]. In early 1985, a small bipolar probe was used to measure the dissipation factor of biological tissues over the range of frequencies between 5 Hz and 13 MHz, as an indicator of physiological state[36]. This variable presented many advantages, among them reduction of sensitivity to implantation variations and elimination of polarization artefacts. The scope of these early observations has been expanded considerably in a technique labelled electrical impedance spectroscopy (EIS). The technique may be capable of giving information on diverse aspects of a specific pathology. Its scope is wide since it senses biological tissue using charged ions mobility. It also has the potential of being fast and simple to execute.

In 1988, the Electric Power Research Institute joined the Canadian Electrical Association and Institut de Recherche d'Hydro-Québec in supporting at the Royal Victoria Hospital a second project on the treatment of electrical burns which has given new impetus to the development of this novel technique. The project has the following four goals.

1 Development of a method of tissue assessment based on the measurement of electrical impedance, EIS.
2 Better definition of the anatomy of electrical burns.
3 Perfecting EIS to the point where it can be a practical tool for the surgeon.
4 Improvement of general understanding of the electrical wound and of electro-biological interactions.

The research is being carried out in the MicroSurgical Laboratories by a group consisting of technologist Yves Brissette, technician Jean Dumas, Hilary Rowland, engineer Michel Bourdages, surgeons Carolyn Kerrigan and Lucie Lessard, and the author.

The project proceeds in two streams. One uses *in vivo* experimentation on rats with the aim of developing a burn assessment method. The main object is the determination of the state of living muscle using electrical measurements over a wide range of frequencies obtained from thin, short electrodes inserted into tissue. The other attempts, through experimentation with primates, to increase knowledge of the electrical wound itself, and to apply the EIS method in a realistic clinical setting.

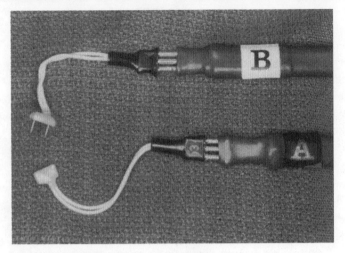

Fig. 11.14. EIS probe.

### EIS probes

Applying small electrical potentials within living tissues allows substantial information to be retrieved on their physiological state from careful analysis of the circulated currents if many measurements of conductivity and permittivity are carried out at closely spaced frequencies. The electronic instrumentation yielding precise measurements of resistance and reactance in such a situation is sophisticated and must be highly automated to be of practical use. If a high degree of automation is realized, however, the technique allows rapid, minimally invasive probing of muscle in real-time and *in vivo*, which is essential to support surgical application.

The potentials are applied using minimally invasive probes consisting of two electrodes 3.5 mm in length and 0.16 mm in diameter, 5 mm apart. Some percutaneous probes to reach underlying tissues are also under development. Actual probes are shown in Fig. 11.14.

### Automated techniques

To support the development of the method, an experimentation module specifically built for long-term (as much as 72 hours) monitoring of 12 EIS probes inserted in the tissue (EIS) of six anaesthetized rats, all under computer control, was developed (Fig. 11.15).

The experimentation module presents as a 1 m² table mounted on rubber wheels. It includes a display screen for the controller, a switching and

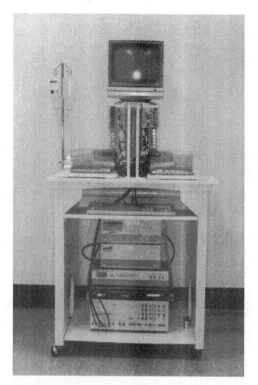

Fig. 11.15. EIS experimentation module.

control unit, a computer keyboard, a mass storage unit (hard-disc, 20 Mbyte and floppy drive), a controller, a data acquisition-control unit and an impedance analyser. Also included are power supplies, a general purpose interface bus data network, bottles for the administration of fluids and anaesthetics, custom electronics, control switches, metering pumps, fluid manifolds, electric valves (administration of anaesthetics and fluids) and six identical floats housing rats individually. Each float consists of a wire mesh cradle, a container for collection of urine, impedance calibration electrical circuits, a foam blanket, mattress, resistive heating pad, thermistor, head support system, piezo-electric detector, tubes for anaesthetics and support fluids and two coaxial cable pairs for impedance measurements.

The automated system described above has been put to use in assembling a database to support the usefulness of EIS. So far, basic measurements have been performed to put the method into perspective, and systematic measurements on burned tissues are under way. However, preliminary data confirming the capacity of EIS have been available for some time.

### Tissue specificity and interspecies similarity

As periodic structures of cytoplasm bounded by insulating membranes and traversed by a circulatory system, all animal tissues have many characteristics in common. However, various tissues differ from one another by characteristics such as perfusion rate and the existence of intercellular channels. Ideally, EIS curves, expected to reflect in their overall appearance the similarities between tissues, would also show smaller variations revealing of the microanatomical differences. Strong variations between the signatures of different organs would support the notion that smaller changes observed in a given tissue following burns are a reflection of post-traumatic physiological changes. 'Tissue specificity' is therefore a desirable attribute of EIS.

A corollary of tissue specificity is that, within the restricted range of mammals, for example, signatures across species should be similar for the same organs. This interspecies similarity is expected because in this group, microanatomical structures are generally similar for the same organ. Interspecies similarity is also important to support the relevance of developing an experimental base using rats for ultimate application to human pathology.

We have data in hand which support both interspecies similarity and tissue specificity (Figs 11.16 and 11.17).

### Pathology

In order to study the pathology of thermal and electrical burns in muscle, the experimentation module is used to monitor the evolution of wounds produced in the gluteus of rats using microwave energy and 50–60 Hz currents.

The wounds are also monitored by conventional means, including haematoxylin and eosin histology, tetrazolium staining and sodium fluorescein for perfusion. These more conventional methods are compared with the information gathered from EIS monitoring.

EIS is of interest not only because it is fast, but also because it will likely yield a multifaceted account of what is happening in tissue as competence in interpreting the dielectric data increases. The dielectric information likely contains many physiologically relevant parameters. Efforts at interpreting the various compartments of the EIS signal and its microstructure are continuing.

At present it seems that EIS can, in approximately a minute, or

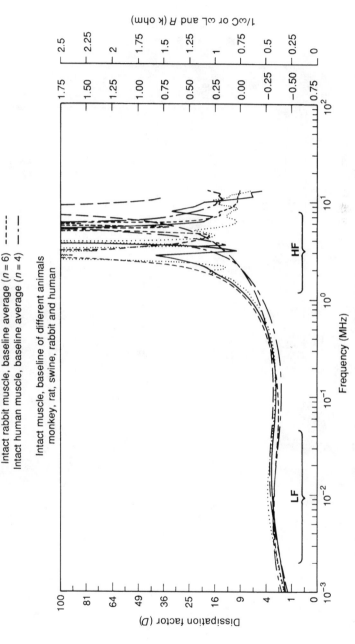

Fig. 11.16. Graphs of the dissipation factor versus frequency show similar curves for the muscles of various species including man.

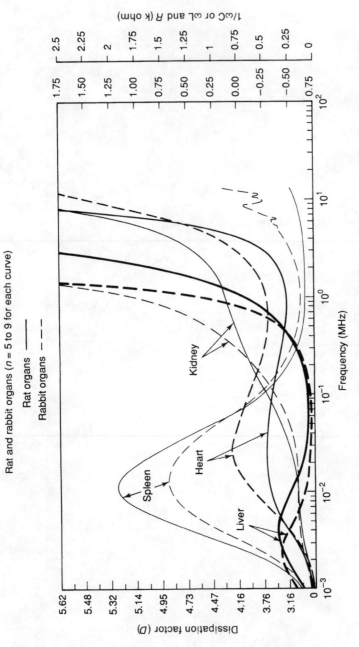

Fig. 11.17. Graphs of the dissipation factor versus frequency show curves specific to various organs but similar across species.

continuously, monitor oedema and yield information on the integrity of cell membranes. Experimental data is mainly from rats, although a sizeable amount of information was gathered from cats, pigs, primates and humans. Work is continuing and physicians collaborating in the project soon will be in a position to assess the clinical value of this new tool.

### References

1  Thomsen, H.K., Danielsen, L., Nielsen, O., Aalund, O., Nielsen, K.G., Karlsmark, T., Genefke, I.K. & Christoffersen, P. (1983). Epidermal changes in heat and electrically injured pig skin. *Acta Pathologia, Microbiologia, Immunologia, Scandinavia,* **91**, 297–306.
2  Hill, S.A. & Denekamp, J. (1982). Histology as a method for determining thermal gradients in heated tumours. *British Journal of Radiology,* **55**, 651–6.
3  Buckley, I.K. (1972). A light and electron microscopy study of thermally injured cultured cells. *Laboratory Investigation,* **26(2)**, 201–9.
4  Hahn, G. (1974). Metabolic aspects of the role of hyperthermia in mammalian cell inactivation and their possible relevance to cancer treatment, *Cancer Research,* **34**, 3117–23.
5  Lemasters, J.J., Diguiseppi, J., Nieminen, A.L. & Herman, B. (1987). Blebbing, free $Ca^{2+}$ and mitochondrial membrane potential preceding cell death in hepatocytes. *Nature,* **325**, 78.
6  Coss, R.A., Dewey, W.E. & Bamburg, J.R. (1982). Effects of hyperthermia on dividing Chinese hamster ovary cells and on microtubules *in vitro. Cancer Research,* **42**, 1059–71.
7  Crile, G. (1963). The effects of heat and radiation on cancers implanted on the feet of mice. *Cancer Research,* **23**, 372–80.
8  Law, M.P., Ahier, R.G. & Field, S.B. (1978). The response of the mouse ear to heat applied alone or combined with X-rays. *British Journal of Radiology,* **51**, 132–8.
9  Overgaard, K. & Overgaard, J. (1972). Investigations on the possibility of a thermic tumor therapy I. Short-wave treatment of a transplanted isologous mouse mammary carcinoma. *European Journal of Cancer,* **8**, 65–78.
10  Overgaard, K. & Overgaard, J. (1975). Pathology of heat damage. Studies on the histopathology in tumor tissue exposed '*in vivo*' to hyperthermia and combined hyperthermia and roentgen irradiation. *Proceedings of the International Symposium of Cancer Therapy and Radiation,* Washington, DC 115–27.
11  Zarkowsky, H.A.S. (1982). Membrane-active agents and heat-induced erythrocyte fragmentation. *British Journal of Haematology,* **50**, 361.
12  Gabbiani, G. & Badonnel, M.C., (1975). Early changes of endothelial clefts after thermal injury. *Microvascular Research,* **10**, 65–75.
13  Willoughby, D.A. (1973). Mediation of increased vascular inflammation. In Zweifach, Grant, & McCluskey, eds, *The Inflammatory Process,* Academic Press. New York: vol. II, 2nd edn.
14  Song, C.W., Kang, M.S. Rhee, J.G. & Levitt, S.H. (1980). The effect of hyperthermia on vascular function, pH, and cell survival. *Radiology,* **137**, 795–803.

15 Gerweck, L.E. (1977). Modification of cell lethality at elevated temperatures: the pH effect. *Radiation Research*, **79**, 224.

16 Baxter, C.R. (1970). Present concepts in the management of major electrical injury. *Surgery Clinics of North America*, **50(6)**, 1401–16.

17 Meshorer, A., Stavros, D., Prionas, M.S., Fajardo, L.F., Meyer, J.L., Hahn, G.M. & Martinez, A.A. (1983). The effects of hyperthermia on normal mesenchymal tissues. *Archives of Pathology and Laboratory Medicine*, **107**, 328–34.

18 Emami, B. & Song, C.W. (1984). Physiological mechanisms in hyperthermia: a review. *International Journal of Radiation Oncology in Biology and Physics*, **10**, 289–95.

19 Kim, C., Martyn, J. & Fuke, N. (1988). Burn injury to trunk of rat causes denervation-like responses in the gastrocnemius muscle. *Journal of Applied Physiology*, (US), **65(4)**, 1745–51.

20 Kahan, T., Dahlof, C. & Hjemdahl, P. (1985). Influence of acetylcholine, peptides and other vasodilators on endogenous noradrenaline overflow and vasoconstriction in canine blood perfused gracilis muscle. *Acta Physiologia Scandinavia*, **124(3)**, 457–65.

21 Griffith, T.M., Edwards, D.H., Lewis, M.J., Newby, A.C. & Henderson, A.H. (1984). *Nature*, **308(5960)**, 645–7.

22 Segal, S.S. & Duling, B.R. (1986). Communication between feed arteries and microvessels in hamster striated muscle: segmental vascular responses are functionally coordinated. *Circulatory Research (US)*, **59(3)**, 283–90.

23 Ferguson, M.K., Seifert, F.C. & Replogle, R.L. (1982). The effects of thermal injury on rat skeletal muscle microcirculation. *Journal of Trauma*, **22(10)**, 880–3.

24 Daniel, R.K., Ballard, P.A., Héroux, P., Zelt, R.G. & Howard, C.R. (1988). High voltage electrical injury: acute pathophysiology. *Journal of Hand Surgery*, **13A(1)**, 44–9.

25 Héroux, P., Ballard, P.A., Daniel, R.K., Howard, C.R. & Zelt, R.G. (1986). Experimental investigation of electrical burns: analysis of recorded temperatures, *10th Scientific Conference on Electropathology*, Freiburg, W. Germany, September 1986. Published in *Beiträge Zur Ersten Hilfe und Behandlung von Unfällen durch Elektrischen Strom*, Hauf, R. ed., Freiburg, West Germany, 147–180.

26 Edwards, J.A. & Brimijoin, S. (1983). Thermal inactivation of the molecular forms of acetylcholinesterase and butyrylcholinesterase. *Biochimica et Biophysica Acta*, **742(3)**, 509–16.

27 Henle, K.J. (1983). Arrhenius analysis of thermal responses. In *Hyperthermia in Cancer Therapy*, F.K. Storm, ed., pp. 47–53, G.K. Hall Medical Publishers.

28 Valvano, J.W., Allen, J.T. & Bowman, H.F. (1984). The simultaneous measurement of thermal conductivity, thermal diffusivity and perfusion in small volumes of tissue. *Journal of Biomechanical Engineering*, **106**, 192–7.

29 Daniel, R.K. (1987). Pathophysiology and surgical treatment of high voltage electrical injury. *Canadian Electrical Association, Final Report of Project*, **165D**, 286.

30 Geddes, L.A. & Baker, L.E. (1967). The specific resistance of biological material – a compendium of data for the biomedical engineer and physiologist. *Medical and Biological Engineering*, **5**, 271–93.

31 Héroux, P. (1985). Intra-body current probes. In *Electric Shock Safety Criteria*. Bridges, Ford, Sherman, Vainberg, eds, Pergamon Press.
32 Zelt, R.G., Ballard, P.A., Common, A.A., Héroux, P. & Daniel, R.K. (1986). Experimental high voltage electrical burns: role of progressive necrosis, *Surgical Forum*, American College of Surgeons, **37**, 624–6.
33 Quinby, W.C., Burke, J.F., Trelstad, R.L. & Caulfield, J. (1978). The use of microscopy as a guide to primary excision of high-tension electrical burns. *Journal of Trauma*, **18(6)**, 423–31.
34 IEEE (1989). Impedance techniques. In *Engineering in Medicine and Biology Magazine*, **8(1)**.
35 Crile, G., Hosmer, H.R. & Rowland, A.F. (1922). The electrical conductivity of animal tissues under normal and pathological conditions. *American Journal of Physiology*, **60**, 59–106.
36 Héroux, P., Ballard, P.A., Daniel, R.K. & Howard, C.R. (1985). Studies on electrical burns. *Seventh Annual Meeting of the BioElectroMagnetics Society*, San Francisco.
37 Henriques, F.C. (1947). Studies of thermal injury. *Archives of Pathology*, **43**, 489–502.
38 Henriques, F.C. & Mortiz, A.R. (1947). Studies of thermal injury. I. The conduction of heat to and through skin and the temperatures attained therein. A theoretical and experimental investigation. *American Journal of Pathology*, **23**, 531–49.
39 Welch, A.J. & Polhamus, G.D. (1984). Measurement and prediction of thermal injury in the retina of the rhesus monkey. *IEEE Transactions in Biomedical Enginering*, **BME–31(10)**, 633–44.
40 Emami, B., Nussbaum, G.H., Tenhaken, R.K. & Hughes, W.L. (1980). Physiological effects of hyperthermia: response of capillary blood flow and structure to local tumor heating. *Radiology*, **137**, 805–9.
41 Emami, B., Nussbaum, G.H., Hahn, N., Piro, A.J., Dritschilo, A. & Quimby, F. (1981). Histopathological study on the effects of hyperthermia on microvasculature. *International Journal of Radiation in Biology and Physics*, **7**, 343–8.
42 Stoll, A.M. & Greene, L.C. (1959). Relationship between pain and tissue damage due to thermal radiation. *Journal of Applied Physiology*, **14**, 373–82.
43 Reinhold, H.E., Blachiewicz, B. & Berg-Blok, A. (1978). Decrease in tumor microcirculation during hyperthermia. In *Cancer Therapy by Hyperthermia and Radiation*, Streffer, ed., Baltimore: Urban & Schwarzenberg.

# 12

# Evaluation of electrical burn injury using an electrical impedance technique

MICHAEL A. CHILBERT

## Introduction

The unique characteristics of electrical burn injury can make initial assessment of trauma very difficult. Techniques that are more deterministic could greatly enhance treatment and reduce morbidity. One technique that is potentially valuable is to measure the complex electrical impedance of the tissue. To understand fully the evaluation of electrical injury by measuring tissue impedance one must be familiar with the concepts of electrical impedance. To this end, this chapter will present first the general theory of complex electrical impedance, then the fundamental properties of tissue impedance and its relationship to electrical injury. The final segment of this chapter will describe the impedance technique and the results of experimental work using this technique.

## Theory

The basis for the electrical impedance technique relies on the application of Ohm's law to the passage of current through tissue. This law is expressed as the electromotive force (voltage, $V$) needed to push electrons (current, $I$) through a media is directly proportional to the quantity of electrons being pushed and the resistance ($R$) of the media to the movement of electrons; more simply expressed as $V = I \times R$. The term resistance here is used in a broad sense, however, it will be defined more strictly in the following paragraph.

To correctly define the term 'impedance' one expresses the resistance of the media to the flow of current in terms of the utilization of energy. Electrical energy is either dissipated (converted to heat) or stored (in an electrostatic field or a magnetic field). The part of impedance that converts electrical energy to thermal energy is now defined as 'resistance' or real

216

Tissue impedance plot

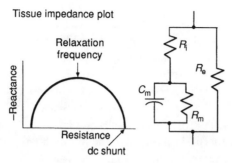

Fig. 12.1. Impedance plot of the resistive (real) and reactive (imaginary) impedance of the circuit on the right. Note that the reactance for a capacitive circuit is plotted on the negative half of the imaginary axis. The DC shunt resistance occurs when a direct current flows through the circuit after the capacitor is at a constant voltage. The relaxation frequency occurs at the maximum reactance level. The circuit represents a uniform region of tissue with an extracellular fluid resistance ($R_e$), an intracellular fluid resistance ($R_i$), a cell membrane resistance ($R_m$) and a cell membrane capacitance ($C_m$). Each electrical element represents the contributions of all the combined cellular components in the tissue region.

impedance. It is this part that heats tissue by a process called joulean heating, which is expressed as the square of the current multiplied by the resistance (joules $= I^2 \times R$). The part of impedance that stores energy in a magnetic or electrostatic field is called the 'reactance' or imaginary impedance. The reactance is represented by capacitance (related to electrostatic energy) and inductance (related to magnetic energy). The capacitive reactance is important here since the tissue has the ability to store electric charge (or ionic charge) across cell membranes. The reactance is represented as the imaginary part of a complex number where the capacitance is defined in the negative half of the imaginary axis and inductance in the positive half. Also associated with complex impedance is a phase shift seen in an oscillating signal. Given a sinusoidal current passing through a material, the measured voltage will be out of phase with respect to the current, or the peak values of measured voltage will not occur at the same time as the peak values of the current. The magnitude of impedance is frequency dependent for a given voltage and alternating current (ac) in tissue and is represented by the phase angle, which is the inverse tangent of the reactance divided by the resistance. Frequency dependent impedance is usually presented graphically on a phase plane (or impedance) plot (Fig. 12.1). Important features of the phase plane plot are the zero frequency intercept (or dc shunt) resistance and the relaxation frequency. The zero frequency intercept resistance is the combination of resistances of the circuit in Fig. 12.1 exclusive of the capacitance. The relaxation frequency is the frequency at which the greatest reactance occurs and is indicative of the quantity of boundaries in the material. Therefore, the impedance of tissue can be expressed in terms of resistance, reactance and relaxation frequency.

To help understand the impedance characteristics of tissue a simple electrical model is given in Fig. 12.1. This model represents a continuous section of tissue where the contributions of cells and other structures are lumped into specific elements of the model. The model has three resistances and one capacitance that represent the compartments and boundaries of tissue. The extracellular fluid resistance is a parallel component to the cellular impedance since this pathway can be separated from cellular contributions. The cellular impedance consists of the intracellular fluid resistance and the resistance and capacitance of the cell membranes.

Changing the tissue structure or its content will alter the tissue impedance. Cellular degradation and oedema alter the tissue impedance differently[1]. Oedema simply alters the extracellular and intracellular resistances of the model in Fig. 12.1. Since the membrane capacitance and resistance are not affected grossly, then the reactance and relaxation frequency will change minimally. However, with cellular degradation the membrane capacitance and resistance are directly affected and large changes in the reactance and relaxation frequency are observed. The clinical relevance of these changes and the ability to measure them will be detailed later in this chapter.

### Clinical aspects

Reviewing current clinical procedures for electrical burn trauma management emphasizes the need for adjunct techniques and delineates the present difficulties in treatment. The immediate care of surgical patients includes fluid replacement, management of acidosis and treatment of burn myoglobinuria[2,3]. Electrical trauma secondary to contact with high-voltage circuits often presents a limited cutaneous burn associated with deep tissue damage of variable and unknown extent[4-16], with clinical features similar to crush injuries[17]. The underlying tissue may produce life-threatening sepsis and loss of limbs. Devastating destruction of fat, tendons, vessels, muscle, nerves and bone is frequent. Determination of the extent of trauma is usually by visual inspection. It is often difficult to determine the demarcation between viable and nonviable tissues following injuries. The two major approaches to surgical management of electrical injury are a gradual debridement of necrotic tissue requiring multiple procedures, which is in contrast to early excision and early grafting of the injured area[3,4,13,18,19-22]. Others have recommended a modified approach which melds the two procedures[4]. Clearly, determination of the optimal time for excision of limited areas of tissue necrosis is difficult. Luce and associates[10] suggest repeat exploration and debridement at 48 hours after injury with particular attention given to periosseous muscle groups, nerve trunks and tendons. The inherent problem with debridement at present is the lack of a deterministic method for identifying nonviable tissue; questions concerning the existence of progressive necrosis also complicate this problem.

Recently, Zelt *et al.*[23] have presented a thorough experimental evaluation of the anatomical changes resulting from high-voltage electrical injury. One important result of this work was that their results found no progressive necrosis over a 10-day period. The extent of nonviable tissue at onset was essentially the same as that after 10 days. The clinical implication is that initial tissue trauma determines the complete extent of injury and that initial surgical removal of all nonviable tissue could reduce morbidity. Present surgical techniques need to be augmented so that all necrotic tissue is located and removed in a single procedure.

Hunt *et al.* used technetium-99m stannous pyrophosphate (99mT-PYP) scintigraphs to identify perfused injured muscle tissue in 14 electrical injury patients. This clinical study shows one qualitative method of identifying regions of muscular necrosis and can potentially aid in the surgical removal of nonviable tissue. It is also consistent with the findings of Zelt *et al.*[23] on the distribution of injury in the limb. Indications of progressive necrosis were not noted by the authors, which would have been evident on the serial scintigraphs.

## Experimental studies of resistance and impedance

To understand fully the application of the impedance technique for determining tissue viability, the following section will present experimental information from electrical injury studies. This information will better define the mechanisms of electrical injury and also impart general concepts to the clinical situation based on experimental results. This section will review the results of experiments done at high and low voltages to measure tissue current densities, and to measure tissue resistivity and impedance.

High-voltage burns were studied by Sances *et al.* to determine the general characteristics of these electrical accidents[16]. The studies were performed at

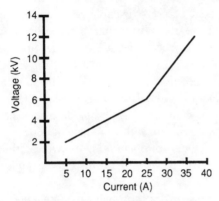

Fig. 12.2. Voltage vs. current for first contact between the forelimb and the hindlimb of the hog. The discontinuity at 6 kV reflects a decrease in the contact impedance with increasing voltage.

voltages up to 14.4 kV and measured the applied voltage and current to the experimental preparation. Results from this study show that the voltage/current relationship is not linear (Fig. 12.2). In terms of total body resistance, calculated from the voltage and current, the resistance decreases with an increase in voltage. Also, the resistance changes with time; here the change was noted as an increase in the resistance from the beginning to the end of the voltage application. This is explained by arcing through desiccated or charred tissue and by the increase in the arcing distance. It should be noted that the increase in resistance with time was over a 16 s application period.

Following this study were experiments that evaluated the electrode contact in high-voltage injuries[13,14]. The results showed that skin initially has a very high resistance which decreases as the dermal interface breaks down (or current pathways are established). The rate of interface breakdown is proportional to the applied voltage. Figure 12.3 shows the typical contact characteristics of current vs. time at low voltages. The first phase is mostly attributed to establishment of the current path through the skin or the breakdown of the skin's capacitance[14,24]. The second phase occurs until the tissue beneath the contact desiccates or chars. There is a slow increase in current that is caused by local heating of tissue. This heating decreases the tissue resistance. The third phase occurs when the tissue under the contact dehydrates and becomes highly resistive. At higher voltages, some arcing at the electrode edge occurs until the tissue is charred. The same type of curve occurs for voltages above 1 kV; however, the first two phases last less than one second, and the last phase requires severe charring or traumatic amputation before the current is interrupted[16].

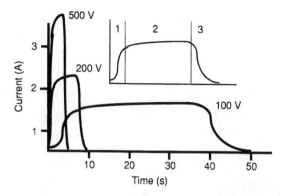

Fig. 12.3. The relationship of current to time for a 5 cm disc in contact with the skin of a hog. The triphasic nature of the current is illustrated in the insert; phase one occurs during the contact interface breakdown, phase 2 occurs during the time of good electrical contact and phase 3 occurs when the contact is disrupted due to desiccation or charring of tissue under the electrode. Note that an increasing voltage results in a decrease in the effective application time.

For short duration current applications at voltages between 500 V and 6 kV[14,24,25], the resistance decreases with application time and applied voltage. The results support earlier findings at low and high voltages. From these studies, one notes that resistance changes with time affect the total current and its distribution in the body. This change in resistance is mainly due to heating of the tissue at the contact site, evidenced by thermal trauma. However, the resistance changes of tissue are not limited to the contact region, but extend to all tissue being heated by the current. Thus, current pathways become important in the analysis of electrical injury.

The distribution and effect of current in the body have been analysed by direct measurement of current densities in the limbs and body of hogs[6,7,13,15,26]. The time of contact, the current density and the resistivity determine thermal energy and resultant temperature in the tissue, where the peak temperature is related to the level of trauma[13,24]. Unfortunately, the time of contact and actual current are seldom known in electrical accidents.

From experimental studies in the hog[13] current densities in the hindlimb have been measured. Figure 12.4 shows the cross-section of the limb where the measurements were taken as well as the potential distribution on the skin for current passing between the hindlimbs. The electric field is approximately uniform so that the current in the tissue is distributed according to tissue resistivities and cross-sectional areas (Table 12.1). Consequently, the current densities, which are inversely proportional to the resistivities, can be estimated in all tissues. The resulting current densities

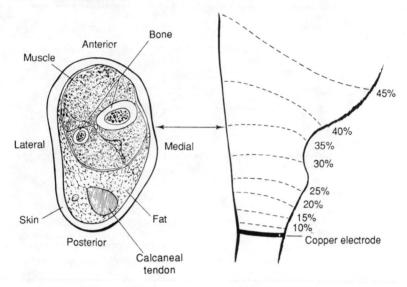

Fig. 12.4. Cross-section of the measurement region and equipotential lines for current density studies in the hog hindlimb. The equipotential lines are for currents passed between the hindlimbs and are given as the percentage of the applied voltage. The copper electrode shown is for application of electricity to the hog and the reference electrode for the equipotential measurements. From Chilbert *et al.*[6]

vs. applied current is shown graphically in Fig. 12.5 for various tissues in the limb. Note that vessels and nerves have the highest average current densities followed by muscle, fat, bone marrow and bone cortex[13]. Table 12.1 gives values for resistivity, current density, total tissue current, total tissue resistance and the tissue cross-sectional area for a typical experiment. Note that muscle tissue at this level carries 46% of the total current, followed by interstitial fat, dermal tissue layers, calcaneal tendon, bone marrow, bone cortex, blood vessels and peripheral nerves.

Observations from current density measurements important to injury evaluation are that muscle heats faster than bone, current density in muscle is typically higher near the bone than away from it[13,15], current density changes with temperature and tissue heating alters the current distribution in the tissue[7]. The energy density in muscle is six times greater than in bone. Peri-osseous muscle damage is due to direct heating of the muscle, which occurs from a higher current density in these muscle groups. The resistivity of muscle decreases with increasing temperature and with trauma[6,7] allowing a greater current density, causing an increase in the energy density which increases temperature. This results in a self-perpetuating injury

Table 12.1. *Typical values for the hog cross-section of Fig. 12.4*

| Tissue | Tissue resistivity (ohm cm) | Tissue resistance (ohm) | Current density (ma/cm²) | Tissue current (ma) | Tissue area (cm²) | Energy density (Joules/cm³) |
|---|---|---|---|---|---|---|
| Vessel | 155 | 911.76 | 51.61 | 8.77 | 0.17 | 412.90 |
| Nerve | 200 | 1666.67 | 40.00 | 4.80 | 0.12 | 320.00 |
| Muscle (L) | 290 | 19.24 | 27.59 | 415.72 | 15.07 | 220.69 |
| (T) | 650 | — | | | | |
| Fat | 380 | 31.77 | 21.05 | 251.79 | 11.96 | 168.42 |
| Bone marrow | 550 | 495.50 | 14.55 | 16.15 | 1.11 | 116.36 |
| Bone cortex | 1850 | 898.06 | 4.32 | 8.91 | 2.06 | 34.59 |
| Tendon | 398 | 196.19 | 20.09 | 40.78 | 2.03 | 160.70 |
| Dermal layers | 432 | 50.94 | 18.52 | 157.04 | 8.48 | 148.15 |
| Average/total | 363 | 8.85 | 22.05 | 903.95 | 41.00 | 176.3 |

*Notes:*
The applied voltage between the hindlimbs was 400 V, with a current of 0.9 A. The electric field strength at this level was 8 V/cm. Resistivity and current density were measured experimentally. The cross-sectional tissue resistance is calculated from: Resistivity × Tissue area/length = 1 cm; tissue current from: Current density × Tissue area; tissue energy from: Current density × Current density × Resistivity × Time = 1 s. The tissue cross-sectional area was determined by digitization of a frozen limb section taken through the measurement region.

mechanism where the temperature rise increases the current density, which further increases the temperature. These studies also revealed a qualitative change in the resistance related to the extent of trauma.

Tissue resistivities and impedances have been observed to change for various experimental conditions[1,6,7,25,27-31]. Typically, tissue is anisotropic, which means that the structure of the tissue differs in one or both cross-sectional planes. This anisotropic organization of tissue causes differences in tissue impedance and usually requires orthogonal measurements to characterize the impedance[28,31,32]. Muscle tissue depicts this anisotropic character with its longitudinal (along the muscle fibres) resistivity being 2.5 to 3 times less than its transverse (across the muscle fibres) resistivity. Additionally, an excellent summary of the use of impedance techniques for detection of physiological events has been published by Geddes and Baker[29]; however, the majority of these studies have used a single measurement frequency. Impedance is also affected by the extracellular and intracellular fluid changes[1,30]. Although many factors alter the tissue impedance, each factor is identifiable by causing a unique change in the impedance.

Temperature changes in tissue change tissue resistivity and are inversely

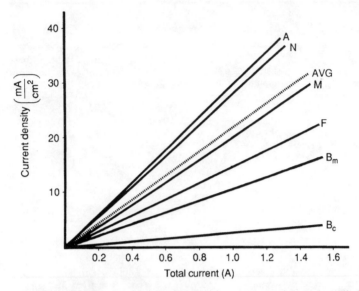

Fig. 12.5. Current densities in tissue with respect to the total applied current measured in the hindlimb of the hog. Measurements were made in arteries (A), nerves (N), muscle (M), interstitial fat (F), bone marrow (Bm) and bone cortex (Bc). AVG is the average current density in the cross-section of the limb.

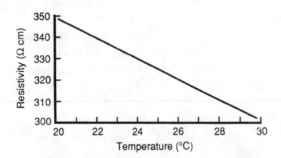

Fig. 12.6. Changes in resistivity with temperature *in vivo* in cat muscle. The rate of change is $-5$ ohm cm/°C, or a 1.7%/°C decrease in resistivity.

proportional to the resistivity. Figure 12.6 shows the resistivity change with temperature measured in the anaesthetized cat. The decrease in resistivity with increasing temperature indicates that there will be a decrease in tissue resistance as the tissue is heated as long as no structural changes occur in the tissue. Further studies show a continued decrease in resistivity when associated with tissue destruction[6,7]. Figure 12.7 shows the temperature

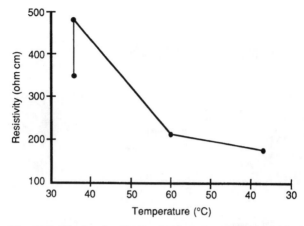

Fig. 12.7. The longitudinal resistivity of muscle measured during, and after, the application of 1 A of 60 Hz current. Current was applied for 15 min at which time the tissue temperature reached 60 °C. The resistivity continued to decrease as the muscle cooled, indicating that tissue injury had occurred. The initial rise in resistivity was due to gross muscular contraction.

change vs. resistivity of muscle as severe trauma is established in the tissue. It is important to note that the tissue resistivity continues to decrease as the temperature decreases indicating a continued change in tissue structure. The resulting resistivity changes have been followed in time for four hours (Fig. 12.8) and show that changes remain constant for that time.

Since the resistivity of muscle at 60 Hz is only one part of the impedance, characteristic studies were performed to investigate the effect of electrical trauma on muscle impedance. To perform a complete analysis, the study was done over a 4-day period. The results of this study indicate that measurement of tissue impedance can be valuable in the determination of tissue destruction.

### Methods

To investigate the alterations in tissue impedance secondary to electrical burn injury, studies were conducted in ten anaesthetized and intubated 30–50 kg mongrel dogs over a 24-hour period. A current of 1 A of 60 Hz current flowed with 400–500 V applied between the distal aspects of the hindlimbs until the distal gracilis muscle reached 60 °C. Impedance and local tissue temperature were measured along the gracilis muscle at 2 cm increments. Impedance measurements were made prior to, and at 1, 4 and 24 hours, following the electrical insult. Figure 12.9 shows a system for measuring the

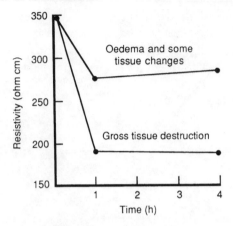

Fig. 12.8. The longitudinal resistivity of muscle measured after the application of 1 A of 60 Hz current. The resistivity decreases correspond to the severity of trauma.

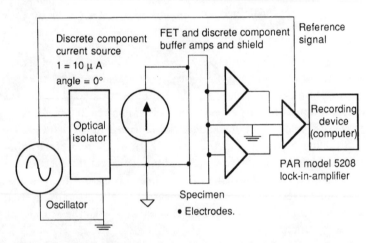

Fig. 12.9. Block diagram of the instrumentation for measuring the complex impedance of tissue.

real and reactive impedance components over the frequency range from 30 Hz to 100 kHz that has been developed using a lock-in amplifier with specialized circuitry. The system is described in detail elsewhere[1,7].

Additional studies were conducted to determine longer-term changes in impedance. Six dogs (15 kg) were sedated with sodium pentobarbital and titrated with barbiturates to maintain a sufficient anaesthetic level and a sufficient analgesic level following arousal to suppress pain. Current was applied through only one hindlimb to localize the burn. The dogs were kept alive for periods of 2, 3 and 4 days to monitor longer-term changes in impedance. Antibiotics were administered daily. Impedance measurements and NMR samples were taken at the end of each study to minimize intrusion and infection.

All of the dogs underwent sequential haematological evaluation to monitor their health and stability. Blood was drawn prior to surgical exposure of the muscle, immediately preceding the burn, and at 1 hour, 4 hours and daily following the burn. NMR spectroscopy was performed on muscle samples taken from proximal, transitional and distal areas using standard techniques published elsewhere[7,33]. Four animals had sections of muscle removed from the three burn areas for histological analysis. Following formalin fixation, slides were made using haemopexin and eosin (H & E) stains. All studies conformed to regulations on standard procedures and care for laboratory animals.

### Results

Immediately following current interruption, systemic arterial pressure and heart rate increased 10–20%. The core temperature was elevated 3 to 5 °C. The amount of change in systemic physiological measurements appeared to be related to the extent of tissue damage. Arterial pressure returned to control levels within 1 to 2 hours. Haematology demonstrated characteristics compatible with the consumptive coagulopathy associated with significant tissue injury produced by burns.

Following the injury, the most distal muscle impedance measurement sites decreased to 25% of control and did not recover (Fig. 12.10). With successive proximal measurements, a transition region was located where the impedance markedly changed. Proximal to this area, a muscle twitch could be elicited. Below this area, muscle was unexcitable. Immediately above the transition zone, muscle impedance was reduced only 20% to 40% and increased toward control values thereafter. The impedance was within physiological limits in the unburned forelimb.

Figure 12.11 shows micrographs of normal and electrically injured muscle. Histological analysis of muscle tissues removed from control areas were all unremarkable (Fig. 12.11(a)). Sections taken from the proximal area showed local oedema between muscle bundles and some loss of cross striations (Fig. 12.11(b)). In the transition zone the changes were similar, but more severe (Fig. 12.11(c)). In the distal area, there were significant generalized oedema, local haemorrhage, and loss of architecture (Fig.

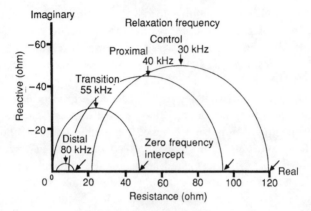

Fig. 12.10. Plots of complex impedance of dog gracilis muscle prior to, and following, electrical burn. Burn severity in proximal tissue was limited to some loss of structure and oedema histologically, middle or transition zone tissue showed a greater loss of structure with oedema and the distal tissue showed a complete loss of structure and was obviously nonviable. Notable changes in impedance are in the zero frequency intercept, the maximum amplitude of the reactive component and the significant increase in the relaxation frequency with trauma.

12.11(*d*). Phosphorylated metabolites, ATP, ADP, NAD and phospho-creatine (determined by [$^{31}$P]-NMR spectroscopy), had slightly reduced peaks in the proximal tissue and peaks further decreased as tissue damage increased through the transition zone and had no metabolite peaks in the distal tissue (Fig. 12.12).

The long-term impedance of muscle decreased two to four times in the hindlimb where the temperature exceeded 50 °C. In areas adjacent to the above regions, the resistivity decrease was proportional to the peak temperature initially. As time progressed, impedances associated with temperatures below 45 °C approached control values and impedances associated with higher temperatures continued to decrease. However, the actual temperature causing nonviability could not be directly determined. The width of the transition region, between viable tissue of increasing impedances and obviously necrotic tissue of very low impedance, decreased so that by the fourth day the transition region was very abrupt. Phosphorylated metabolites were observed in tissue with near normal impedance, whereas these metabolites were not detected in tissues with low impedance. Transition region tissues had reduced metabolite peaks consistent with reduced impedance and histology.

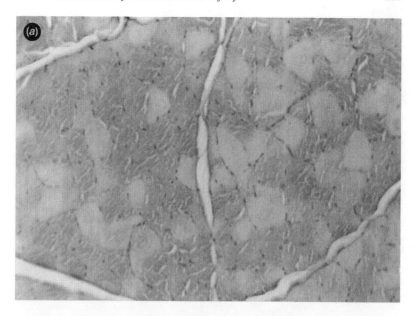

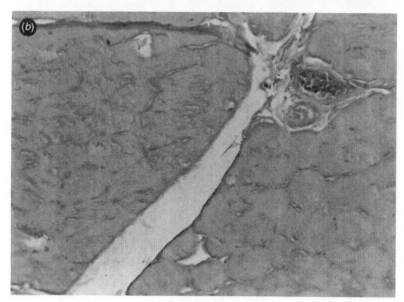

Fig. 12.11. Photomicrographs of muscle tissue: (*a*) normal tissue from control region; (*b*) tissue from the proximal muscle: the tissue is intact with oedema; (*c*) tissue near the transition region: greater oedema and early fibre changes observed; (*d*) tissue from the distal muscle; gross destruction of the tissue is evident. From Chilbert *et al.*[10].

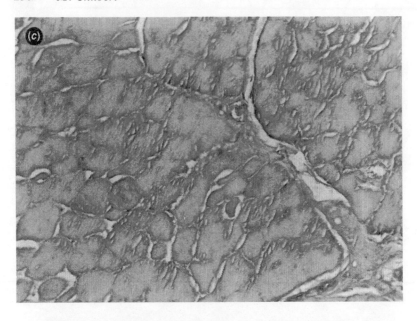

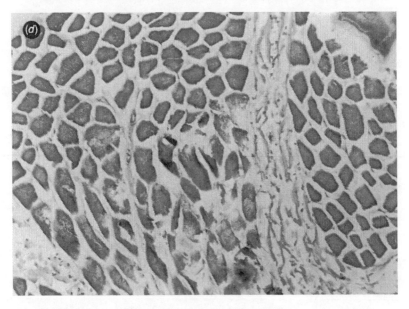

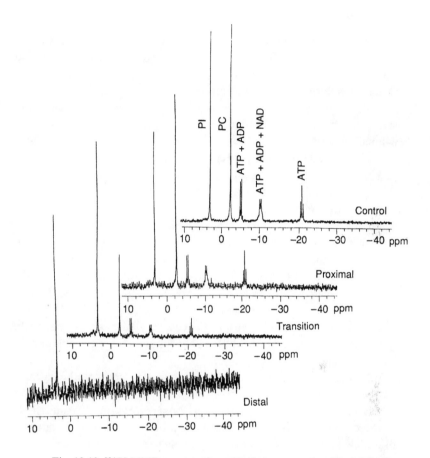

Fig. 12.12. [$^{31}$P]-NMR spectra of perchloric extracts of muscle following electrical injury. The proximal region is associated with a peak temperature of 42 °C, the transient region with a peak of 45 °C and the distal region with a peak of 60 °C. Phosphate peaks of the spectra are ATP (adenosine triphosphate), ADP (adenosine diphosphate), NAD (nicotinamide-andenine-dinucleotide), PC (phosphocreatine) and PI (inorganic phosphate). When compared to the control spectra, the burned tissue exhibits reduced concentrations of the phosphate metabolites (ATP, ADP, NAD, PC) with a concomitant increase in the concentration of inorganic phosphates. The concentration of metabolites correlates to the severity of trauma.

### Discussion

The measurement of biological impedance has been used for a variety of applications. The multifrequency techniques involve measurement of both real and reactive components of impedance over a wide frequency range, along with plotting and analytical methods. For a biological system, the advantages of these methods over conventional, single-frequency measurements are that changes in material properties can be distinguished from volumetric changes, and that the percentage of current in various pathways can be estimated from electric circuit models such as the one shown in Fig. 12.1. This method permits a discrimination of intravascular blood volume changes from those of interstitial fluids.

Multifrequency measurements have been used for the study of electrical properties of cell membranes. Multifrequency studies of more complex systems have been somewhat more limited. However, Lofgren[30] demonstrated both theoretically and experimentally that changes in relaxation frequency occur with oedema in the rat kidney. Ranck[31] conducted studies in the rabbit cerebral cortex and postulated an equivalent circuit model. A number of studies have also been performed on muscle fibre[7,28]. These studies suggest that local tissue impedance measurements may be a reliable indicator of tissue integrity and that changes in tissue micro-anatomy are measurable.

Validation of the impedance technique depends on the accurate reproduction of the injury in the laboratory. Physiological parameters monitored in this study were the same as those reported in 1985[6] and similar to those in pathophysiologically significant burns. Histological evaluation of muscle tissue in this study is comparable to the previous study and the study of Zelt et al.[23]. The long-term observations revealed tissue improvement or tissue necrosis. The [31P]-NMR spectroscopy was consistent with histology with respect to burn severity and changes in time. One should note that changes in [31P]-NMR spectroscopy is different for electrical burns and ischaemia. Spectroscopic changes associated with electrical burns show all metabolites decreasing at the same rate, and the levels are related to burn severity. Since all the metabolite peaks remain at the same relative level, the change from control levels is an indication of the quantity of viable cells that remained in the tissue. Spectroscopic changes associated with ischaemia show that the phosphocreatine peak decreases first, indicating that the tissue is utilizing this metabolite first[33].

In the long-term dog study, changes in the zero frequency intercept on the real axis from control to the postburn proximal region data probably indicate that a DC shunt path has developed secondary to some oedema (Fig. 12.10). However, the relaxation frequency has remained essentially the same between the control and postburn proximal curves indicating minimal alteration in the structural characteristics of the tissue. Corresponding histological sections and NMR spectroscopy support these findings as seen in Figs. 12.11(*b*) and 12.12[6,23]. In contrast, the postburn middle region demonstrates an increase in relaxation frequency which suggests an alteration in structural characteristics. A concomitant change in the low frequency intercept is consistent with increased oedema, and histology of this region (Fig. 11(*c*)) shows more extracellular space and cell destruction. This also corresponds to NMR spectroscopy reductions in the metabolite peak amplitudes (Fig. 12.12). Finally, the postburn distal region demonstrates changes which are more marked than the postburn middle area. The relaxation frequency in this region is approximately 80 kHz with a ten times change in the low frequency intercept. The histological specimen of this region (Fig. 12.11(*d*)) shows substantial cell destruction with a marked increase in extracellular space, and NMR spectroscopy shows no metabolites in this tissue (Fig. 12.12). The most striking changes shown by the impedance data is the marked increase in relaxation frequency which is indicative of the level of gross cellular destruction. The decrease in the zero frequency intercept correlates to an increased extracellular space and oedema.

The results of the 4-day study show that the transition region where tissue changes from oedematous to severely burned reduces in size with time (Fig. 12.13); indicating that this region of tissue either continues to necrose or remains viable. Correlation of peak tissue temperature to tissue trauma did not suggest progressive necrosis. However, the bounds of the transition region were determined only at the end of each experiment. The transition region can be located initially using the impedance technique, and tissue that is necrotic can be identified and removed. Further investigation is needed to define changes better in this region.

The separation of viable and nonviable tissue by impedance and relaxation frequency is illustrated in Fig. 12.14. Comparison of impedance changes to phosphate metabolite content reveals that viable tissue has impedance levels above 70% of control values with a normal quantity of metabolites. Tissue that is nonviable has impedance values less than 50% of control. Transition region tissue has increased levels of inorganic phosphates and decreased levels of metabolites, which indicates cellular degradation. The quantity of lost metabolites correlates to the level of trauma and is reflected in the measured impedance. Similarly, the

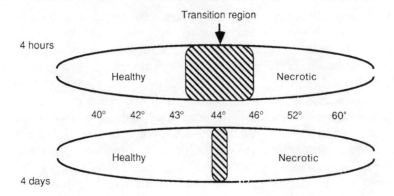

Fig. 12.13. Changes in the transition region with time in muscle. The temperatures (°C) are peak values measured along the muscle immediately following cessation of current. The extent of the transition region was determined by impedance measurement.

relaxation frequency change compares well with the tissue metabolite content. A greater change is observed in the relaxation frequency when compared to the impedance, and it is more indicative of cellular destruction (since oedema affects it minimally). Using both impedance and relaxation frequency, one can directly discriminate between severely damaged tissue and minor tissue damage, which may not be visibly apparent. The changes in impedance and relaxation frequency are substantial. However, the technique used here is slow. By modifying this technique or using other impedance measuring techniques, the development of a clinically useful instrument is possible.

### Conclusions

Experimental electrical injury studies have delineated the distribution and effects of electric current in the body[6,7,12 16,27,34]. It was noted in one study that resistivity changed significantly following tissue trauma and was associated with elevated temperatures[7]. The use of animal models show immediate tissue involvement that is comparable to other forms of injury, which suggests that impedance changes may be useful in other types of trauma. The model can be localized and involves both deep and superficial structures. The resulting electrical burns produced were consistent with clinical findings and required treatment similar to clinical situations[6].

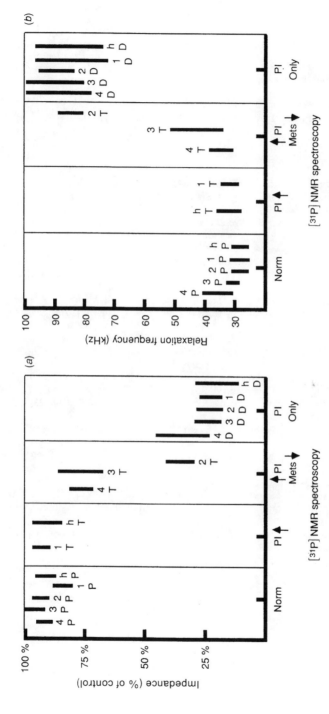

Fig. 12.14. Comparison of [³¹P] NMR spectroscopy with changes in (a) impedance change in % of control and (b) relaxation frequency. Vertical bars indicate the range of values, 1–4 is days after burn, **h** is 1 h after burn. Measurements were made in the proximal (P), transition (T) and distal (D) regions of the gracilis muscle in dog. NMR spectra were divided into normal (Norm), increased inorganic phosphates (PI), increased inorganic phosphates with reduced metabolites (Mets) and only inorganic phosphate present (PI only) in the sample.

Impedance measurements correctly identify the severity of tissue trauma when compared to histology and [$^{31}$P]-NMR spectroscopy.

### Acknowledgements

The author's research was supported in part by NIH Grant GM38456 and Veterans' Administration Medical Center Research Funds.

### References

1 Ackmann, J.J. & Seitz, M.A. (1984). Methods of complex impedance measurements in biologic tissue. *CRC Critical Revision in Bioengineering*, **11(4)**, 281–311. (Appendix III).
2 Baxter, C.R. (1970). Present concepts in the management of major electrical injury. *Surgery Clinics of North America*, **50(6)**, 1401–18. (Review).
3 Wang, X.W., Lu, C.S., Zhang, Z.M., Wong, C.Y., Tu, D.K. & Zapata-Sirvent, R.L. (1984). Verdoglobinuria phenomenon in severe electrical burns. *Burns Including Thermal Injury*, **10(3)**, 188–92.
4 Boswick, J.A. Jr. (1974). The management of fresh burns of the hand and deformities resulting from burn injuries. *Clinics in Plastic Surgery*, **1**, 621.
5 Burke, J.F., Quinby, W.C. Jr. & Bondoc, C. *et al.* (1977). Patterns of high tension electrical injury in children and adolescents and their management. *American Journal of Surgery*, **133**, 492.
6 Chilbert, M., Maiman, D., Sances, A. Jr., Myklebust, J., Prieto, T.E., Swiontek, T., Heckman, M. & Pintar, K. (1985). Measure of tissue resistivity in experimental electrical burns. *Journal of Trauma*, **25(3)**, 209–15.
7 Chilbert, M., Swiontek, T., Prieto, T., Sances, A. Jr., Myklebust, J., Ackmann, J., Brown, C. & Szablya, J. (1985). Resistivity changes of tissue during the application of injurious 60 Hz currents. In *Symposium on Electric Shock Safety Criteria*, Bridges, J.E. & Arnot, S. eds, pp. 193–201, Toronto, Ontario.
8 Davies, J.W.L. (1975). The fluid therapy given to 1027 patients during the first 48 hours after burning. I. Total fluid and colloid input. *Burns*, **1**, 319.
9 Janzekovic, Z. (1975). The burn wound from the surgical point of view. *Journal of Trauma*, **15**, 42.
10 Luce, E.A., Dowden, W.L., Su, C.T. & Hoopes, J.E. (1978). High tension electrical injury of the upper extremity. *Surgery, Gynecology and Obstetrics*, **147**, 38.
11 Mills, W. Jr., Switzer, W.E. & Moncrief, J.A. (1966). Electrical injuries. *Journal of the American Medical Association*, **195**, 164.
12 Sances, A. Jr., Larson, S.J., Myklebust, J. & Cusick, J.F. (1979). Electrical injuries. *Surgery, Gynecology and Obstetrics*, **149(1)**, 97–108. (Review).
13 Sances, A. Jr., Myklebust, J.B., Larson, S.J., Darin, J.C., Swiontek, T., Prieto, T., Chilbert, M. & Cusick, J.F. (1981). Experimental electrical injury studies. *Journal of Trauma*, **21(8)**, 589–97.

14 Sances, A. Jr., Myklebust, J.B., Szablya, J.F., Swiontek, T.J., Larson, S.J., Chilbert, M., Prieto, T. & Cusick, J.F. (1981). Effects of contacts in high voltage injuries. *IEEE Transactions on Power Apparatus and Systems*, **PAS–100**, (6), 2987–92.

15 Sances, A. Jr., Myklebust, J.B., Szablya, J.F., Swiontek, T.J., Larson S.J., Chilbert, M., Prieto, T., Cusick, J.R. & Pintar, K. (1983). Current pathways in high voltage injuries. *IEEE Transactions on Biomedical Engineering*, **30(2)**, 118–124.

16 Sances, A. Jr., Szablya, J.F. Morgan J.D., Myklebust, J.B. & Larson, S.J. High voltage powerline injury studies. *IEEE Transactions on Power Apparatus and Systems,*, **PAS–100**, (2), 552–8.

17 Artz, C.P. (1967). Electrical injury simulates crush injury. *Surgery, Gynecology and Obstetrics*, **125(6)**, 1316–17.

18 Barnard, M.D. & Boswick, J.A. Jr. (1976). Electrical injuries of the upper extremity. *Rocky Mountain Medical Journal*, **73**, 20.

19 Wang, X.W., Bartle, E.J., Roberts, B.B., Cheng, H.H., Wu, W.A. & Wang, X.Z. (1987). Free skin flap transfer in repairing deep electrical burns. *Journal of Burn Care and Rehabilitation*, **8(2)**, 111–14.

20 Wang, X.W. & Zoh, W.H. (1983). Vascular injuries in electrical burns – the pathological basis for mechanism of injury. *Burns Including Thermal Injury*, **9(5)**, 335–8.

21 Wang, X.W., Roberts, B.B., Zapata-Sirvent, R.L., Robinson, W.A., Waymack, J.P., Law, E.J., MacMillan, B.G. & Davies, J.W. (1985). Early vascular grafting to prevent upper extremity necrosis after electrical burns. Commentary on indications for surgery. *Burns Including Thermal Injury*, **11(5)**, 359–65.

22 Wang, X.W., Lu, C.S., Wang, N.Z., Lin, H.C., Su, H., Wei, J.N. & Zoh, W.Z. (1984). High tension electrical burns of upper arms treated by segmental excision of necrosed humerus. An introduction of a new surgical method. *Burns Including Thermal Injury*, **10(4)**, 271–81.

23 Zelt, R.G., Daniel, R.K., Ballard, P.A., Brissette, Y. & Heroux, P. (1988). High-voltage electrical injury: chronic wound evolution. *Plastic and Reconstructive Surgery*, **82(6)**, 1027–39.

24 Prieto, T., Sances, A. Jr., Myklebust, J. & Chilbert, M. (1985). Analysis of cross-body impedance at household voltage levels. In *Symposium on Electric Shock Safety Criteria*, Bridges, J.E. & Arnot, S. eds, pp. 151–60, Toronto, Ontario: Pergamon Press.

25 Chilbert, M.A., Swiontek, T., Myklebust, J.B., Prieto, T., Sances, A. Jr., Leffingwell, C. & Henderson, J.D. (1989). Fibrillation induced at powerline current levels. *IEEE Transactions in Biomedical Engineering*, **36**, 565–8.

26 Laberge, L.C., Ballard, P.A. & Daniel, R.K. (1984). Experimental electrical burns: low voltage. *Annals in Plastic Surgery*, **13(3)**, 185–90.

27 Chilbert, M., Sances, A. Jr., Myklebust, J., Swiontek, T. & Prieto, T. (1983). Postmortem resistivity studies at 60 Hz. *Journal of Clinical Engineering*, **8(3)**, 219–24.

28 Fatt, P. (1964). An analysis of the transverse electrical impedance of striated muscle. *Proceedings of the Royal Society of London (Biology)*, **B159**, 606–51.

29 Geddes, L.A. & Baker, L.E. (1975). Detection of physiological events by impedance. In *Principles of Applied Biomedical Instrumentation*, New York: Wiley.

29a  Hunt, J., Lewis, S., Parkey, R. & Baxter, C. (1979). The use of technetium-99m stannous pyrophosphate scintigraphy to identify muscle damage in acute electric burns. *Journal of Trauma*, **19**, 409–13.

30  Lofgren, B. (1951). The electrical impedance of a complex tissue and its relation to changes in volume and fluid distribution. A study on rat kidneys. *Acta Physiologia Scandinavia*, **23(81)**, 5–51.

31  Ranck, J.B. Jr. (1964). Specific impedance of cerebral cortex during spreading depression, and an analysis of neuronal, neuroglial, and interstitial contributions. *Experimental Neurology*, **9**, 1–16.

32  Rush, S. (1962). Methods of measuring the resistivities of anisotropic media *in situ*. *Journal of Research National Bureau of Standards*, **66C(3)**, 127–32.

33  Brown, C.E., Battocletti, J.H. & Johnson, L.F. (1984). Nuclear magnetic resonance (NMR) in clinical pathology: current trends. *Clinical Chemistry*, **30**, 606–18.

34  Chilbert, M.A., Moretti, D.J., Swiontek, T., Myklebust, J.B., Prieto, T., Sances, A. Jr. & Leffingwell, C. (1991) Instrumentation design for high voltage electrical injury studies. *IEEE Transactions in Biomedical Engineering*, **35**, in press.

# 13

# Impedance spectroscopy: the measurement of electrical impedance of biologic materials

ROBERT SCHMUKLER

## Introduction

Measuring the electrical impedance of biologic materials over a wide frequency range (Hz–MHz) either *in vitro* or *in vivo* presents some unique difficulties. The aqueous environment, necessary for physiologic conditions, is the main source of these difficulties. First, in order to pass currents or measure voltages, electrodes must be used, so that electrochemical processes at electrodes are present. Second, conduction through an aqueous environment is ionic, not electronic, so that ionic current conduction is present. Third, the heterogeneity of biologic materials increases the complexity of measurement. And lastly, there are instrumentation problems, which are a result of inherent component limitations and interactions with electrodes. All of these problems must be considered, and methods must be employed to reduce or eliminate them. Some of the problem solutions can only be compromises, and, in order to produce meaningful measurements, limitations should be recognized. However, it should also be noted that electrical impedance of tissue has been used diagnostically, and its use in detecting tissue damage from electrical injury shows great promise.

This chapter will cover, from a bioelectrochemistry viewpoint, three primary areas in looking at the problems or difficulties in biological impedance measurements.

## Electrodes

The most commonly used electrodes in biology are produced when an electrical conductor, commonly a metal, but it may be any conducting material, is immersed in a fluid solution, usually water containing ions (electrolyte). Due to free energy differences between the electrode and the solution, certain molecular structures are formed at the interface between the two phases (electrode, solution). Kinetic processes dependent on ionic mobility in solution, surface adsorption, and charge transfer can also be present. The discussion which follows is not a comprehensive treatment of electrodes[1-12,14,24,25], but covers some of electrode phenomena from an electrochemistry standpoint to provide a basic understanding. The final equivalent circuit representation of an electrode as seen in Fig. 13.1 and discussed below is a linear small-signal model *only*.

The Stern model[1] of an electrode interface is a synthesis of the Helmholtz–Perrin double-layer model with the Gouy–Chapman diffuse-layer model (see also refs[2,3,9,10,12]). The equivalent circuit representation of this model is two capacitors in series. The Helmholtz–Perrin double-layer capacitance ($C_D$) is formed by the alignment of ions and primarily water dipoles that balance or compensate the charges on the aqueous surface of the electrode. The Gouy–Chapman diffuse-layer capacitance ($C_d$) is formed by the distribution of ions in solution in thermal disarray, an ionic cloud, that compensates the electrode charge. The distribution of ions (concentration variation) is an exponential one, based on the potential, starting from the interface to the bulk solution (Poisson–Boltzmann distribution)[1,12]. In physiological solutions, the ionic strength of the solution is sufficiently large that the thickness of the diffuse layer is small and the capacitance seen at the interface is equal to the Helmholtz–Perrin double-layer capacitance alone, $C_D < < C_d$. Conduction through the electrolyte is purely resistive over a wide frequency range[1,4,13], and is represented by $R_E$. Currents which flow strictly due to double-layer charging are displacement currents and do not require an electron transfer. As the surface area of an electrode increases, the $C_D$ capacitance of the electrode increases, because the area of $C_D$ increases. Figure 13.1 is an equivalent circuit representation of the electrode–electrolyte interface. All circuit components are defined in the following sections.

Once $C_D$ is fully charged, current can only pass through kinetic processes, e.g. Faradaic charge transfer and specific adsorption of ions. Faradaic charge transfer involves a chemical reaction, whereby electrons are transferred between the electrode and ions in solution. This produces what is commonly called oxidation or reduction, depending on whether an electron is donated or accepted. In a simple case, if a positive ion in solution accepts (an) electrons, undergoing reduction, it becomes a neutral (zero charge) atom or molecule. Conversely, if a metallic atom on the electrode donates (loses) an electron, undergoing oxidation, it becomes an ion in solution. Since all nonspontaneous chemical reactions require some

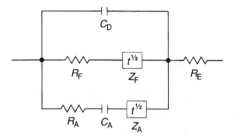

Fig. 13.1. An equivalent circuit representation of an electrode interface including $R_E$ (bulk solution). Commonly called a Randles Diagram.[2]

activation energy, the equivalent circuit for a Faradaic process is a resistor $(R_F)$, in parallel to $C_D$ (see Fig. 13.1). Basically, the magnitude of $R_F$ is proportional to the magnitude of the activation energy.

Faraday's Law describes the magnitude of current in a Faradaic process: 'The magnitude of the chemical effect, in chemical equivalents, is the same at each of the metallic–electrolyte boundaries in an electric circuit and is determined solely by the amount of electricity passed'[13]. One important point about Faraday's Law: the amount of electricity (current) determines the total number of chemical equivalents reacting and not simply the number from a single reaction[13]. In a heterogeneous electrolyte, the potential (voltage) on an electrode determines which ionic species will undergo a reaction via a Faradaic process. This is demonstrated by the production of gas from water at about one volt from a platinum (Pt) electrode[15]. If the voltage is negative (cathodic), hydrogen is produced; if positive (anodic) oxygen is produced.

When the concentration of the reacting species in a Faradaic process is low, a concentration gradient eventually results. The concentration gradient starts at the electrode surface, extends a distance into the bulk solution, and exists in series with the Faradaic resistive impedance. A concentration gradient of reacting species can be present even in high ionic strength solutions. The impedance due to a concentration gradient is called a Warburg Diffusion Impedance[2,3,12]. This impedance can be represented by either a semi-infinite or infinite transmission line representing either semi-infinite or infinite diffusion ($Z_F = f(t^{\frac{1}{2}})$), as seen in Fig. 13.1. The diffusion may involve either products diffusing away from the electrode surface or reactants diffusing to the electrode surface.

There are two classifications of electrodes with respect to Faradaic processes: reversible (nonpolarizable) and irreversible (polarizable) electrodes. A reversible electrode is an electrode which is in equilibrium with an ion in solution, e.g. silver/silver chloride (Ag/AgCl), as described by the Nernst equation[1,12,13]. Since, for a reversible electrode, the activation energy for the electron transfer is relatively low, the resistor, $R_F$, of small magnitude is a good representation. A reversible electrode can usually carry larger currents than a polarizable (irreversible) electrode before an appreciable overpotential develops (see below). The larger current-carrying ability, without a potential (voltage) shift, of a reversible electrode is mostly a function of the fact that ions are produced from the electrode material and the electrode is in equilibrium with the electrolyte. This is why reversible electrodes make good reference electrodes. In the case of an irreversible electrode, e.g. Pt, there are no ions in solution which are in equilibrium with the electrode. Since the activation energy for electron transfer is relatively high compared to a reversible electrode, the resistor, $R_F$, of large magnitude is a good representation. An overpotential reduces the effective voltage at the interface of an electrode due to dissipative (nonequilibrium) irreversible processes[1,9,12]. Polarization produces a nonlinear[6-9] voltage drop (overpotential) from the Nernst equilibrium potential, which is a function of current density (not total current) at the electrode interface[6-9,14,15]. Polarization also varies nonlinearly as a function of frequency[6-8,14]. As the surface area of an electrode increases for a given current, the Faradaic resistance, $R_F$, decreases because the number of reaction sites increases[10]. Current density also decreases for a given current as electrode surface area increases.

Another kinetic process which occurs as a result of current at electrode interfaces is that of adsorption. In adsorption an ion binds to a site on the electrode surface. When the binding involves a chemical affinity similar to a metal–ligand interaction, the process is called specific adsorption[1,3,9,12]. The concentration of a specifically adsorbed ion at an interface generally exceeds the ion's bulk concentration in the electrolyte. There is an activation energy associated with the binding of the ion in specific adsorption, resulting again in an equivalent circuit representation of a resistor, $R_A$. Since the charge density at the interface usually increases with ion adsorption, so does the interfacial electrode capacitance. The equivalent circuit representation for this specific adsorption process is usually a series resistor–capacitor. The resistor ($R_A$) represents the energy of binding, and the capacitor ($C_A$), the added charge storage (see Fig. 13.1) associated with specific adsorption. The specific adsorption capacitance is sometimes called a pseudocapacitance[1,3,12]. If the concentration of adsorbing species in solution is low, a diffusion impedance ($Z_A$), a Warburg impedance, will then exist in series with the series $R_A - C_A$[1,3]. As the surface area of the electrode increases, $C_A$ increases and $R_A$ decreases, because the number of binding sites increases.

If electrode effects (polarization) are so small as to be negligible, then measurements of impedance can be done by one-port electrode measurements. Unfortunately, polarizable electrodes cannot be used in one-port measurements at low frequencies due to polarization[14]. In one-port measurements, the biological material to be measured is placed between the two electrodes, a current applied and measured, and the voltage measured. From these measurements tissue impedance can be determined. A four-terminal, one-port Kelvin measurement with a guard provides the greatest frequency and amplitude range. The only electrodes that have a negligible impedance at low as well as high frequencies are reversible electrodes. However, within the biologic environment, reversible electrodes present physiologic problems. Ag/AgCl is the most common reversible electrode and can carry substantial currents. However, silver ions are toxic to most biological materials[16,17]. Sometimes stainless steel (SS) electrodes are used; however, these too produce Faradaic ions (ferrous) that may induce inflammation in the body[16,17].

Salt bridges[1,9,12,13,15,18] are one remedy used to prevent undesirable ions from contacting living tissue. Salt bridges can be of several designs, but, in general, are electrolyte-filled channels placed between the electrode and tissue that serve to isolate the (usually reference) electrode. The electrode is placed in a solution as the tissue but in a different vessel from the tissue, the fluid heights are equalized, and the salt bridge is used to connect the two vessels electrically. One design is an Agar– or Agarose–electrolyte salt bridge, where the Agar or Agarose gel produces the necessary isolation. Another is a tube filled with electrolyte and a fritted glass end. Salt bridges that use physiological solutions as an electrolyte have an undesirable liquid junction potential associated with them due to differences in mobilities of ions and low ionic strength[12,18]. The salt bridge for measurements that produces the best results is a saturated potassium chloride (KCl) salt bridge[12,18]. Over long periods of time there may be mixing of the electrolyte of the KCl bridge with the physiological solution because of diffusion, pressure gradients, currents, iontophoresis, etc, which could alter the ionic composition of the physiological solution.

A technique to reduce polarization errors at low frequencies in impedance measurements, when using polarizable electrodes, is the four-electrode technique[4,11] (two port). By using different electrodes to pass currents (current electrodes) and measure voltage (voltage electrodes), several advantages are obtained. The first is that the currents carried by the

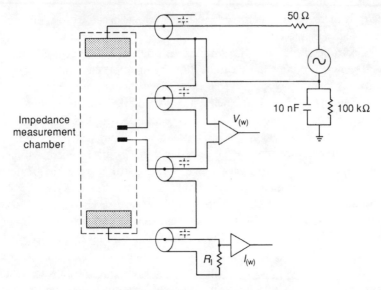

Fig. 13.2. Schematic of four-electrode impedance chamber measurement system for frequency domain measurements.

electrodes that measure voltage are very low, so their polarization is much lower. Second, though the current passed by the current electrodes decreases as frequency decreases because the current-passing electrodes carry a higher current and do polarize, the measured voltage concomitantly decreases. Since the electrolyte can be thought of as a pure resistance ($R_E$), any change in current I, is reflected proportionally in the voltage measured $V (= IR_E)$, see Fig. 13.2.

One problem that exists with Pt, the most commonly used polarizable electrode, is that of the adsorption of oxygen ($O_2$) and hydrogen ($H_2$) on Pt[1,15,19] at potentials below gassing potentials. This can change the concentration of $O_2$ and or the pH of the physiological solution. When carbon (C) electrodes were used to pass pulses into physiologic solutions containing Phenol Red, at 10 mV[20], pH shifts could be seen near the

Cyclic voltammetry studies on electrodes, i.e. Pt, tantalum (Ta), titanium (Ti), and SS in various physiological buffers, demonstrated that Ti and Ta had the largest inert voltage range[19]. The lack of Faradaic and nonFaradaic processes on Ti and Ta provides the largest stable potential range for reproducibility and accuracy. Pt, Ti, and Ta have been found to be nontoxic to tissue as an implant material[17]. If the surface area of the polarizable electrode can be increased so that $C_D$ is increased (neglecting decreases in $R_F$), measurements at a much lower frequency are possible (see Fig. 13.1) by

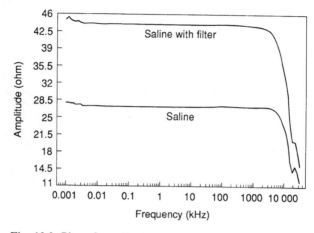

Fig. 13.3. Plot of amplitude vs. log frequency for phosphate buffered Ringer's (saline) alone and with a Nuclepore filter (saline with filter).

coupling through $C_D$[12,22-26]. One way of increasing surface area is by platinizing the surface[13] of a Pt electrode (Pt black). A much larger increase in surface area can be achieved by using powder metallurgy techniques to produce porous electrodes[24,25]. Porous platinum black electrodes with surface areas on the order of 10 m$^2$/gm can be made[10,24-26]. Small porous Ta (metallurgical grade, Cabot Corp., Boyertown, Pa) electrodes (cylinders, 0.9 mm D × 1 mm H) with capacitances between 15–25 $\mu$F have been used successfully down to 10 Hz in a four-electrode technique[20,22,23] (see below and Figs 13.2–4). The four-electrode technique has been the primary method for electrically evaluating tissue damage from electrical injuries[27-30] *in vivo* because of its lower frequency limit. The following sections will focus on this technique to measure impedance.

### Current distribution

In order to make accurate and precise measurements of biological impedance, volume conduction effects on current distribution in electrolytes and tissue must be considered. These points have been addressed from theoretical and experimental considerations[31-35]. The inherent heterogeneity in tissue, and its effects on current distribution[35], cannot be avoided, but can be somewhat minimized if the proper techniques are used. *In vivo* measurements are less defined with respect to conduction volumes than *in vitro* measurements because of a more complex geometry. Some common problems can be addressed through insights gained from *in vitro* measure-

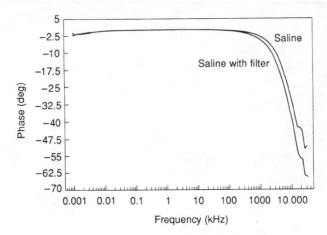

Fig. 13.4. Plot of phase vs. log frequency for phosphate buffered Ringer's
(saline) alone and with a Nuclepore filter (saline with filter).

ments. The principles of the four-electrode technique learned from *in vitro*
measurements, which are discussed here, can provide the basis for *in vivo*
measurements.

In the development of a higher sensitivity four-electrode *in vitro*
impedance chamber[20,22,23], two problems first emerged: nonuniform
current distribution and distortion of current distribution by the voltage-
measuring electrodes. The polycarbonate chamber forms a cylindrical
electrolyte column 2 cm long and 1 cm in diameter[23] (see Fig. 13.2). The
current electrodes are porous C electrodes that form the top and bottom of
the cylinder. The voltage-measuring electrodes are porous Ta electrodes, as
described above, separated by 0.3 cm centre to centre, at the cylinder
midline and recessed into the chamber wall.

A uniform current distribution, such that the measured potential only
depends on the axial distance, produces the least artifacts[22]. In the
development of the *in vitro* impedance chamber[22,32-34], electrode
placement to achieve uniform current distribution at the point of voltage
measurement was evaluated. In the case of point electrodes, if the distance
from a current electrode to voltage electrode is equal to the diameter of the
conducting cylinder, the current flux distribution at the voltage electrode is
uniform[33]. For transients, Rall[32] showed theoretically that, when the
length-to-diameter ratio for a conducting cylinder is large, uniform current
distributions result within a few microseconds. For a homogeneous
conducting cylinder, when the distance between the current electrodes (in
this case, C disc electrodes as described above) is twice the diameter of the
cylinder, a uniform current distribution is achieved[22,23].

The distortion of the current flux distribution by the voltage-measuring electrodes was first recognized by Schwan[4]. In the first version of the chamber described above[22], it was found that when one voltage electrode was placed near and directly over the other voltage electrode in a uniform current distribution, an interaction resulted. This distortion (seen primarily at higher frequencies) could be eliminated by placing the electrodes on opposite walls of the chamber[22]. In the latest version of the chamber, the electrodes are recessed into the walls of the chamber so that they lie completely outside of the current conduction pathways[4,23]. Removing the voltage electrodes from the current conduction path might not be possible for *in vivo* measurements, but displacing the electrodes, as in the earlier chamber design, should provide improvement.

### Measuring instruments

Measuring the impedance of biological materials requires that both the current applied to the tissue (input) and the resulting voltage change (output) be determined. Usually the current is determined by using an ammeter or by measuring the voltage across a known series resistance. The voltage response is determined by measuring the voltage change of the tissue directly. In order to utilize equivalent circuits in evaluating tissue impedance, the perturbation to the tissue should be small[11,22]. Low-level perturbation also produces minimal tissue interaction[11,22,35]. One of two types of amplifiers that are generally used (the electrometer and the instrumentation amplifier) is usually the first stage in most measurement instruments. A brief instrumentation review will be presented that will cover areas of importance to biological impedance measurements.

Electrometer amplifiers, such as the type used in pH and pX (ion specific) measurements, are single-ended, very high input impedance ($10^{12}$–$10^{15}\Omega$), very low input bias current (5–300 fA) amplifiers[36-38]. Generally, the bandwidth of electrometer amplifiers is less than 100 kHz[37,38]. Electrometer amplifiers can be connected directly to electrodes because of their extremely low input bias currents. These amplifiers produce negligibly small electrode polarization because of their extremely high input impedance.

Instrumentation amplifiers, such as those used in oscilloscopes and impedance analysers, are differential, high input impedance ($10^6$–$10^8\Omega$), low bias current (1–100 nA) amplifiers[36,39-41]. Generally, the bandwidth of instrumentation amplifiers can be up to 100 MHz[12,39,40]. One problem is the higher level of input bias current. This current leaving the input of the amplifier can slowly charge $C_D$, resulting in a dc drift and eventually

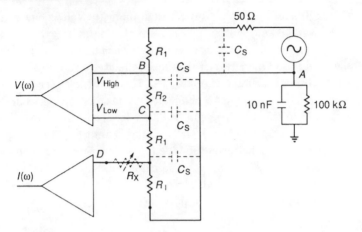

Fig. 13.5. Equivalent circuit representation for the impedance chamber and measurement system (see text for definitions of symbols).

complete charging of $C_D$, producing signal clipping[41]. By using a decoupling series capacitor in the input of the amplifier and an input resistor to ground, a low-frequency cutoff of $< 1$ Hz can be attained with an input resistance of $10^8 \Omega$[42,43], $10^7 \Omega$[22], or $10^6 \Omega$[23,39]. Shield drives based on negative capacitance compensation[44] can reduce inherent stray capacitances and increase the high-frequency limit[39,44-46].

Calibration measurements on the impedance chamber described above[23], filled with phosphate-buffered Ringer's alone and with a Nuclepore filter present, are shown in Figs. 13.3 and 13.4. The Nuclepore filter is used here to simulate the presence of a thin piece of tissue. Since the filter pores are cylindrical, the filter impedance is a resistance with just a small parallel capacitance ($\sim 200$ pF)[20,22,23]. The amplitude and phase data shown were obtained using a Solartron 1260 Impedance Analyser. Both the current and voltage amplifiers were AC coupled ($-3$ dB @ 1 Hz). The input voltage level was 10 mV from 1 Hz–32 MHz (at 30 $\mu$A input). As can be seen in Fig. 13.3 and 13.4, the amplitude response is flat from 10 Hz–2 MHz. The phase shift is: saline, less than $0.4°$ at 10 Hz–150 kHz increasing to $6.6°$ at 2 MHz; saline with filter, less than $0.4°$ at 10 Hz–71 kHz increasing to $8.4°$ at 2 MHz.

A source of measurement error at higher frequencies (note: where electrode polarization is minimal) is imbalance in the source impedance[47], Rs at the measurement points (see Figs. 13.2 and 13.5). The output of a differential amplifier is proportional to the voltage difference between the positive and negative inputs. The voltage difference is the quantity measured. The source impedance at the point of measurement and the total stray capacitance ($Cs = \Sigma C_s$) of the system determine the bandwidth at the point of measurement. The voltage at each point is the voltage with respect to the reference plane. When there is an imbalance in the source impedance between two points of measurement, the measured voltage at each point has a different frequency dependence. Therefore the voltage difference between the two points becomes a function of frequency ($\omega$) and source impedance ($Rs$). Assuming an equivalent circuit model for the chamber and measurement system (see Fig. 13.5) demonstrates this effect. The source impedance between points B ($Rs^B$), C ($Rs^C$), D ($Rs^D$), and point A is as follows:

$$Rs^B = (R_1 + 50\Omega)//(R_2 + R_1 + R_1) \tag{1}$$

$$Rs^C = (R_2 + R_1 + 50\Omega)//(R_1 + R_1) \tag{2}$$

$$Rs^D = \{R_x\} + (R_1//(R_1 + R_2 + R_1 + 50\Omega)) \tag{3}$$

where:

$R_1$ = the electrolyte resistance between the current electrodes and the voltage electrodes.

$R_2$ = the electrolyte resistance between the two voltage electrodes.

$R_1$ = the current measuring resistance.

$R_X$ = the source impedance compensation resistor (see below).

and

$//$ = added as a parallel resistance.

As can be seen from Equations (1) and (2), the source impedance at the high ($B$) and low ($C$) inputs to the differential voltage amplifier is different. When $Rs^B > Rs^C$, at frequencies above the roll-off frequency determined by $Rs^B C_s$, an additional capacitive effect is seen ('paradoxical' capacitance). If the reverse is true, $Rs^B < Rs^C$, then an additional inductive effect is seen ('paradoxical' inductance) above the roll-off frequency determined by $Rs^C C_s$. This is illustrated by Fig. 13.6. In Fig. 13.6, amplitude and phase curves (dotted lines) similar to the ones in Figs. 13.3 and 13.4 are shown. For this measurement, $R_1$ is kept constant at 2 $\Omega$ for the entire frequency range. For the other curves (solid line), $R_1$ was set at 110 $\Omega$ up to 10 MHz and then changed from 110 $\Omega$ to 2 $\Omega$ for frequencies > 10 MHz. As can be seen, there is an anomalous peak between the 9.4 and 11.2 MHz points. This peak disappears when $R_1$ remains constant at 2 $\Omega$ throughout the entire frequency range of measurement (dotted line). When $Rs^B$ and $Rs^C$ are calculated, to a first-order approximation with the usual values for $R_1$ (100 $\Omega$), $R_2$ (25 $\Omega$), and either 2 or 110 $\Omega$ for $R_1$ the following can be seen. When

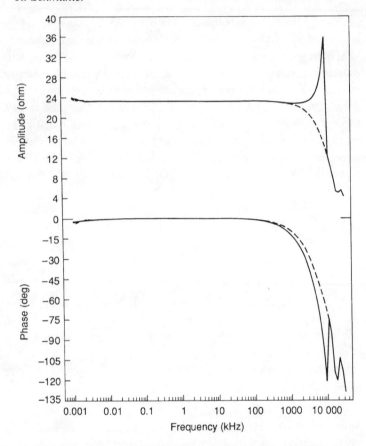

Fig. 13.6. Plots of amplitude and phase vs. log frequency for phosphate-buffered Ringer's for different values of the current measuring resistance.

$R = 110\,\Omega$, $Rs^B < Rs^C$; when $R_1 = 2\,\Omega$, $Rs^B > Rs^C$. This would seem to explain the apparent amplitude peak that appears in the lower curve. A simple solution to the problem is to make the circuit symmetric by always using a resistance for $R_1$ that matches the output impedance of the signal source, in this case 50 $\Omega$. The source impedance at point D (see Fig. 13.5) can also be made to match, though not exactly, the source impedance at points B and C by using an adjustable trimpot $R_X$.

### Conclusion

The measurement of tissue impedance can be accomplished over a large frequency range. In spite of inherent problems in the measurement, if care is taken to minimize sources of errors, precise measurements are possible. The promise of using tissue impedance to evaluate tissue viability in electrical trauma is attainable. From earlier measurements by Schwan[4,48], tissue impedance exhibits distinct relaxations. Measurements by Pauly and Schwan[49], in which the impedance of cells at high frequencies ($>\beta$ relaxation) when the cell membranes are electrically shorted, compares to low-frequency measurements of cells with chemically disrupted membranes. Therefore, membrane integrity can be assessed by comparing the impedance of tissue above the $\beta$ relaxation (MHz), with impedance at low ($<100$ Hz) frequency. If the tissue is damaged and the membranes are permeable, then the impedances should be similar at both points and should not show the normal frequency dependence and impedance differences.

The mention of commercial products, their sources, or their use in connection with material reported herein is not to be construed as either an implied or actual endorsement of such products by the Department of Health and Human Services.

### Acknowledgements

The author would like to thank T. Whit Athey for his help in the preparation of this manuscript, and Jianzhong Bao for the data presented.

### References

1 Bockris, J.O'M. & Reddy, A.K.N. (1970). *Modern Electrochemistry*, Plenum Press.

2 Macdonald, J.R. ed. (1987). *Impedance Spectroscopy*, J. Wiley and Sons.

3 Macdonald, D.D. (1977). *Transient Techniques in Electrochemistry*, Plenum Press.

4 Schwan, H.P. (1963). Determination of biological impedances. In *Physical Techniques in Biological Research*, Nastuk, W.L., ed. Academic Press, p. 323.

5 Schwan, H.P. & Onaral, B. (1985). Linear and nonlinear properties of platinum electrode polarization III: equivalence of frequency- and time-domain behavior. *Medical and Biological Engineering and Computing*, **23**, 28–32.

6 Sun, H.H. and Onaral, B. (1983). A unified approach to represent metal electrode polarization. *IEEE Transactions BME*, **BME–30**, 7.

7 Onaral, B., Sun, H.H. & Schwan, H.P. (1984). Electrical properties of bioelectrodes, *IEEE Transactions BME*, **BME–31**, 12.

8 Onaral, B. & Schwan, H.P. (1982). Linear and nonlinear properties of platinum electrode polarization. Part 1: frequency dependence at very low frequencies. *Medical and Biological Engineering and Computing*, **20**, 299–306.

9  Bauer, H.H. (1972). *Electrodics*, Georg Thieme Verlag.

10  DeRosa, J.F. & Beard, R.B. (1979). Linear AC electrode polarization impedance at smooth noble metal interfaces. *IEEE Transactions BME*, **BME–24 (3)**, 260.

11  Schanne, O.F. & P.-Cerriti, E.R. (1978). *Impedance Measurements in Biological Cells*, J. Wiley and Sons.

12  Bard, A.J. & Faulkner, L.R. (1980). *Electrochemical Methods Fundamentals and Applications*, J. Wiley and Sons.

13  MacInnis, D.A. (1961). *The Principles of Electrochemistry*, Dover Publications Inc.

14  Schwan, H.P. (1966). Alternating current electrode polarization. *Biophysic*, **3**, 181–201.

15  Hoare, J.P. (1968). *The Electrochemistry of Oxygen*, J. Wiley and Sons.

16  Barold, S.S. ed. (1985). *Modern Cardiac Pacing*, Futura Publishing.

17  Feinberg, B.N. & Fleming, D.G. eds, (1978). *Handbook of Engineering in Medicine and Biology*, Sect. B. CRC Press.

18  Koryta, J. ed., (1980). *Medical and Biological Applications of Electrochemical Devices*, J. Wiley and Sons.

19  Pilla, A.A. (1974). Electrochemical Information Transfer. *Annals New York Academy of Sciences*, **238**, 149–69.

20  Schmukler, R., Kaufman, J.J., Maccaro, P.C., Ryaby, J.T. & Pilla, A.A. (1986). Transient impedance measurements on biological membranes: application to red blood cells and melanoma cells. In *Electrical Double Layers in Biology*. Blank, M., ed., Plenum Press.

21  Schmukler, R. (1985). Unpublished observations.

22  Schmukler, R. (1981). A New Technique for Measurement of Isolated Cell Impedance, Eng Sc D Thesis, Columbia University.

23  Schmukler, R. (1989). Measurements of the electrical impedance of living cells in the frequency domain. In *Charge and Field Effects in Biosystems II*, Allen, M.J., Cleary, S.F. & Hawdridge, F.M., eds, Plenum Press, in press.

24  Beard, R.B., DeRosa, J.F., Koerner, R.M., Dubin, S.E. & Lee, K. (1972). Porous cathodes for implantable hybrid cells. *IEEE Transactions BME*, **BME–19**, 233–8.

25  DeRosa, J.F. (1974). Linear AC Electrode Polarization Studies on Solid and Porous Noble Metals, PhD Thesis, Drexel University.

26  Schmukler, R. (1976). Characterization Studies for an Optimal Hybrid Fuel Cell Cathode, MS Thesis, Drexel University.

27  Lee, R.C. (1990). Physical mechanisms of tissue injury in electrical trauma. *IEEE Transactions Education*, **34**(3), 223–30.

28  Bhatt, D.L., Gaylor, D.C. & Lee, R.C. (1990). Rhabdomyolysis due to pulsed electric fields. *Plastic and Reconstructive Surgery*, **86**(1), 1–11.

29  Chilbert, M., Maiman, D., Sances, A., Myklebust, J., Prieto, T.E., Swiontek, T., Heckman, M. & Pintar, K. (1985). Measure of tissue resistivity in experimental electrical burns. *Journal of Trauma*, **25**(3), 209–15.

30  Chilbert, M.A. Evaluation of electrical burn injury using an electrical impedance technique, this volume.

31  Plonsey, R. (1969). *Bioelectric Phenomena*, McGraw-Hill Inc.

32  Rall, W. (1969). Distributions of potential in cylindrical coordinates and time constants for a membrane cylinder. *Biophysical Journal*, **9**, 1509–41.

33  Eisenberg, R.S. & Johnson, E.A. (1970). Three dimensional electric field problems, part A, *Progress in Biophysics and Molecular Biology*, **20**, 5–65.

34  Robillaird, P. & Poussart, Y. (1979). Spatial resolution of four electrode array, *IEEE Transactions BME–*26(8), 465–70.

35  Geddes, L.A. & Baker, L.E. (1975). *Principles of Applied Biomedical Instrumentation*, J. Wiley and Sons.

36  Christian, G.D. (1971). *Analytical Chemistry*, Ginn and Co.

37  Green, R. (1985). For sensitive measurements, use a good electrometer, *Research and Development*, 88–93.

38  Keithley Instruments, Inc., 1985–86 Catalog and Buyer's Guide.

39  Solartron Instruments, 1987–88 Catalog, Model 1260 Impedance Analyzer.

40  Tektronix Instruments, Inc., 1988 Catalog.

41  Riskin, J.R. (6/1979). A user's guide to IC instrumentation amplifiers, *Application Note Analog Devices*.

42  (1977). Grass Medical Instruments, Manual P15 Differential Microelectrode Preamplifier.

43  (1988). EG&G Princeton Applied Research Catalog, Model 113 pre-Amplifier.

44  Amatniek, E. (3/1958). Measurement of bioelectric potentials with microelectrodes and neutralized input capacity amplifiers, *IRE Transactions on Medical Electronics*, PGME–10.

45  Analog Devices, Isolation and Instrumentation Amplifiers Designers Guide, G351a–12.5–11/78.

46  Ott, W.E. (8/1978). Instrumentation amplifiers versatile differential input gain blocks, AN–75, Burr-Brown Corp.

47  Hewlett-Packard Product Note 1726A–3 (2/1983). Bandwidth, probing and precise time interval measurements.

48  Schwan, H.P. (1981). Dielectric properties of biological tissue and biophysical mechanisms of electromagnetic-field interaction. In *Biological Effects of Nonionizing Radiation*, Illinger, K.H., ed., American Chem. Soc., 109–31.

49  Pauly, H. & Schwan, H.P. (1966). Dielectric properties and ion mobility in erythrocytes. *Biophysical Journal*, **6**, 621–39.

# 14

# Analysis of heat injury to the upper extremity of electrical shock victims: a theoretical model

BRADFORD I. TROPEA
RAPHAEL C. LEE

## Introduction

Studies have estimated that 3% of all admissions to hospital burn units are for electrical trauma[1] and most of these injuries are work-related. Based on data accumulated by the Edison Electric Institute[2], the majority of contact voltages for surviving electric utility linemen range from 1 to 10 kilovolts (kV), with the hand-to-hand circuit path being the most frequent path through the body. A 'high-voltage' electric shock can produce massive destruction of tissue and major physiologic imbalances. In electrical trauma victims, extensive injury to peripheral nerve and skeletal muscle is very common, with resultant upper extremity amputation rates as high as 65%[3].

The large electric fields produced by a 'typical' high-voltage shock can produce injury either from heat generated by electrical currents (joule heating)[3,4], cell membrane electroporation[5,6] or both. In the medical community, it is generally believed that the cellular injury is largely mediated by joule heating. The circumstances surrounding electrical shock accidents are so variable that it is nearly impossible to precisely determine the tissue exposure in the majority of cases. The amount of heat generated at a point along the current path depends on the quality and duration of contact, the contact voltage, the properties of the tissue and other variables. Usually, only the contact voltage is known accurately. But even that is not enough because the voltage across the body depends on clothing, shoes, gloves and whether the contact was mediated by an arc. As a result, the amount of heat generated in any one case is very difficult to estimate. The purpose of this project was to perform a worst-case analysis of the heating dynamics of electrical shock and to estimate the resulting tissue damage.

### Thermotolerance of cells

It is known that cells exposed to supraphysiological temperatures cause injury by denaturing macromolecules[7], disrupting cell membranes[7,8] and producing other effects that are potentially fatal to cells. Nearly four decades ago, Moritz and Henriques[9] demonstrated that the heat tolerance of cells was dependent on both temperature and duration of exposure. Henriques[10] demonstrated that the reaction kinetics leading to skin damage resembles a simple first-order chemical rate process described by the Arrhenius equation:

$$k = \frac{d\Omega}{dt} = \Gamma e^{-\frac{E}{RT(t)}}$$ (1)

where $k$ is the rate of accumulation of cell damage, $\Gamma$ is an empirical frequency factor describing the rate of cell damage when $T = \infty$, and $R$ is the universal gas constant. This expression can be used to describe the rate at which cell damage accumulates when exposed to temperature history $T(t)$. $\Omega$ is an arbitrary function of cellular injury which varies from 0 to 1 representing the range from no cellular damage to all cells exposed, respectively. Henriques[10] found that the earliest histologic sign of skin damage (first-degree burn) corresponded to an $\Omega = 0.53$ when he defined full-thickness damage to the epidermis (second-degree burn) as an $\Omega = 1.0$. Figure. 14.1 replots Henriques data indicating the duration of exposure of porcine skin to constant supraphysiologic temperatures needed to cause complete epidermal necrosis ($\Omega = 1.0$).

Over the past two decades, the temperature–time tolerance curves for isolated fibroblasts[7,1], red blood cells[12] and skeletal muscle cells[13] in culture have been reported. Some of these data are replotted in Fig. 14.1. In each case, the kinetics of heat damage could be adequately described by the Arrhenius equation with a single energy of activation. As a result, when the temperature history is known, the Arrhenius equation can be used to predict the kinetics of cellular damage. An expression for the accumulation of heat damage ($\Omega$) can be derived by integrating Equation (1) over the time course of exposure to damaging supraphysiological temperatures to obtain

$$\Omega(t) = \Gamma \int_0^\tau e^{-\frac{E}{RT(t)}} dt$$ (2)

which has been called the 'heat-death equation'.

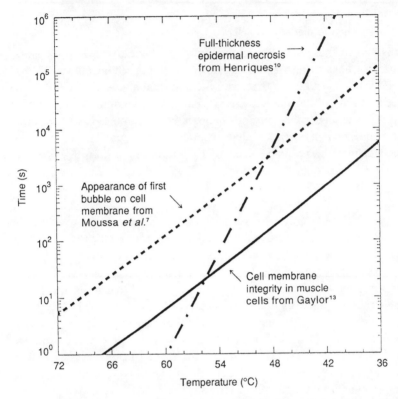

Fig. 14.1. Comparison of the time required to produce irreversible changes in various biomaterials versus temperature. Moussa *et al.*[7] determined the endpoint to be when the appearance of the first bubble occurred on cell membrane of fibroblasts. Gaylor[13] measured a 5% reduction of a carboxyfluorescein diacetate dye in skeletal rat muscle cells. Henriques[10] histologically determined epidermal necrosis. Each of these histological endpoints defines $\Omega = 1.0$. All of these data can be described by the Arrhenius equation. The thermal injury constants ($E$ in KJ/mole, $\Gamma$ in 1/s) for the three protocols: Gaylor ($\Gamma = 2.9 \times 10^{37}$, $E = 244$), Henriques ($\Gamma = 3.1 \times 10^{98}$, $E = 628$), and Moussa ($\Gamma = 9.09 \times 10^{36}$, $E = 249$).

Diller and Hayes[14] and Palla[15] exploited this mathematical description of cellular heat damage kinetics to predict the distribution of burn injury to skin and subcutaneous tissues caused by heating the skin surface. They solved the bioheat equation for the temperature distribution in the tissue as a function of time. They convolved the tissue time–temperature history curves for preselected points in the subcutaneous tissue with Equation (2) to predict the distribution of tissue damage. This led to valuable insight into the factors determining the severity of burns.

In this theoretical study, a quasi three-dimensional finite element model of the human upper extremity was formulated to solve the equations which describe the effects of joule heating on tissue temperature during and following high-voltage electrical shock. The model considered the anatomical distribution and physical properties of the four most abundant tissues (bone, muscle, fat and skin), their respective blood flow rates and boundary air convection. The results from these simulations were utilized along with the heat–death equation to predict the accumulation of cellular damage due only to the effects of joule heating.

### Theoretical model formulation

Because the contact voltage is the only variable accurately known for most electrical trauma cases, the input for the model was a voltage source. Hand-to-hand contact is assumed, as illustrated in Fig. 14.2. As a result of instantaneous breakdown of the epidermal skin barrier in high-voltage shock[16,17], this highly resistive barrier to current passage can be ignored in the calculation of body resistance. The metal–electrolyte contact impedance is a strong function of current frequency and density[18]. For practical purposes, an average contact impedance of 100 ohm may be used as a representative value assuming an interfacial capacitance of 1 $\mu F/cm^2$ and a contact area of 5 $cm^2$. The spreading resistance may be another 150 ohm. The arms and legs have electrical resistances which can be estimated first by assuming a tissue resistivity of 250 ohm/cm and then by solving for the total limb resistance. Reasonable agreement between theory and published experimental values can be obtained[19].

Current distribution in the body will be dependent on location. The current density will be highest at the contact points; the maximum power density is dissipated there. Once the current travels away from the contact points into the subcutaneous tissues, it spreads across the extremity tissues so that the electric field is nearly constant in any cross-sectional plane perpendicular to the current path. Consequently, once away from the contact points, the tissues with the least resistance (i.e. muscle, nerve and blood vessels) will carry the largest current density.

As the first step, the electric field strength in the tissues was calculated. The current path was assumed to be hand-to-hand in an adult male victim in contact with a 10 000 V ac power line, as illustrated in Fig. 14.2. A three-dimensional finite element model of the human arm was constructed to solve for the electrical potential distribution (voltages). ADINAT was chosen as the finite element program[20]. The three-dimensional mesh was based on

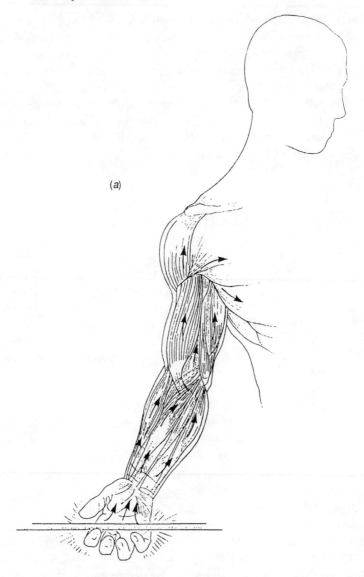

*(a)*

Fig. 14.2. Schematic representation of the current path through the upper extremity in an adult male.

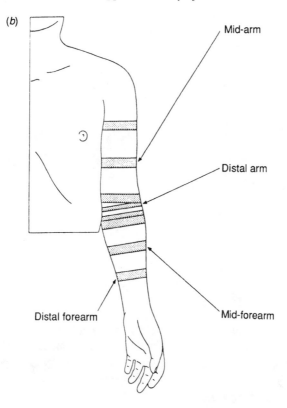

life-size photographs of anatomical cross sections published by Paterson[21], but only incorporated the structure and properties (Table 14.1) of the most abundant tissues: bone, skin, muscle and fat. A 33.5 cm portion of the upper extremity centred about the elbow was based on eight anatomical transverse cross sections, as shown in Figs. 14.2(*b*) and 14.3.

The Laplace equation ($\nabla^2 \Phi = 0$) was solved for the electrical potential distribution throughout the selected arm segment with the boundary conditions:

$$\Phi(x,y,z) = \begin{cases} V \text{ if } z = 0 \\ 0 \text{ if } z = 33.5 \end{cases} \tag{3}$$

where *z* represents the longitudinal axis of the upper extremity, $\Phi$ is the electric potential (voltage) and *V* is the voltage defined as the ratio of the impedance of the modelled segment to the impedance of the total current path multiplied by the input voltage. $z = 0$ is the cross-section located

Table 14.1. *Electrical and thermal properties of human tissues*

| Tissue | Electrical conductivity (s/m) | Thermal conductivity (watt/m °C) | Heat capacity (Joule/m³ °C) |
|---|---|---|---|
| Saline | 1.3 | 0.59–0.66 | $4.13 \times 10^6$ |
| Skin (dry) | $\sim 10^{-4}$ | 0.2 | $3.2 \times 10^6$ |
| Skin (normal) | 0.038 | 0.5–0.6 | $3.6 \times 10^6$ |
| Fat | 0.05 | 0.1–0.4 | $1.98 \times 10^6$ |
| Muscle | 0.4 (L) | 0.385 | $3.8 \times 10^6$ |
|  | 0.14 (T) |  |  |
| Major nerve | 0.47–0.72 (L) | — | — |
|  | 0.083 (T) |  |  |
| Bone cortex | 0.054 | 2.2 | $(4.13 \times 10^6)$ |
| Bone marrow | 0.180 | 0.385 | $\sim 4.14 \times 10^6$ |
| Blood | 0.65 | 0.53 | $\sim 4.14 \times 10^6$ |

*Notes:*
L: Longitudinal to the long axis of the fibres.
T: Transverse to the long axis of the fibres.

approximately 8 cm proximal to the wrist, and at $z = 33.5$ cm is located in the upper arm approximately 5 cm distal to the shoulder. The electric field strength was calculated by linearly interpolating the electrical potential distribution, then calculating the negative gradient of the electrical potential ($\vec{E} = -\Delta\Phi(x,y,z)$).

To avoid modelling the complex geometry of the hand and wrist, they were considered to be 150 ohm lumped resistances in series with the arm and forearm. (The electrical impedance of the tissues at 60 Hz is almost entirely real.) While the electrical properties of muscle are anisotropic[22,23], only the longitudinal conductivity was considered because it was assumed that the current was flowing roughly parallel to the muscle fibres. The voltage drop across the detailed segment of the arm could be calculated from the ratio of its resistance to that of the entire current path.

To determine the thermal response in the upper extremity, the electric field solution described above was used to solve for the temperatures in eight three-dimensional cross sections (Fig. 14.3). The electrical power that is dissipated as heat during ohmic conduction is called joule heating. The joule heating rate per unit volume ($p$, watts/m³) can be calculated from

$$P = J \cdot E \tag{4}$$

where $J$ is the current density (A/m²), and $E$ is the electric field (V/m). Substituting Ohm's law ($J = \sigma E$) into Equation (4),

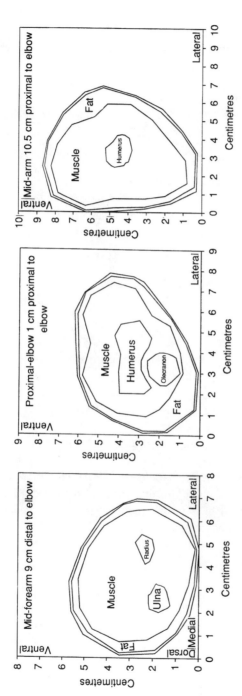

Fig. 14.3. Detailed sketches of three of eight cross sections located in the modelled segment of the human upper extremity are shown. Cross-sectional anatomy is taken from Paterson.[21] Only muscle, fat, bone and skin were included because they represent the bulk of the tissue volume.

$$P = \sigma E^2 \tag{5}$$

where $\sigma$ is the electrical conductivity (mhos/m). The joule heating term is used as the source term in the heat energy balance equation for tissues *in vivo*[24].

The effect of blood flow on the cooling of the tissues was modelled assuming that the blood will leave the control volume essentially at the tissue temperature using the following expression:

$$q_b = \rho_b c_b \omega_b (T_b - T(x,y,t)) \tag{6}$$

where $q_b$ is the convective transport of heat energy per unit volume, $\rho_b$ and $c_b$ are the specific heat and mass density of blood, respectively, and $\omega_b$ is the volumetric blood flow rate through 1 cm$^3$ of tissue. The blood flow rates specific to each tissue[36] were assumed to be constant during, and after, shock.

The addition of the joule heating term (Equation (5)) to the bioheat equation leads to the following heat energy balance equation:

$$\rho c \frac{dT(x,y,t)}{dt} = k \nabla^2 T(x,y,t) + \rho_b c_b \omega_b (T_b - T(x,y,t)) + q_m + \sigma E^2 \xi(t_h) \tag{7}$$

In this expression, $T(x,y,t)$ is the temperature distribution in the various tissues contained in a two-dimensional cross section. $k$ is the tissue specific thermal conductivity (watt/m K), $\rho$ is the tissue specific mass density (kg/m$^3$), $c$ is the specific heat (J/kg) for the respective tissues (Table 14.1). The subscript $b$ refers to blood, and $\omega_b$ is the volume rate of blood perfusion in the respective tissues: muscle, fat, skin and bone (Table 14.2). The third term in this equation describes the convective heat transport of the blood flow. The term $q_m$ represents heat metabolism and $\xi(t_h)$ defines a pulse for $t_h$ seconds so that the cooling phase (postburn) can be modelled. The joule heating term is multiplied by a pulse function, $\xi(t_h)$, which defines the duration of electrical contact, where

$$\xi(t_h) = u(t) - u(t - t_h) \tag{8}$$

ADINAT was used to solve Equation (7) for $T(x,y,t)$ for each of the eight cross sections. Heat conduction in the axial direction, even for bone, was considered negligible, which is justified by considering the relatively long heat conduction time between cross sections in comparison to the calculated temperature dynamics.

Heat flux at the skin–air interface ($q^s$) is the other mechanism of heat

Table 14.2. *Blood flow rates for various tissues*

| Tissue | Blood perfusion rate constant (ml/100 g min) |
|---|---|
| Skin | 9.8–22.0 |
| Fat | 3.75 |
| Muscle | 2.71 |
| Bone cortex | — |
| Bone marrow | 2.71 |

convection away from the extremity. It was assumed to occur at a constant rate at the skin–air interface. Heat flux across the interface has been empirically derived:

$$q^s = h(T_s - T_{air}) \qquad (9)$$

where $T_s$ is the temperature of the surface of the skin and $T_{air}$ is the temperature of the air. The heat transfer coefficient $h$ is $2 \times 10^{-4}$ watts/cm$^2$ °C and was determined originally from experimental measurement of convective transport of heat in air under normal wind conditions[25].

An outline of the boundaries of different tissues for the mid-forearm, proximal elbow and the mid-arm are shown in Fig. 14.3. Only the spatial variation of the tissues and their respective electrical conductivities were pertinent to the three-dimensional potential solution. To establish the mesh used to solve the Laplace equation, sets of 15 nodes were placed at the tissue boundaries and an additional two sets of 15 nodes were placed in the skeletal muscle for a total of 105 nodes for each cross section. A mesh generator created three cross sections between each of the eight original ones to form 29 cross sections. There were 2880 three-dimensional curved elements to satisfy the steady-state potential solution. The electric field for each of the nodes was calculated from this. ADINAT[1] was also used to solve Equation (7) for the upper extremity as previously formulated. However, for this problem 855 nodes were used per cross section (Fig. 14.4). Such a high element density was required because ADINAT does not permit direct solution of Equation (7); it requires the volume convective cooling term (i.e. Equation (6)). This was approximated by choosing small elements and allowing line heat convection. In the limit of infinitesimally small elements, the result would be the same. In practice the approximation is valid as long

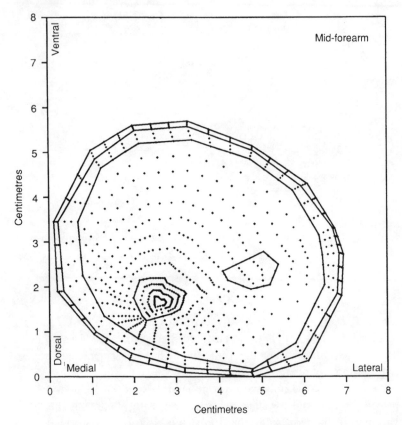

Fig. 14.4. Placement of nodes in one cross section of the forearm. Nodes were placed systematically so that a 3-D model could be formulated.

as the elements are small enough to allow thermal conduction equilibration to occur more quickly than line convection cooling[35,26].

The calculations were carried out for both the heating phase (during electrical contact) and the cooling phase (postburn), which was examined for up to one hour. In the heating phase there were 100 times steps and typically the solution advanced by time step intervals of 0.01 seconds; however, in the cooling phase, the time interval was set to 0.1 seconds for over 35 000 time steps. The duration of each time step was limited to a maximum of 0.1 seconds, because the interval had to be less than the characteristic heat conduction time between the two closest nodes[26]. The closest two nodes in the skin gave a conduction time of 0.26 seconds.

Upon obtaining a solution for $T(x,y,t)$ for each node in the eight cross-

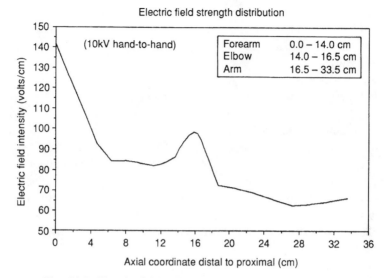

Fig. 14.5. Electric field strength distribution in the upper extremity induced by a 10 kV hand-to-hand contact. Values probably represent worst case predictions.

sections, the duration of electrical contact required to cause an $\Omega = 1.0$ was determined for a node centrally located in the muscle of each cross section. Based on experimental data[27], it was assumed that temperatures at or below 42 °C were not damaging to cells. The two constants ($E$ and $\Gamma$) of Equation (1) for muscle cells were taken from Gaylor[13] and Rocchio[28], who measured the tolerance of mammalian skeletal muscle cells to supraphysiologic temperatures. A modified trapezoidal rule for numerical integration was used to perform the integration of Equation (2). The duration of electrical contact required to produce an $\Omega = 1.0$ was defined as the LT time, meaning the lethal contact time for cell damage. This calculation was performed only for skeletal muscle tissue because of the clinically recognized significance of rhabdomyolysis in the electrical injury problem.

### Results

For a relatively thin adult male electrically in contact with 10 kV from hand-to-hand (Fig. 14.2), this model predicted a variation of the electric field magnitude in the arm between 65 V/cm and 140 V/cm, as shown in Fig. 14.5. Such strong electric fields can cause rapid tissue heating to damaging temperatures in a matter of seconds or cause direct cell damage by electroporation. The field strengths were highest near the wrist and in the elbow where the current density was highest and the resistance was greatest, respectively.

The model predicted that for a 10 kV shock the thermal response of muscle and bone was nearly adiabatic throughout the contact time. This occurs because the joule heating term dominates the heating conduction and correction terms in Equation (7). This is noted in Fig. 14.7 by the constant rate of temperature rise during the 1 second of current passage, where the temperature at the end of 1 second is simply the product of the joule heating term and the duration of current flow divided by the heat capacity, an approximation which would be valid until boiling occurred. The heating in both the skin and fat is not necessarily adiabatic because these tissue layers are much thinner. On the basis of these results, it would appear that joule heating of muscle and bone would be adiabatic for durations exceeding 10 seconds.

It should be noted that the predicted temperature of skeletal muscle is nearly uniform (Fig. 14.6) immediately following the cessation of current flow and that large temperature gradients between both the muscle–bone and muscle–fascia layers are predicted to exist. As expected, the predicted peak temperatures in the muscle varied with the square of the electric field and linearly with the duration of current flow. The model predicts that the peak temperature of the muscle exceeds that of adjacent bone in each cross section. Thus, it appears that, in most cross sections, muscle heats adjacent bone, rather than vice versa as had been commonly believed[29]. Because nerve and blood are the most highly conductive tissues, they would be expected to reach the highest temperatures, were they included in the model. However, they would not get significantly higher because they have small dimensions and would rapidly equilibrate with surrounding tissues. At sufficient distance from the sites of skin contact, the skin temperature does not rise appreciably despite substantial heating of tissues below. This is consistent with the clinical picture that many electrical burn victims manifest. Figure. 14.7 illustrates the relative thermal changes in the centre of muscle tissue at different cross sections of the upper extremity. The distal forearm experiences the most rapid heating. In all of the simulations the blood perfusion rate was maintained constant. Kinetically, the blood flow rate is the single most important variable determining the rate of cooling as illustrated in Fig. 14.8.

The most meaningful insight into the pathogenesis of tissue injury in electrical trauma can be gained by evaluating the prediction of the damage

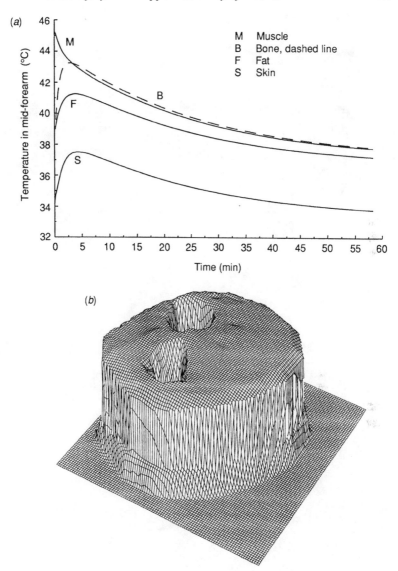

Fig. 14.6(*a*). The dynamics of temperature change in the tissues of the forearm during and following a 1 s, 10 kV pulse. (*b*) Surface plot of the temperature distribution in the mid-forearm at the end of the 1 s current pulse through the arm.

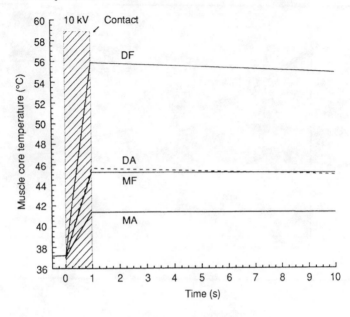

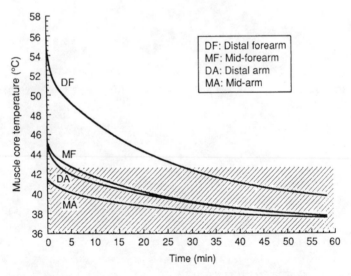

Fig. 14.7. Core muscle temperature of different levels of the upper extremity with a 1 s, 10 kV pulse. The temperature reaches its highest temperature at locations of strong electric field strengths.

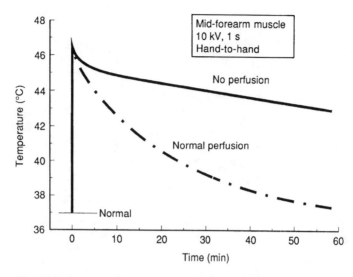

Fig. 14.8. Core muscle temperature of the mid-forearm with a 1 s 10 kV pulse. Comparison of basal blood perfusion (P) versus no perfusion (NP). Without blood flow, it would take significantly longer for the tissues to cool down.

accumulation expression. The lethal contact time (LT) is the duration of exposure to a specified voltage necessary to cause an $\Omega = 1.0$ based on data from Gaylor[13] and Rocchio[28]. They measured the change in membrane permeability which was observed as a 5% decrease in cell fluorescence of a carboxyfluorescein diacetate dye in rat skeletal muscle cells ($\Omega = 1.0$). Their data are replotted in Fig. 14.1. The LT predicted by the model for skeletal muscle tissue in the different anatomical cross sections is shown as a function of contact voltage in kilovolts in Fig. 14.9(a). Thus at a 10 kV hand-to-hand contact, approximately 0.5 second is required to cause muscle damage in the distal forearm, 1.1 seconds in the mid-forearm and more than 1.9 seconds in the mid-arm. Contacts with 20 kV or more would cause almost instant thermal destruction of cells in the distal forearm. Empirically, the LT appears to vary inversely with the voltage squared. Predictions obtained using data from our laboratory[13,28], Moussa *et al.*[7] and Henriques[10] are graphically compared in Fig. 14.9(b). Moussa *et al.* measured the time it took for a bubble to first appear when fibroblasts were exposed to constant elevated temperatures ($\Omega = 1.0$). Their data are also replotted along with Henriques'[10] and Gaylor's[13] in Fig. 14.1. The LT values clearly depend on the thermal injury rate constants. The rate of cellular injury using the results from Gaylor is approximately twice that

(a)

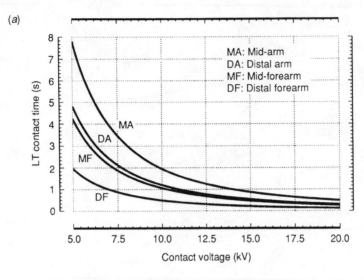

(b)

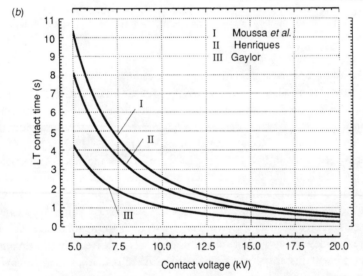

Fig. 14.9(*a*). The LT (lethal contact time) curves for skeletal muscle located in selected cross sections. At times greater than the LT, substantial muscle damage can be expected from heat alone. Thermal injury parameters taken from Gaylor.[13] (*b*) Comparison of the LT curves utilizing the data from Henriques,[10] Gaylor[13] and Moussa *et al.* for skeletal muscle in the mid-forearm.[7]

predicted by Moussa *et al.* or Henriques. However, measurement of dye leakage from cell membranes is more sensitive than the histological endpoints defined by Moussa or Henriques.

### Discussion

Sances *et al.*[30,31] suggested that 10 A was probably the upper limit for a 10 kV to 20 kV contact. Perhaps in most cases of high-voltage electrical accidents there is current passage prior to mechanical contact by arcing from the power source. The muscle contractions generated by the current can set the victim in motion away from the power source[3]. The upper limit to physiological muscle excitation–contraction coupling is in the range of 0.1 seconds. It seems reasonable that typical contact times would be in this range for those victims who never grasp the power source. These complexities add to the difficulty in estimating the magnitude of current flow as well. Perhaps in many, if not most, instances the magnitude is less than that predicted by Sances[31] because the victim may never actually make direct mechanical contact with the power source.

The insight into the pathophysiology of electrical trauma provided by this numerical simulation is clinically useful for understanding the common patterns of injury. Readily appreciated is the similarity between the electric field strength variation and the pattern of tissue injury commonly seen in humans[1,3,29] and in primates[32]. Also, the maximum field strength corresponds to where the current density is highest or where the electrical resistance is greatest, as expected from basic physical laws.

The model appears to be valid as a worst-case approximation of the electric field strength and joule heating magnitude in the human upper extremity during hand-to-hand electric shock. The calculations were performed assuming good electrical contact. It has been demonstrated in animals that, for certain voltage ranges, there is a marked diminution in current over time when current is applied continuously. In one experiment using pigs as an animal model[17], the current precipitously diminished soon after turn-on at voltages below 1000 volts. The higher the voltage, the less time it took for the current to precipitously drop; however, the initial current was proportional to the voltage. This phenomenon is consistent with an earlier publication[33] and can be explained because the charring and drying of the skin at the electrode contact point increase the series resistance to current flow. These same investigators[31] also applied 2100 to 14 400 volts across the hind limbs; however, with these higher voltages, the current did

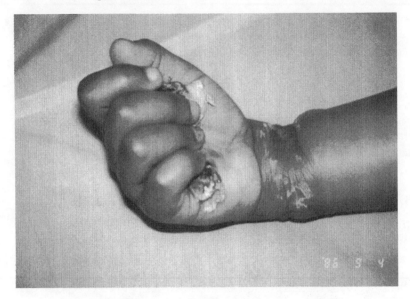

Fig. 14.10. Obvious thermal damage to the skin of the hand and wrist of a child. Note that the skin overlying the muscles which are in spasm (clenched fist) is apparently unharmed.

not precipitously decrease. The skin was vaporized and the current was able to follow a lower resistive pathway.

In addition to joule heating, conduction and convection mechanisms determine the temperature distribution. Because muscle typically occupies the largest cross-sectional area in the upper extremity, its thermal properties dominate other tissues in governing the thermal response. In fact, it appears that heat conduction from muscle to bone is more likely than vice versa. However, it is the bone temperature that remains elevated the longest, because it has the highest thermal capacity. For example, the temperature of the ulna in the mid-forearm continues to rise for approximately 3 minutes following cessation of the current (Fig. 14.6(*b*)). In the same cross section, the temperature in the centre of the fascia continues to rise for almost 4 minutes, primarily due to the conductive effects of the skeletal muscle.

Proximal to the contact point, the temperature of the skin does not rise appreciably and this model predicts that the skin would not be as damaged as the underlying tissues. This is consistent with the clinical picture that some shock victims (see Fig. 14.10) have little skin damage proximal to the contact point, yet there is underlying muscle cell necrosis[1,3]. In many of the simulations, the temperature rise in the skin did not exceed a few degrees and the primary cause was from the conduction of the hotter tissues. A factor inhibiting the temperature elevation of the outer skin was boundary convection, though its effect on the thermal distribution of the deeper tissues was minimal compared to blood perfusion.

Blood flow through tissue is the most important mechanism for transporting heat away from tissues. Traditionally, it had been assumed that the equilibration of the blood temperature with that of the tissues occurs predominantly in the capillaries and small arterioles; however, recent studies have shown that exchange occurs primarily by an incomplete countercurrent heat exchange in arterioles[34]. Blood flow is critical for cooling deep subcutaneous tissues following a high-voltage electrical injury[4,35], (Fig. 14.8). If perfusion is restricted, it will take several hours for the arm to return to basal temperatures. Because there is no conclusive evidence concerning joule heating effects on perfusion rates, the simulation was carried out with normal blood flow rates.

While large arteries influence the rate of heating in their immediate vicinity, they were not included in the model because they do not contribute significantly to general heat flow in the tissue. If there is total occlusion of blood flow, the rate of heat transport out will slow to the point when the arm would probably take many hours to return to normal temperatures. But, if the blood flow is unaltered by the heat, this model predicts normal temperatures are restored in approximately 1 hour. Since the extent of skin damage has been shown to be both time and temperature dependent[9], maintenance of blood flow to the tissues is essential to minimize the damage. There is little information concerning the changes in blood flow following high-voltage injury. The muscle blood flow time constant was assigned to be on the order of 20 minutes, consistent with published resting values[36]. Factory workers and linemen are probably not resting so that the perfusion rate may exceed resting level, which may reduce the amount of damage. In one study of muscle blood flow response to microwave diathermy[37], there was a precipitous increase in blood flow by approximately one order of magnitude when the tissue temperature reached 42–45 °C. In another study, it was shown that the muscle blood flow decreased in rabbit thighs following an electrical shock[38].

It has been shown in many studies that the relationship among thermal tissue injuries can be defined by a simple rate process, an Arrhenius equation[7,10,13]. Henriques determined the degree of epidermal injury by histological methods[10], whereas Moussa *et al.*[7] assumed that damage occurred in HeLa cells about the time when blebs appeared. Investigators in our laboratory[13,28] measured the change in membrane permeability which was observed as a decrease in cell fluorescence of a carboxyfluorescein diacetate dye in rat skeletal muscle cells. Because rhabdomyolysis is such an important clinical feature of major electrical trauma, the magnitude of thermally mediated cellular damage in the upper extremity has been estimated by considering the data of Gaylor[13]. The constants experimentally determined did not investigate the damage response to temperatures below 44 °C, and it may not be appropriate to extrapolate Arrhenius's equation down to basal temperatures. It has been shown in studies that below 42 °C the metabolism of organs is not inhibited, but at temperatures above 42 °C there is progressive decrease in metabolism[27]. Therefore, it was assumed that there was no additional effect on cell necrosis once the temperature fell below 42 °C in all of the simulations.

The LTs are rather disparate in a comparison of both experimental protocols (Fig. 14.9(*b*)); however, it should be noted that in Gaylor's experiment, a 5% reduction in dye fluorescence probably represents a change in the cell permeability, but does not necessarily indicate any permanent sequelae[13]. On the other hand, bleb formation following heat conduction probably represents the cells in a state of irreversible injury, or close to it[7]. Overall, the LT's range between 0.5 and 2 seconds in the upper extremity if a victim comes in contact with a 10 000 V line. In summary, for electrical contacts greater in duration than the LTs, thermal injury to tissue can be anticipated to accompany nonthermal membrane breakdown. For shorter durations, joule heating may not be important other than at the contact points. Further studies using this approach will consider the thermotolerance of other cell types as well as take into account heat conduction in the axial direction.

### Acknowledgements

The authors would like to thank Ms. Teresa Raffaelli for her editorial assistance in the preparation of this manuscript, and Dr Lawrence J. Gottlieb for use of the photograph in Fig. 14.10. This work has been partly supported by The Electrical Power Research Institute; Empire State Electric Energy Research Corporation; EUA Service Corporation; Northeast Utilities Service Corporation; Pacific Gas & Electric Company; Pennsylvania Power & Light Company; the Public Service Company of Oklahoma and the Public Service Electric and Gas Company of New Jersey. Finally, the authors wish to express their gratitude for the excellent care provided to these patients by the residents and fellows of the University of Chicago Hospitals.

**References**

1 DiVincenti, F.C., Moncrief, J.A. & Pruitt, B.A. Jr. (1969). Electrical injuries: a review of 65 cases. *Journal of Trauma*, **9**, 497–505.
2 Edison Electric Institute Safety and Industrial Health Committee Summary Report (1979). *Non-Fatal, Contact Electric Shock and Burn Accidents*, Prepared by: AB Vimont and WB Rich, Kentucky Utilities Company.
3 Butler, E.D. & Grant, T.D. (1977). Electrical injuries with special reference to the upper extremities. *American Journal of Surgery*, **134**, 95–9.
4 Lee, R.C. & Kolodney, M.S. (1987). Electrical injury mechanisms: dynamics of the thermal response. *Plastic and Reconstructive Surgery*, **80**, 663–71.
5 Lee, R.C., Gaylor, D.C., Bhatt, D. & Israel, D.A. (1988). Role of cell membrane rupture in the pathogenesis of electrical trauma. *Journal of Surgical Research*, **44**, 409–19.
6 Lee, R.C. & Kolodney, M.S. (1987). Electrical injury mechanisms: electrical breakdown of cell membranes. *Plastic and Reconstructive Surgery*, **80**, 672–9.
7 Moussa, N.A., McGrath, J.J., Cravalho, E.G. & Asimacopoulos, P.J. (1977). Kinetics of thermal injury in cells. *ASME Journal of Biomechanical Engineering*, **99**, 155–9.
8 Gershfeld, N.L. & Murayama, M. (1968). Thermal instability of red blood cell membrane bilayers: temperature dependence of hemolysis. *Journal of Membrane Biology*, **101**, 62–72.
9 Moritz, A.R. & Henriques, F.C. (1947). Studies of thermal injury II: the relative importance of time and surface temperature in the causation of cutaneous burns. *American Journal of Pathology*, **23**, 695–720.
10 Henriques, F.C. Studies of thermal injury V. *Archives of Pathology*, **43**, 489–502.
11 Mixter, G. Jr., Delhery, G.P., Derksen, W.L. & Monahan, T.I. (1963). The influence of time on the death of HeLa cells at elevated temperatures. In *Temperature: Its Measurement and Control in Science and Industry*. Hardy, J.D. ed. New York: Reinhold.
12 Moussa, N.A., Tell, E.N. & Cravalho, E.G. (1979). Time progression of hemolysis of erythrocyte populations exposed to supraphysiologic temperatures. *ASME Journal of Biomechanical Engineering*, **101**, 213–17.
13 Gaylor, D.C. (1989). Physical Mechanisms of Cellular Injury in Electrical Trauma PhD Thesis, Massachusetts Institute of Technology.
14 Diller, K.R. & Hayes, L.J. (1983). A finite element model of burn injury in blood-perfused skin. *Transactions of the ASME Journal of Biomechanical Engineering*, **105**, 300–7.
15 Palla, R.L. (1981). A heat transfer analysis of scald injury. US Dept. of Commerce NBSIR 81–2320.
16 Hunt, J.L., Sato, R.M. & Baxter, C.R. (1980). Acute electric burns: current diagnostic and therapeutic approaches to management. *Archives of Surgery*, **115**, 434–8.
17 Sances, A., Myklebust, J.B., Larson, S.J., Darin, J.C., Swiontek, T.S.,

Prieto, T., Chilbert, M. & Cusick, J.F. (1981). Experimental electrical injury studies. *Journal of Trauma*, **21**, 589–97.

18  Bard, A.J. & Faulkner, L.R. (1980). *Electromechanical Methods: Fundamentals and Applications*. New York: John Wiley & Sons.

19  Freiberger, H. (1933). The electrical resistance of the human body to d.c. and a.c. currents (Der elektrische Widerstand des menschlichen Korpers gegen technischen Gleich und Wechelstrom). *Electrizitatswirtschaft*, Berlin **32(17)**, 373–5, 442–6.

20  *ADINAT – Automatic Dynamic Incremental Nonlinear Analysis of Temperatures* (1984). Report ARD 84–2, ADINA Engineering, Massachusetts.

21  Paterson, R.R. (1980). *A Cross-sectional Approach to Anatomy*, Chicago: Yearbook Medical Publishers, Inc.

22  Geddes, L.A. & Baker, L.E. (1967). The specific resistance of biological material – a compendium of data for the biomedical engineer and physiologist. *Medical and Biological Engineering*, **5**, 271–93.

23  Poppendieck, H.F., Randall, R., Breeden, J.A., Chambers, J.E. & Murphy, J.R. (1966). Thermal and electrical conductivities of biological fluids and tissues, Reports under Contract No. ONR 4095(00), Geoscience Ltd., Solana Beach, California, specifically: DDC No. Ad 630 712.

24  Pennes, H.H. (1948). Analysis of tissue and arterial blood temperatures in the resting human forearm. *Journal of Applied Physics*, **1**, 93–105.

25  Shitzer, A. & Eberhart, R.C. (1985). Heat generation, storage and transport processes. In *Heat Transfer in Medicine and Biology*. Shitzer, A. & Eberhart, R.C. eds, vol. I, pp. 137–52. New York: Plenum Press.

26  Tropea, B.I. & Lee, R.C. (1992). Thermal injury kinetics in electrical trauma. *ASME Journal of Biomechanical Engineering* (in press).

27  Dickson, J.A. & Calderwood, S.K. (1980). Temperature range and selective sensitivity of tumors to hyperthermia: a critical review. *Annals of the New York Academy of Sciences*, **335**, 180–201.

28  Rocchio, C.M. (1989). *The Kinetics of Thermal Damage to an Isolated Skeletal Muscle Cell*. SB Thesis, Massachusetts Institute of Technology.

29  Bingham, H. (1986). Electrical burns. *Clinics in Plastic Surgery*, **113**, 75–85.

30  Sances, A., Larson, S.J. Mykleburst, J.B. & Cusick, J.F. (1979). Electrical injuries. *Surgery, Gynecology and Obstetrics*, **149**, 97–108.

31  Sances, A., Szablya, J.F., Morgan, J.D., Myklebust, J.B. & Larson, S.J. (1981). High voltage power-line injury studies. *IEEE Transactions Power Apparatus and Systems*, **PAS–100**, 552–7.

32  Daniel, R.K., Ballard, P.A., Héroux, P., Zelt, R.G. & Howard, C.R. (1988). High-voltage electrical injury: acute pathophysiology *Journal of Hand Surgery*, **13(A)**, 44–9.

33  Carter, A.O. & Morley, R. (1969). Effects of power frequency voltages on amputated human limb. *British Journal of Industrial Medicine*, **26**, 224–230.

34  Chen, M.M. (1985). The tissue energy balance equation. In *Transfer in Medicine and Biology*, Shitzer, A. & Eberhart, R.C. eds, vol. I, pp. 193–205, New York: Plenum Press.

35  Tropea, B.I. (1987). A Numerical Model for Determining the Human

Forearm Thermal Response to High Voltage Injury. SB Thesis, Massachusetts Institute of Technology.

36 Eberhart, R.C. (1985). Thermal models of single organs. In *Heat Transfer in Medicine and Biology*, Shitzer, A. & Eberhart, R.C. eds, vol. I, pp. 261–273, New York: Plenum Press.

37 Sekins, K.M. & Dundore, D., Emery, A.F., Lehmann, J.F., McGrath, P.W. & Nelp, W.B. (1980). Muscle blood flow changes in response to 915 MHz diathermy with surface cooling as measured by Xe133 clearance. *Archives of Physical Medicine and Rehabilitation*, **61**, 105–13.

38 Clayton, J.M., Hayes, A.C., Hammel, J., Boyd, W.C., Hartford, C.E. & Barnes, R.W. (1977). Xenon-133 determination of muscle blood flow in electrical injury. *Journal of Trauma*, **17(A)**, 293–8.

# Nomenclature

**Terms**

$c =$ specific heat
$h =$ empirical heat transfer coefficient
$k =$ thermal conductivity of muscle, skin, fat or bone
$q_m =$ heat metabolism
$q^s =$ heat flux at skin–air interface
$t =$ time
$x, y =$ Cartesian coordinates of transverse cross section
$z =$ longitudinal coordinate
$A =$ amperes
$E =$ energy of activation, electric field
$J =$ current density
$LT =$ contact time needed to cause cellular injury
$P =$ power per unit volume
$Q_b =$ convective transport of heat due to blood flow
$R =$ universal gas constant
$T =$ temperature of the tissues
$T_{air} =$ temperature of the air
$T_b =$ temperature of blood
$T_s =$ temperature of surface skin
$V =$ volts
$u(t) =$ step function
$\rho =$ mass density
$\sigma =$ electrical conductivity
$\xi(t_h) =$ pulse for $T_h$ seconds
$\omega_b =$ volume rate of perfusion
$\Phi =$ electric potential
$\Omega =$ arbitrary function of damage accumulation
$\Gamma =$ rate of cell membrane damage at temperature equal to infinity

**Subscripts**

air $=$ air
b $=$ blood
c $=$ conduction
h $=$ heating phase
m $=$ membrane
s $=$ surface
t $=$ tissue

# Part IV:

Biophysical mechanisms of cellular injury

# 15

# Response of cells to supraphysiological temperatures: experimental measurements and kinetic models

ERNEST G. CRAVALHO
MEHMET TONER
DIANE C. GAYLOR
RAPHAEL C. LEE

## Introduction

As shown in Chapter 14, along the track of current flow, there are measurable changes in temperature due to the effect of joule heating. That is, the tissue in the current path presents a finite resistance to the flow of current which, in turn, leads to a local dissipation of electrical energy given by $I^2R$ where $I$ is the local current and $R$ is the electrical resistance measured at the same point. According to the first law of thermodynamics, this energy appears as an increase in the internal energy of the tissue and manifests itself as a rise in the local temperature. Tropea and Lee (Chapter 14) show that these temperature increases can be substantial depending upon proximity to the point of entry and the type of tissue. Because of these elevated temperatures, it is highly likely that the injury experienced by tissue, and hence, the cells that make up the tissue, has two components, one *electrical* and the other *thermal*. It is also just as likely that these two modes of cellular injury can be uncoupled and addressed independently of one another. The only coupling that exists is a consequence of the fact that all the thermodynamic and electrical tissue properties depend upon the local temperature.

In order to develop therapeutic protocols for the treatment of tissue damaged by either of these modes of injury, it is essential to understand both the fundamental mechanisms and the time progression of the injury, i.e. the kinetics of the damage processes. Accordingly, the present chapter attempts to focus on the damage processes associated with elevated temperatures and to develop some models for the description of the dynamics of these processes based upon experimental observations under carefully controlled conditions.

### Background

There have been surprisingly few attempts in the literature to quantify the thermal injury process in spite of the many situations in which cells are exposed to elevated temperatures. Perhaps the earliest attempt to quantify thermal injury was due to Henriques and co-workers who published a series of articles that culminated in a paper describing the cumulative injury to a cell population exposed to elevated temperatures[1]. Henriques and co-workers postulated that the reaction leading to cell death should conform to the well-known Arrhenius description of rate processes. Because they were concerned with injury of the cutaneous surface resulting from elevated environmental temperatures produced by a variety of weapon systems, the results of their study are not directly applicable in the present instance. More recent studies that have focused on populations of cellular suspensions are more relevant[2-9].

All of these studies were similar in that the experimental protocols basically consisted of exposing a suspension of cells to a step change in temperature and then following the time course of cell viability. Cellular injury was assessed according to some previously selected criterion which was often based upon some readily observable feature of the cell (blistering, ghosting, haemolysis, dye permeability) or upon the ability of the cell to grow into colonies. In attempting to apply the results of such studies to a given situation, there is always the problem that different studies use different cell types so that the results of a particular study may not apply in the case of another cell type. Furthermore, even for a given cell type, the results of different studies may not be comparable since the choice of damage criterion is somewhat arbitrary and different studies use different damage criteria.

Although these studies used a wide variety of cell types and damage criteria, all of the data emanating from these studies can be characterized in the Arrhenius format as shown in Table 15.1, namely:

$$\frac{1}{\tau} = Ae^{-E/RT} \tag{1}$$

where $\tau$ is the time in seconds required to satisfy the specific damage criterion used in the particular study, $A$ is the frequency factor in units of $s^{-1}$, $E$ is the activation energy for the damage process in units of kcal/mole, $R$ is the universal gas constant (1.986 kcal/mole K), and $T$ is the thermodynamic temperature in Kelvin.

In spite of the wide variation of cell types and damage criteria, the data of Table 15.1 do show some common features. If the data of Westra and

Table 15.1. *Thermal injury to cells* $\frac{1}{\tau} = Ae^{-E/RT}$

| Cell type | Damage criterion | Temperature range | $A$ (1/s) | $E$ (kcal/mol) (kJ/mol) | References |
|---|---|---|---|---|---|
| HeLa S-3 | Blister formation | 36–68 °C | $9.09 \times 10^{+36}$ | 59.50 (249) | 6 |
| HeLa S-3 | 50% eosin Y-stain | 48.2–65 °C | $8.80 \times 10^{+59}$ | 92.64 (388) | 2 |
| Erythrocytes (Human) | Haemolysis (1%) | 37–45 °C | $4.16 \times 10^{+13}$ | 30.00 (126) | 8 |
| Erythrocytes (Human) | Haemolysis (5%) | 44–60 °C | $7.57 \times 10^{+27}$ | 46.31 (194) | 7 |
| Erythrocytes (Human) | Ghosting | 60–76.6 °C | $1.79 \times 10^{+30}$ | 50.38 (211) | 5 |
| Skeletal muscle | Increased permeability to FADH (5% dye leakage) | 45–60 °C | $1.6 \times 10^{+37}$ | 57.59 (241) | 9 |
| Chinese hamster cells | Grow into colonies (37% reduction in survival) | 43.5–46.5 °C | $3.8 \times 10^{+96}$ | 141 (59) | 4 |
| Pig kidney cells | Grow into colonies (90% reduction in survival) | 45–47 °C | $1.1 \times 10^{69}$ | 105 (441) | 3 |

Dewey[4] and Harris[3] are set aside because of the special nature of their damage criterion compared with criteria used in other studies (cloning ability vs. some measure of membrane behaviour) and the data of Gershfeld and Murayama[8] for reasons that will become apparent shortly, it is noted that the activation energy for the thermal damage process is of the order of 50 kcal/mole (average value of 53.4 kcal/mole) for all the other experiments. The data of Mixter *et al.*[2] are not included since they used a staining technique in which injured cells take up a stain that is excluded by healthy cells. Since the transport of stain through the cell membrane is itself a dynamic process of uncertain kinetics which might possibly obscure the kinetics of the injury process, the large value of 92.64 kcal/mole obtained by Mixter *et al.* is probably misleading. Thus, among diverse experiments that use some sort of measure of membrane integrity as a damage criterion, there is remarkable agreement, particularly with respect to the activation energy of the damage process.

If the data for erythrocytes is considered in detail, it is apparent that the damage due to elevated temperature can be related to some sort of phase transition in membrane proteins. Figure 15.1 shows the summary of erythrocyte injury data reported in the literature[5,7,8,10]. The first two studies reveal an activation energy of approximately 50 kcal/mole, whereas the latter two studies reveal an activation energy of approximately 29 kcal/mole. There also appears to be a transition from the latter to the former at approximately 45 °C.

Kumamoto *et al.*[11] have shown that temperature 'breaks' in Arrhenius plots of this type of data are a consequence of a phase change in the system, the plasma membrane in this case. The observations of Raison and co-workers[12,13] and Chapman *et al.*[14] have confirmed this hypothesis for mitochondrial membranes. Studies of the effects of heat treatment on the elasticity of human red cell membranes by Rakow and Hochmuth[15] have shown that there is, in fact, an irreversible phase transition between 46 °C and 50 °C attributable to irreversible protein denaturation. These findings support the hypothesis that thermal injury (at least in erythrocytes) can be attributed to a phase transition in membrane proteins in the neighbourhood of 45 °C and that for temperatures above this, the membrane has been irreversibly altered in a manner which will lead to cell damage at a rate which increases with temperature according to the Arrhenius formulation.

### Thermal injury in skeletal muscle cells: membrane permeability

Based upon these findings for various cell types, it is reasonable to assume that similar results would be obtained in the case of skeletal muscle cells.

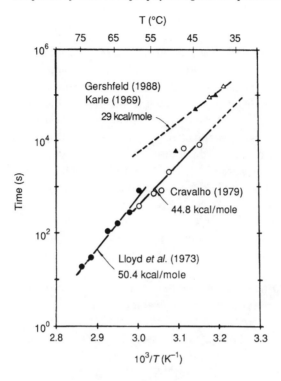

Fig. 15.1. Arrhenius relationship for thermal injury. $A$ is the frequency factor, and $E$ is the activation energy as given by

$$= A \exp - \frac{E}{RT}$$

The value $A = 4.16 \times 10^{13}$ was calculated based on Gershfeld and Murayama results[8] (Fig. 15.2 and $E = 29$ kcal/mole). Haemolysis of 5% of erythrocytes was obtained from Moussa *et al.*[7] (see Fig. 15.1). $A$ and $E$ were predicted by least-squares analysis. Lloyd *et al.*[5] reported their data as an exponential function rather than as the well-known Arrhenius plot. Experimental data were obtained from Fig. 15.4 of Lloyd *et al.* and least-squares analysis was used to predict $A$ and $E$. The value of the frequency factor, $A$, was not reported in Westra and Dewey[4]. This value was estimated from Fig. 15.3 of Westra and Dewey. $A$ and $E$ were determined for 90% mortality data given in Table 15.1 of Harris[3] between 45 °C and 47 °C. Data for 44 °C were not included in the curve fit as suggested by Harris.

Accordingly, an experimental model was developed by Gaylor[9] in which skeletal muscle cells were harvested from the *flexor digitorum brevis* muscle of the hind foot of adult female Sprague–Dawley rats. Muscles excised from sacrificed rats were placed in Dulbecco's modified eagle's medium (DMEM) supplemented with antibiotics. Cells were loosened from the intact muscle with collagenase and washed four times in the supplemented DMEM. Tendons were teased apart and agitated mechanically. The resulting cell suspension was pipetted into petri dishes and cultured at 37 °C in 5% $CO_2$–95% air at 99% humidity.

The isolated cells were 600 to 1200 $\mu$m in length and 15 to 30 $\mu$m in diameter. Several hundred cells were obtained from each digested muscle and could be maintained in culture for at least 1 week. As will be shown subsequently, cells subjected to thermal protocols tended to contract, but this contraction could be prevented by suspending the cells in hypertonic solutions (2 to 3 × normal toxicity). Accordingly, cells were suspended in phosphate-buffered saline with an isotonic concentration of 280 mOsm increased to 840 mOsm by the addition of sucrose which does not penetrate the plasma membrane. In order to assay the integrity of the plasma membrane, cells were loaded by simple diffusion with carboxyfluorescein diacetate (CFDA). The nonfluorescent CFDA penetrates the cell and is hydrolysed in healthy cells to form anionic carboxyfluorescein (CF) which fluoresces brightly and is impermeable to the cell membrane.

The thermal response of cells was measured by placing the cells on a specially designed stage as shown in Fig. 15.2. The temperature of the cell suspension was monitored by means of a thermocouple immersed in the suspension. Temperature was regulated by refrigerant flowing through the chamber at a constant rate and simultaneously dissipating electrical energy at a controlled rate in a heater in thermal communication with the cell suspension. By adjusting the amount of electrical energy dissipated in a programmed fashion, the temperature and rate of change of temperature could be maintained precisely.

As cell membranes became altered structurally by thermal injury, CF leaked from the cells. Hence, by monitoring the intensity of the fluorescent image with the aid of a video image processor as shown in Fig. 15.3, the kinetics of cellular injury could be determined. In a typical experiment, a given cell was monitored at room temperature for 5 minutes to establish baseline levels of cell intensity loss due to natural leakage and bleaching. The temperature of the cell was then raised in 5 seconds to a temperature of 37°, 45°, 50°, 55°, or 60 °C, and the cell was monitored until it lost all, or nearly all, fluorescent activity (cf. Fig. 15.4). From video recordings of the

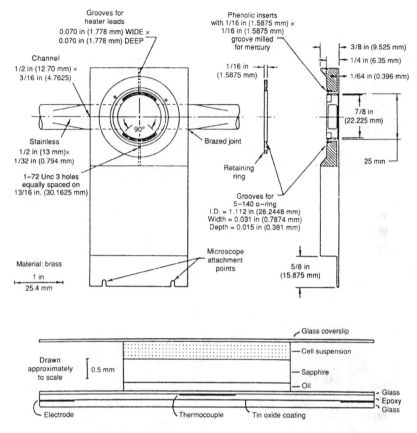

Fig. 15.2. Chamber used to expose isolated skeletal muscle cells to controlled temperature elevations. A flow of cold nitrogen gas cools the chamber. Feedback from thermocouple is used to control the resistive heater. The transparent windows allow real-time observation of the cells.

cell during the protocol, image intensity was measured as a function of time. The data thus obtained are shown in Fig. 15.5 normalized with respect to the intensity at the time the temperature first reached its maximum value.

From the data of Fig. 15.5, an Arrhenius plot can be constructed for the time required for the intensity of the image to reach 50% of its initial value. The results are shown in Fig. 15.6 along with the earlier results of Moussa *et al.*[7]. The results show that the activation energies of the two experiments are identical at 59.50 kcal/mole thereby indicating that the mechanisms of damage are similar and consistent with the hypothesis of irreversible denaturation of membrane proteins.

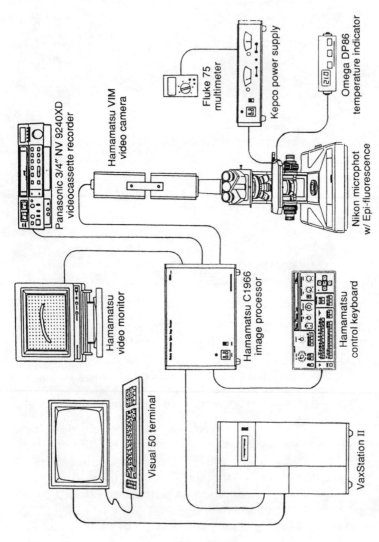

Fig. 15.3. Schematic overview of the system used to observe the response of isolated skeletal muscle cells to elevated temperatures.

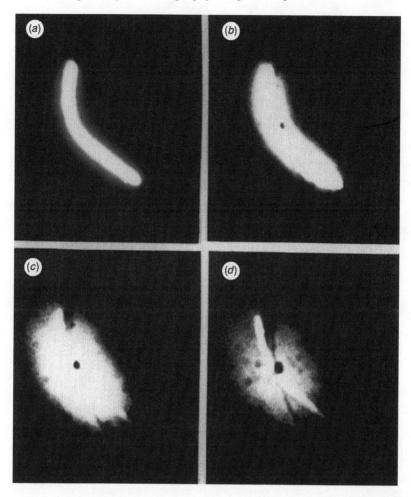

Fig. 15.4. Diffusion of CFDA across a cell membrane of thermally induced increased permeability. The cell was raised to 60 °C in 5 seconds. The high-contrast sequence of photographs shows the dye leakage before the temperature rise, and every 10 seconds for the 30 seconds following the temperature rise. The cell lost all fluorescence intensity within 60 seconds. (*a*) Intact cell at start. (*b*) Dye leakage begins. (*c*) Dye leakage continues. (*d*) Nearly all dye is lost.

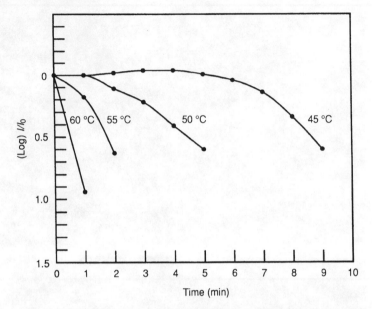

Fig. 15.5. Cell fluorescence intensity as a function of time for cells elevated from room temperature to 45°, 50°, 55° and 60 °C in 5 seconds at the 5-minute mark. The effects of natural dye leakage and bleaching have been subtracted off; thus, a slope of zero indicates the normal membrane permeability.

If it is assumed that the intensity of the fluorescent activity is directly proportional to the number of dye molecules, the intensity can be written as:

$$I = aVc_i \tag{2}$$

where $c_i$ is the concentration of dye inside the cell in moles per unit volume, $V$ is the volume of the cell, and $a$ is a proportionality constant that is a measure of the efficiency with which the dye fluoresces. As the membrane becomes altered, and dye is able to diffuse through it, the intensity of the image changes as the concentration of dye inside the cell changes with time. Thus:

$$\frac{dI}{dt} = aV\frac{dc_i}{dt} \tag{3}$$

But the concentration of dye inside the cell is governed by a conservation equation, namely:

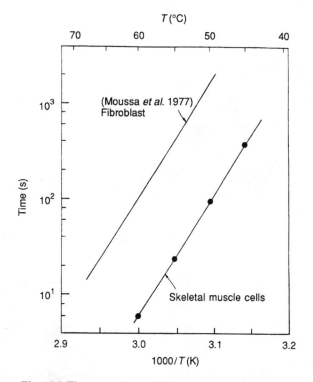

Fig. 15.6. Time to produce 50% dye leakage from isolated muscle cells as a function of the inverse absolute temperature. Fibroblast data are included for comparison[7] and refer to the membrane bleb formation.

$$V\frac{dc_i}{dt} = -PA(c_i - c_o) \tag{4}$$

where $A$ is the plasma membrane surface area, $c$ and $c_o$ are, respectively, intra- and extracellular dye concentrations, and $P$ is the membrane permeability in cm/s. If it is assumed that $c_o < < c$ and that both $V$ and $A$ are constant, the internal concentration of dye becomes:

$$\frac{c_i(t)}{c_o} = \exp\left[-\frac{AP}{V}t\right] \tag{5}$$

Since $A$ and $P$ are constants, an increase in permeability leads to an increased rate of dye loss. If Equation (2) is substituted into this last equation, the behaviour of the intensity with time is obtained:

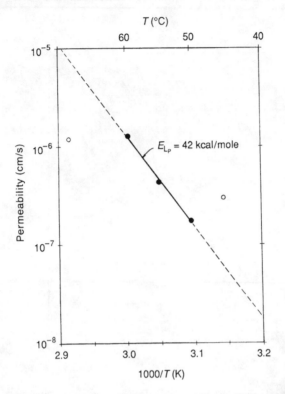

Fig. 15.7. Plasma membrane permeability to CFDA for isolated skeletal muscle cells as a function of the inverse absolute temperature. $E_{L_p}$ is the activation energy for the altered membrane permeability reaction. The open circles represent values which do not fit behaviour of majority of measurements. $L_p$ is the cell membrane filtration coefficient in cm/s.

$$\frac{I(t)}{I_o} = \exp\left[-\frac{AP}{V}t\right] \tag{6}$$

Thus, from the data shown in Fig. 15.5, the value of $P$ at each temperature can be obtained. If a least-squares regression analysis is used on these data, the results depicted in Fig. 15.7 as a function of temperature are obtained. If the permeability is assumed to be of the form:

$$P = P_o \exp\left[-E/RT\right] \tag{7}$$

then, in the temperature range between 45 °C and 60 °C, $P_o = 7.3 \times 10^{21}$ cm/ s and $E = 42.3$ kcal/mole.

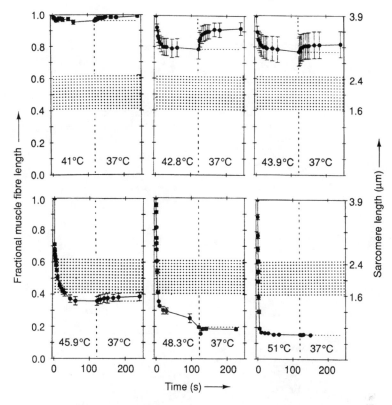

Fig. 15.8. Fractional length of isolated skeletal muscle cells as a function of time at different temperatures between 41° and 51 °C. Also included is the recovery of length change at 37 °C following an elevated temperature treatment for 120 seconds.

## Thermal injury in skeletal muscle cells: mechanical damage

As mentioned previously, it was necessary to suspend the cells in hypertonic sucrose in order to prevent contraction of the cells during thermal insult. Since the contraction itself could be a possible mechanism of damage at elevated temperatures, a series of experiments was conducted to investigate this possibility. Accordingly, cells were suspended in isotonic media containing calcium but no sucrose. The temperature was increased rapidly to its final value in approximately 0.1 s. The ensuing cellular contraction was then recorded and analysed using an image analysis system designed specifically for this purpose.

Figure 15.8 summarizes all of the experiments between 37 °C and 51 °C.

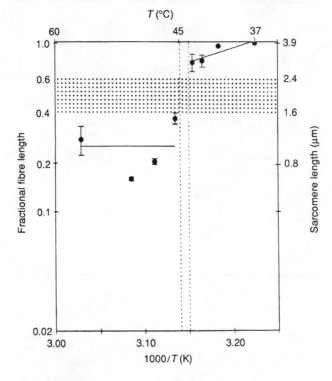

Fig. 15.9. Fractional length of isolated skeletal muscle cells at the end of heat treatment for 120 seconds as a function of the inverse absolute temperature.

This figure shows the time history of the fractional muscle fibre length, i.e. the length of the muscle cell at any instant of time divided by its original length. Each plot is divided into a left half and a right half. On the left half of the figure is plotted the fractional length for a step change in temperature from 37 °C to the temperature shown. On the right half of the figure is plotted the fractional length for a step change in temperature back to 37 °C. Thus, these data for a thermal cycle provide an indication of the ability of the cell to recover from thermal insult.

From these data, it is clear that the kinetic behaviour of contraction is temperature dependent. When the final temperature was in the range of 41 °C to 44 °C, the contraction was reversible, and the cell returned to its original length, either wholly or partially when the temperature was returned to its original value of 37 °C. For final temperatures of 45 °C and above, the contraction was irreversible and no recovery of length was experienced

experienced when the temperature of the cell was returned to 37 °C. If the logarithm of the fractional length is plotted as a function of reciprocal thermodynamic temperature as in Fig. 15.9, it is clear that this kinetic process of contraction exhibits some sort of biphasic behaviour with a break point at approximately 45 °C.

In order to interpret these results, consider a single sarcomere as shown in Figs. 15.10 and 15.11. The resting length of a sarcomere for skeletal muscle cells is 3.19 $\mu$m. At the sarcomere level, this is $L_o$, the initial length. Typically, at a sarcomere length of 2.39 $\mu$m, the thin filaments of the sarcomere will interfere with one another. This situation occurs at a fractional length of $L/L_o = 0.62$. If the sarcomere contracts further to 1.62 $\mu$m, the thick filaments will now become compressed by the Z lines. This occurs at a fractional length of $L/L_o = 0.41$. Thus, for contractions that result in a fractional length in the range 0.62 to 0.41, it is likely that mechanical damage has occurred to the muscle fibre. Certainly, contractions resulting in a fractional length less than 0.41 should be damaged irreversibly.

From Fig. 15.8, it appears that final temperatures in the range 41 °C to 44 °C result in reversible (partially or wholly) contractions. Thus, cells at these temperatures were not damaged mechanically. However, Fig. 15.8 shows that at final temperatures in excess of 44 °C, the cells have contracted beyond the mechanical limit corresponding to the compression of the thick filaments by the Z lines. Thus, cells at temperatures in excess of 44 °C have experienced irreversible mechanical damage.

From the data of Fig. 15.8, those times at which the contraction reached 63% of its maximum value, i.e. the time required for the fractional length to be within 37% of its final value, can be determined. This time is known as the time constant of the contraction process. If the logarithm of the time constant is now plotted as a function of reciprocal temperature as in Fig. 15.10, a linear correlation is obtained with a correlation factor of 0.996. The activation energy for this process is 29 kcal/mole.

How then, does this information relate to the normal excitation–contraction coupling which is usually triggered by an action potential in the plasma membrane of the muscle fibre? As is well known, this action potential triggers the release of calcium ions from the lateral sac of the sarcoplasmic reticulum. The calcium, in turn, binds to troponin, removing the blocking effect of tropomyosin and thereby initiating contraction through the movement of cross-bridges between the actin and myosin filaments (cf. Fig. 15.11). From the point of view of absolute reaction rate theory, the contraction process is modelled as a rate process with two

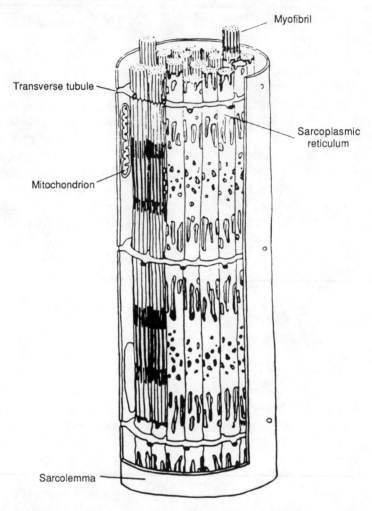

Fig. 15.10. Schematic diagram of internal organelles of an isolated skeletal muscle cell.

energy barriers: the first barrier corresponds to the diffusion of calcium ions from the sarcoplasmic reticulum to the troponin and has an activation energy on the order of 19 to 20 kcal/mole; and the second barrier corresponds to the closing of the bridge, the splitting of ATP, and the conformational transition of tropomyosin and has an activation energy of approximately 15 to 16 kcal/mole. These activation energies do not add simply since the two steps are not simply in series.

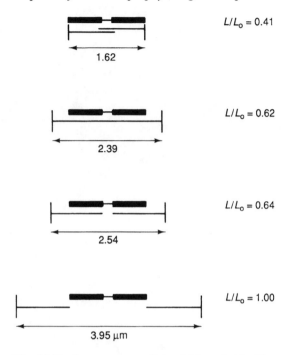

Fig. 15.11. Arrangements of the thick and thin filaments at different sarcomere lengths for skeletal muscle cells.

Thus, the observed activation energy of 29 kcal/mole is of a magnitude which is consistent with this rate model of the contraction process. What is unclear at this time is the reason why the process is irreversible when the stimulus is of thermal origin but reversible when triggered by an action potential. Perhaps the thermal insult has disrupted the carrier-mediated active transport system that pumps the calcium ions from the cytosol into the lumen of the reticulum. On the other hand, the situation may be more akin to *rigor mortis* in that the thermal insult does not provide sufficient energy to complete the calcium transport cycle. That is, once the myosin cross-bridges are bound to the actin, there is not enough ATP to bind the actin and dissociate the cross-bridge from the thin filament. Clearly, further research is required in order to complete the picture.

**Thermal injury in skeletal muscle cells: applications**

Thus far, the work has shown that thermal insult to skeletal muscle cells is a consequence of two injury mechanisms with very different time constants.

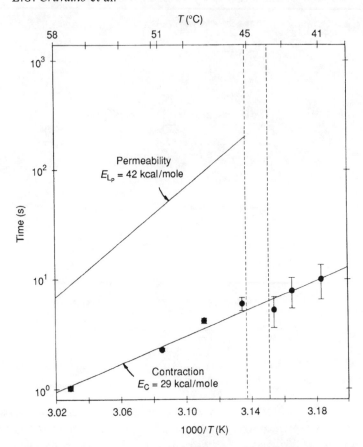

Fig. 15.12. Time to produce 50% contraction of isolated skeletal muscle cells as a function of the inverse absolute temperature. Data from Fig. 15.6 are also included for comparison purposes.

From Fig. 15.12, it is apparent that if the duration of thermal insult is of the right magnitude, say 60 s, only the mechanical damage mechanism associated with contraction will be activated. Thus, isolated skeletal muscle cells will be damaged first by mechanical compression of the thick filaments by the Z lines rather than by membrane protein denaturation. To test this hypothesis, cells were loaded with carboxyfluorescein in isotonic solution at 37 °C and subjected to a step change in temperature to 45 °C. Image analysis showed that there was no dye leakage after the cells collapsed. Thus, the cell membranes were not damaged, but irreversible mechanical damage had occurred.

Finally, the experimental evidence of Figure 15.8 suggests that some of the mechanical damage can be reversed in those situations in which the final temperature was in the range 41 °C to 44 °C. Figure 15.8 shows fractional recovery experienced by isolated skeletal muscle cells upon returning the temperature of the suspension to 37 °C after 2 min of exposure to the elevated temperature. Clearly, total or partial recovery occurred only for maximum temperatures of 41 °C to 44 °C. For maximum temperatures of 45 °C and higher, damage was permanent. The present experimental evidence is not sufficient to quantify the mechanism of partial damage or loss of recovery at temperatures in the range 41 °C to 44 °C. It is possible that, for exposure times long enough to initiate mechanical damage, but too short to produce denaturation of membrane proteins, there is a transition zone such that thermal histories with resulting minimum sarcomere length (normalized) that lie within this zone will experience partial recovery upon return to normal temperatures. Thermal histories outside this zone will result in either complete recovery or no recovery. It must be borne in mind, however, that this sort of behaviour may be singular to isolated skeletal muscle cells. The behaviour of cells *in vivo* may be tempered to a great extent by the support of the extracellular matrix and surrounding cells. Clearly, further research needs to be done in this area.

### Conclusion

Experimental evidence has been presented here that suggests that there is more than one single mechanism responsible for thermal injury to isolated skeletal muscle cells. For exposure temperatures in excess of 45 °C, initial damage is caused by excessive contraction leading to compression of thick filaments by Z lines. At a later time, damage to the plasma membrane occurs by denaturation of membrane proteins. For exposure temperatures in the range 37 °C to 44 °C, mechanical damage is wholly or partially reversible and disruption of the membrane structure with formation of membrane defects may be dominant with disruption of the actin–myosin interaction playing a lesser role. The existence of a break point at 45 °C is consistent with existing data for phase transitions in membrane components.

### References

1 Henriques, Jr., F.C. (1947). Studies of thermal injury. *Archives of Pathology*, **43**, 489–502.
2 Mixter, G., Jr., Delhry, G.P., Derksen, W.L. & Monahan, T. (1963). I. The influence of time on the death of Hela cells at elevated

temperature. In *Temperature: Its Measurement and Control in Science and Industry*, Hardy, J.D., ed., vol.3, Reinhold.

3  Harris, M. (1966). Criteria of viability in heat-treated cells. *Experimental Cell Research*, **44**, 658–61.

4  Westra, A. & Dewey, W.C. (1971). Variation in sensitivity to heat shock during the cell-cycle of Chinese hamster cells *in vitro*. *International Journal of Radiation and Biology*, **19**, 467–77.

5  Lloyd, J.J., Mueller, T.J. & Waugh, R.E. (1973). On in-vitro thermal damage to erythrocytes. *ASME Paper No. 73–WA/Bio. 33, ASME*.

6  Moussa, N.A., McGrath, J.J., Cravalho, E.G. & Asimacopoulos, P.J. (1977). Kinetics of thermal injury in cells. *Journal of Biomechanical Engineering*, **99**, 155–9.

7  Moussa, N.A., Tell, E.N. & Cravalho, E.G. (1979). Time progression of hemolysis of erythrocyte populations exposed to supraphysiological temperatures. *Journal of Biomechanical Engineering*, **101**, 213–17.

8  Gershfeld, N.L. & Murayama, M. (1988). Thermal instability of red blood cell membrane bilayers: temperature dependence of hemolysis. *Journal of Membrane Biology*, **101**, 67–72.

9  Gaylor, D.C. (1990). Electrical Field Effects on Isolated Skeletal Muscle Cells, PhD, Thesis, Dept. of Electrical Engineering, MIT, Cambridge.

10  Karle, H. (1969). Effect on red cells of a small rise in temperature: in-vitro studies. *British Journal of Haematology*, **16**, 409–19.

11  Kumamoto, J., Raison, J.K. & Lyons J.M. (1971). Temperature 'breaks' in Arrhenius plots: a thermodynamic consequence of a phase change. *Journal of Theoretical Biology*, **31**, 47–51.

12  Raison, J.K., Lyons, J.M., Mehlhorn, R.J. & Keith, A.D. (1971). Temperature-induced phase changes in mitochondrial membranes detected by spin labeling. *Journal of Biological Chemistry*, **246**, 4036–40.

13  Raison, J.K., Chapman, E.A. & White, P.Y. (1977). Wheat mitochondria: oxidative activity and membrane lipid structure as a function of temperature. *Plant Physiology*, **59**, 623–7.

14  Chapman, E.A., Wright, L.C. & Raison, J.K. (1979). Seasonal changes in the structure and function of mitochondrial membranes of artichoke tubers. *Plant Physiology*, **63**, 363–6.

15  Rakow, A.L. & Hochmuth, R.M. (1975). Effect of heat treatment on the elasticity of the human erythrocyte membrane. *Biophysical Journal*, **15**, 1095–100.

# 16

# Cell membrane rupture by strong electric fields: prompt and delayed processes

JAMES C. WEAVER

### Introduction

Exposure of cells to strong electric fields can cause both reversible and irreversible cell membrane behaviour through the occurrence of transient pores. Such pores now are believed to occur whenever the transmembrane potential, $U(t)$, reaches values somewhat above normal resting potentials, and have been observed over the range 200 mV $< U(t) < 1500$ mV. Although the terminology relating to strong field effects has changed as understanding has developed, here the term 'electroporation' is used to refer to the occurrence of significant membrane pores due to electric fields. Once formed, the transient pores can have a variety of consequences, including both reversible and irreversible membrane phenomena. The irreversible event of rupture may occur by two quite different processes. A prompt rupture process occurs in planar bilayer membranes. A hypothesis for cell membrane rupture is that a portion of a cell membrane can experience this type of rupture if the boundaries of that portion interact with cell structures such as a cytoskeleton. In an artificial planar bilayer membrane, the prompt rupture of the cell membrane arises from the immediate interaction of an elevated transmembrane potential with transient aqueous pores. The rapidly changing pore population leads to the formation of one or a small number of supracritical pores, i.e. pores with radii greater than a critical radius, $r_c$, which then expand until the membrane is destroyed. The second, a delayed rupture, may arise from physiochemical consequences of persistent smaller pores which arise in a different way from the pore population if reversible electrical breakdown (REB) occurs. Persistent or metastable pores may lead to unrelieved chemical imbalances, and to osmotic pressure differences which rupture the cell membrane. In short, two very different processes may lead to cell membrane rupture due to electroporation. This discussion reviews the

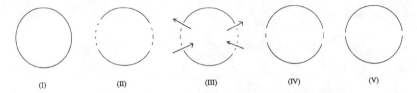

(I)             (II)             (III)           (IV)            (V)

Fig. 16.1. Illustration of qualitative sequence of electroporation events. A brief description of these events is given in the text. An isolated spherical cell is assumed, as this is a good approximation to the usual experimental arrangement of a cell suspension. (I) Cell prior to electrical exposure. (II) Pulse applied; significant pores appear ($\mu$s). (III) Ionic conduction of small ions simultaneously begins, and rapidly discharges the cell transmembrane voltage (reversible electrical breakdown = REB). This concludes within $10^{-4}$ s, and transient pores shrink within ms. (IV) Some pores persist for seconds to hours, allowing uptake of molecules (the transient, but persistent high permeability). Cells begin to swell if in hypotonic medium. (V) An electroporated cell is now highly stressed, may have a few persistent pores, and attempts to recover. Cells either lyse due to processes secondary to pore formation, or repair the perforated membrane and return to their initial state.

present understanding of electroporation mechanism, and describes the two possible rupture mechanisms.

### Electroporation background

Electroporation is believed to be a universal phenomenon, which occurs in bilayer-containing membranes if the transmembrane potential exceeds about 200 mV[1,2]. Much recent emphasis has focused on the use of electroporation to introduce genetic material into cells otherwise difficult to transform[3]. Other interest in electroporation relates to the introduction of other macromolecules into cells[4,5], and to cell killing[6]. Further, although essentially all of the studies to date have emphasized isolated cell electroporation, interest in tissue electroporation has recently emerged, with findings of both damaging behaviour[7,9] and nondamaging behaviour[10].

The essential features of cell membrane electroporation, as presently understood, are summarized in Fig. 16.1, for which electroporation of an isolated spherical cell membrane is illustrated[11]. As suggested by this qualitative sequence, electroporation-related phenomena can be placed into two categories: (a) early events that occur while the transmembrane potential is elevated above normal physiological values, and (b) events that occur after the transmembrane potential has returned to physiological or lower values. It is believed that prompt cell membrane rupture may occur during (a), and that a delayed rupture may occur during (b). In either case, a population of transient aqueous pores is believed to lead to membrane rupture. Before proceeding to discuss these two processes, a brief discussion of the sequence electroporation-associated events is worthwhile.

Broadly, two types of measurements, electrical and molecular transport, are made in studies of electroporation. Electrical measurements are readily made on artificial planar bilayer membranes, and most of the detailed information concerning electrical behaviour derives from them[12-18] (Figs 16.2 and 16.3). The surface-to-volume ratio based on the membrane area and the chamber volume is usually unfavourable for molecular flux studies, as the transported molecules would be diluted by the relatively large volume of liquid which bathes the membrane. The opposite case holds for cells and vesicles, which have large surface-to-volume ratios. Fluxes of molecules and ions result in larger chemical concentration changes within the liquid volumes (intracellular or extracellular), and are more readily measured. For this reason, cells and vesicles are well suited to studies of the movement of molecules and labelled ions across the membranes. In contrast, electrical measurement is difficult, because access to the inside of a cell or vesicle requires penetration by a microelectrode[19], or the use of membrane potential fluorescence dyes[20].

### Brief description of electroporation events in an isolated cell

The following sequence of events is believed to occur for an isolated, spherical cell, starting with the time that a pulse is applied.

1 A 'high voltage' pulse of magnitude $\Delta\phi$ is applied across two electrodes (assumed to be the usual configuration of parallel planes of separation $L$) which contain a cell suspension. The resulting nominal electric field is $E_{nominal} \equiv \Delta\phi/L$, but this is not necessarily the field actually experienced by the cells[21,22]. Instead, an electric current, $I(t)$, flows within the aqueous electrolyte comprising the suspending medium. The corresponding current density is $j(t) \equiv I(t)/A_{electrodes}$ where $A_{electrode}$ is the macroscopic surface area of one of the two electrodes. There is an associated electric field, $E_e = j/\sigma_e$, where $\sigma_e$ is the electrical conductivity of the medium. Generally, $E_e \leqslant E_{nominal}$, because significant potential drops can occur at the electrode–electrolyte interface[23].

2 The transmembrane potential, $U(t)$, increases rapidly, with $U(t)$ having different values at different sites on the cell membrane. For

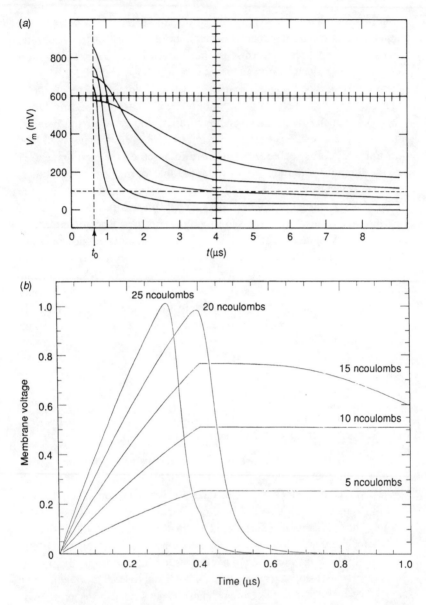

Fig. 16.2. Comparison of experimental and theoretical behaviour for REB caused by charge injection. (*a*) Experimental results showing $U(t)$ *after* the $0.4\,\mu s$ pulse terminates.[12] (*b*) Theoretical behaviour of the transmembrane potential $U(t)$ during REB caused by electroporation as the result of a charge injection protocol that introduced $Q_{inject} = 20$ ncoulomb during a $0.4\,\mu s$ square pulse.[27] The model explicitly involves a dynamic pore

a spherical cell at low values of $U(t)$, the relationship between the applied field and the change in transmembrane potential, $\Delta U(t,\theta)$ at different sites on the membrane is given by the well-known approximate relation[24]:

$$\Delta U(t,\theta) \approx 1.5 E_e(t) R_{cell} \cos\theta \qquad (1)$$

Here $R_{cell}$ is the cell's radius, and $\theta$ is the angle between the direction of $E_e$ and the site on the membrane under consideration. The maximum change occurs at the poles ($\cos\theta \pm 1$), yielding the widely used estimate:

$$\Delta U(t)_{max} \approx 1.5 E_e(t) R_{cell} \qquad (2)$$

If the cell's resting transmembrane potential prior to application of $E_e$ was $U_0$, then $U(t) \approx U_0 + \Delta U(t)$, an estimate which neglects the perturbation of the resting potential by the changes in permeability caused by electroporation. Dramatic electroporation effects are believed to occur if $\Delta U(t)_{max}$ reaches values of about 200 mV to 1500 mV.

3 Some types of membrane openings (pores) rapidly develop in the sense that large numbers and/or large sizes of transient aqueous pores appear if 200 mV $< U(t) <$ 1500 mV. A wide range of pore sizes is likely[25-27]. Such pores are generally capable of passing both ions and molecules, but the specificity and size cutoff change with time as the pore population evolves in response to $U(t)$. In addition to small ions and molecules, macromolecules such as proteins and DNA, or small particles such as latex beads or viruses, may begin to cross the membrane at this stage.

4 If $U(t)$ reaches a larger value, often approximately 500 mV, reversible electrical breakdown (REB) occurs by massive ionic conduction through pores (Fig. 16.2). A very rapid decrease in membrane resistance, $R(t)$, therefore occurs, but the membrane capacitance, C, hardly changes. As a result, the membrane is rapidly discharged, with an approximate RC time constant governed by the changing $R(t)$. Essentially complete discharge is usually obtained within $10^{-3}$ s, often within $10^{-5}$ s[12,25-27].

*Caption for Fig. 16.2 (Cont.)*
population, in which pores of many sizes are transiently present. Five values of $Q_{inject}$ were used (5 ncoulomb to 25 ncoulomb), with the 20 ncoulomb corresponding approximately to a threshold for REB. This result agrees reasonably with experimental results.[12]

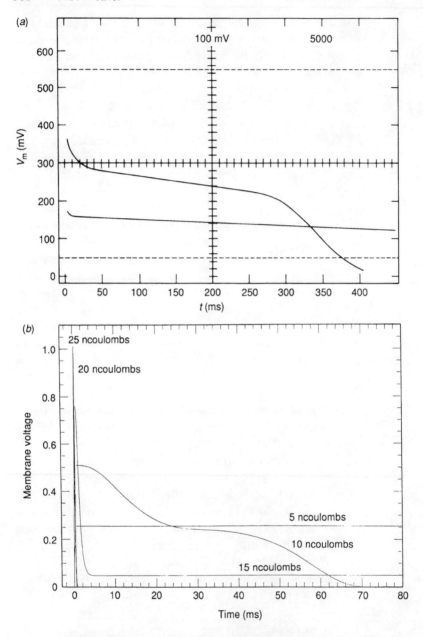

Fig. 16.3. Comparison of experimental and theoretical $U(t)$ for rupture for a moderate 0.4 $\mu$s pulse. (*a*) Experimental behaviour associated with rupture, with the characteristic sigmoidal decay curve for $U(t)$.[12] (*b*) Theoretical behaviour of the transmembrane potential $U(t)$ during rupture, a mechanical destruction of a membrane caused by electro-

5 The temperature, $T$, of the medium rises at a tremendous rate (e.g. of the order of $10^5$ deg $s^{-1}$). However, the actual temperature change is often negligible (e.g. 1 °C), because of the short duration of the applied electric field or current. In this sense, electroporation is a nonthermal event.

6 A transient high permeability state has developed. The elevated permeability persists long after $U(t)$ has decayed to zero, often for seconds or longer, with the time dependence apparently depending on cell type and on temperature. This high permeability appears to allow transport of all types of ions and molecules, ranging from ubiquitous small ions to macromolecules. The maximum size of transported entities is not yet known, nor is the time-range at which high permeability for the larger molecules vanishes. It is also not at all clear whether or not pores alone can account for the transport of small particles, but it is likely that one or a small number of metastable pores can account for considerable macro-molecular transport by hindered diffusion[28,29].

7 Membrane recovery begins to occur as $U(t)$ first begins to decrease, which begins to relieve the expanding pressure associated with $E_m^2$.

*Caption for Fig. 16.3 (Cont.)*
poration.[27] The membrane is that of Fig. 16.2, but with a longer time-scale. Although the time-scale is different, the theoretical behaviour is otherwise in good agreement with experiment.[12] Four distinguishable types of behaviour are evident in Figs. 16.2 and 16.3: (1) For small injected charge (5 ncoulomb) the membrane charges to a moderately low voltage (here 230 mV), which is retained for a long time on the scale of the experiment. This essentially passive membrane charging results because few pores exist which have grown large enough to conduct significantly, and the membrane resistance therefore remains too large to rapidly discharge the membrane. In addition, there are no large pores, so membrane rupture does not occur. (2) For larger $Q_{inject}$ (10 ncoulomb) the membrane develops more larger pores, and an initial slow discharge begins, levels off after about 20 $\mu$s, and then begins again as one or more pores have surpassed the critical size, and have begun to expand until the membrane ruptures. (3) For still larger $Q_{inject}$ (15 ncoulomb), an incomplete REB is found, in which the membrane initially has sufficient pores (and corresponding large conductance) to discharge rapidly, but the pores' sizes and numbers are marginal, so that upon partial discharge enough pores shrink and/or disappear that the conductance diminishes, discharge halts, and the membrane is left with $U > 0$ (in this case about 230 mV). (4) For even larger $Q_{inject}$ (20 and 30 ncoulomb), complete REB occurs as sufficient pores exist transiently to completely discharge the transmem-brane potential to zero, even though all pores shrink and some pores disappear during the discharge. Overall, this description of four dis-tinguishable membrane fates is in good agreement with experimental results.[12]

Initial recovery is believed to be rapid[27], but, after essentially complete discharge of the membrane by REB, some pores shrink and/or disappear much more slowly. As pores shrink, the cell membrane excludes smaller and smaller molecules and ions. Persistent pores, even very small pores which can pass small ions, may cause long-term cell stress and, eventually, cell lysis[30-32].

8  An electroporated cell usually becomes highly stressed, through the loss of vital intracellular compounds, and also through an influx of extracellular compounds. This intracellular and extra-cellular exchange continues, with a time varying molecular cut-off interposed, until membrane recovery is complete. For this reason, the composition of the suspending medium is believed to be important, with minimization of intracellular and extracellular differences relevant. As a result of chemical imbalances, a variety of cellular functions can become temporarily or permanently disrupted. Electroporation-induced cell stress is presently poorly understood, but is crucial to understanding the conditions for cell death and cell survival.

9  Cells often recover completely, so that survival can occur in a significant percentage of electroporated cells. Other cells die, apparently because of delayed effects such as osmotic lysis[30], or the unrelieved demands on metabolic systems because of membrane shunting by persistent pores. Surviving cells can retain the electroporatively introduced molecules if the molecules do not permeate the recovered membrane and are not degraded intracellularly[4,33,34].

Many of the electroporation studies have been carried out on erythrocytes or their ghosts[33,35,36], and it should be noted that RBC ghosts, when osmotically stressed, exhibit unusual recovery[37]. Many other studies have used artificial planar bilayer membranes[12,14 17,38,39] which contain no membrane proteins and are not interacting with other cell constituents. For this reason, inferences made from RBC ghost and artificial planar bilayer membrane experiments may not be applicable to cells generally. Finally, although application of electroporation to gene transfer has involved many types of cells and protoplasts[1-3], these experiments yield only the biological endpoint of transformation, and therefore reveal little about electroporation events themselves (e.g. amount of molecular uptake, kinetics of membrane recovery). Overall, therefore, understanding of electroporation of isolated cells remains incomplete.

## Electroporation of artificial planar bilayer membranes

A typical apparatus consists of a macroscopic (e.g. $10^{-2}$ cm$^2$) membrane separating two chambers, with both sides of the membrane easily accessible to electrodes for stimulating and measuring. One advantage of electrical measurements is their ability to continuously follow rapidly changing behaviour. For this reason, present understanding of early electroporation events derives mostly from electrical measurements of both the transmembrane potential, $U(t)$, and the membrane conductance, $G(t)$ (or its inverse, the membrane resistance, $R(t)$). By use of electrical measurement, behaviour occurring from 100 nseconds to seconds can be determined. The membrane can be regarded as a capacitor, C, which remains unchanged by the altered transmembrane potential, $U(t)$, and a conductance, $G(t)$, which changes dramatically because of electroporation.

Two types of experiments should be distinguished, charge pulse and voltage clamp[27,40]. In charge pulse experiments, a current, $I(t)$, often a square wave pulse, is applied to the electrodes, and at the end of the pulse a switch is opened, disconnecting the current source. The membrane charges because of $I(t)$, but cannot discharge except through the membrane once the switch is opened. The charge accumulated on the membrane results in an altered $U(t)$, which in the case of electroporation rapidly changes due to pores causing $G(t)$ to dramatically change. Charge pulse electroporation studies are particularly well suited to short time scales[12,14,16].

In voltage clamp experiments, a potential difference, $U_i(t)$, often a series of square waves, is applied across the membrane. The resulting current, $I(t)$, is measured, which is the sum of the current which charges the membrane, and the current which flows through the membrane conductance, $G(t)$. Voltage clamp electroporation studies are particularly well suited to relatively long time-scales, e.g. $10^{-3}$ seconds and longer. A theoretical model based on average pore size, and not the complete pore population, is in good agreement with these measurements[13,15,17,18].

The short time-scale charge pulse studies are particularly interesting, because the electrical behaviour is particularly dramatic, and also because a theoretical model involving a complete pore population is needed to describe different types of behaviour in the same membrane. This has provided insight into the behaviour of the transient aqueous pore population, as the pore population cannot itself be observed directly. In charge pulse experiments, four distinguishable membrane fates have been observed (see Table 16.1).

An important aspect of these four possible fates is that they can occur in

Table 16.1. *The four distinguishable fates of artificial planar bilayer membrane as the applied square wave pulse amplitude is increased for fixed pulse width*[12,27].

| General feature | Pulse magnitude |
| --- | --- |
| • Charging of membrane; very slow discharge | Small pulse |
| • Prompt rupture with sigmoidal discharge curve | Moderate pulse |
| • Incomplete reversible electrical breakdown | Large pulse |
| • Reversible electrical breakdown (REB) | Still larger pulse |

the same membrane simply by altering the properties of the applied pulse (Figs 16.2 and 16.3).

### Electrical behaviour: rupture in planar bilayer membranes

Electroporation can cause nonthermal rupture, i.e. prompt destruction, of artificial planar bilayer membranes through runaway expansion of supracritical pores[13,27,41-43]. It is conjectured that partial rupturing of cell membranes may occur similarly. Although the closed membrane of a cell or vesicle is not completely vulnerable to the unbounded expansion of pores[44], if portions of the cell membrane are attached to essentially permanent (on the time-scale of interest) cell structures, then a portion of the cell membrane may behave similarly to a planar membrane. That is, a portion of a cell membrane may rupture, leading to an essentially permanent loss of a portion of the cell's membrane. Alternatively, creation of one or a small number of large pores may result in 'pore trapping', with many of the same, destructive consequences for the cell. Both should cause death. In planar bilayer membranes, the rupture process is prompt (e.g. occurring within about $10^{-3}$ seconds), and has also been termed 'irreversible breakdown' and 'irreversible mechanical breakdown'. Rupture occurs in planar bilayer membranes exposed to a transmembrane potential, $U(t)$, if $U$ is approximately in the range 200 mV $< U(t) <$ 600 mV for times of about $t > 10^{-4}$ s[13,15,17,38,39,41-43,45]. Prompt rupture of planar membranes involves electrical discharges with decay times significantly longer than those of REB (see later section).

This prompt rupture is termed nonthermal, because the bulk temperature rise is generally small. The lack of heating results from the experimental configuration: the high resistance membrane separates the stimulating electrodes, and this prevents significant current from flowing, thereby limiting ohmic dissipation in the medium. In this sense, rupture is not caused by heating. Instead, the existence of $U > 200$ mV for times of order of $10^{-4}$ s or longer leads to pores which expand beyond a critical size. The supracritical pores then expand rapidly, without limit, until a mechanical boundary is encountered, and this effectively destroys the membrane[13,27,41-43]. Another significant attribute of prompt rupture is that the membrane capacitance, $C$, initially changes insignificantly, which rules out significant electrocompression of the entire membrane[45-47] as the mechanism of rupture[15,38]. Another striking attribute of electroporation is that planar membranes often avoid rupture when exposed to the shorter, but significantly larger transmembrane potentials which cause REB.

A characteristic electrical 'signature' of rupture is a sigmoid curve of $U(t)$, in which the destruction phase of the membrane is revealed by $U(t)$ smoothly decreasing over an interval of many microseconds, which is much longer than the very rapid and history-dependent decay of REB[12]. Although early electroporation theories[13,15,38,41-43] correctly predicted the magnitude of a critical transmembrane potential, $U_c$, associated with rupture, they did not describe the kinetics of rupture in a way which gave description of $U(t)$ which could be directly compared to experiments. In contrast, a recent theory involving a dynamic population of pores of many sizes successfully describes $U(t)$ during the rupture process[27].

The behaviour of the membrane conductance, $G(t)$, during rupture is revealing, especially when compared to REB. For clarity, the behaviour of $G(t)$ is shown in Fig. 16.4 for the short time-scale (0 to 1 $\mu$second) of REB. It is immediately clear that while nothing dramatic occurs for a small pulse (e.g. injected charge, $Q_{inject} = 5$ ncoulombs), as the pulse magnitude is increased (for fixed pulse width) for REB, the conductance increases by orders of magnitude in a short time. For the largest pulse shown, an approximately eight order of magnitude increase occurs over an interval of about 200 nseconds. It is achievement of this high conductance in REB that allows the membrane to rapidly discharge before any pore reaches supracritical size, and this protects the membrane against prompt rupture.

With this in mind, the behaviour of $G(t)$ during rupture is particularly interesting. As shown in Fig. 16.5 with a longer time-scale (0 to 80 $\mu$seconds, all four fates are shown in terms of the change of conductance with time. The small pulse results in only slight electroporation, which causes a slight rise in $G(t)$, that persists on this time-scale. The pulse leading to prompt rupture rapidly results in a five order of magnitude increase in $G(t)$, which initially decays, but at $T \approx 30$ $\mu$s begins to increase again as at that time first

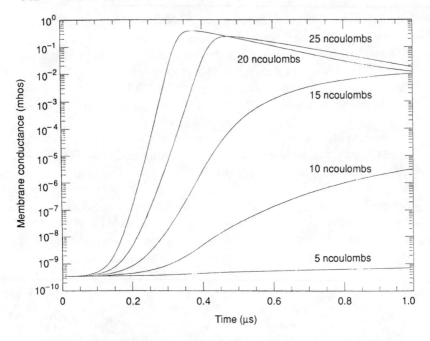

Fig. 16.4. Theoretical behaviour of the membrane conductance, $G(t)$, over the time interval 0 to 1 $\mu$s for the artificial planar bilayer membrane charge–pulse experiment modeled in Fig. 16.2($a$). For a fixed pulse width of 0.4 $\mu$s the smallest pulse ($Q_{inject} = 5$ ncoulomb) a slight increase in conductance occurs, which is due to only a small amount of electroporation. This case is essentially passive charging of the membrane as an ordinary capacitor. The $Q_{inject} = 10$ ncoulomb pulse subsequently will lead to a prompt rupture, but on this time-scale shows only a monotonic, three order of magnitude increase in $G(t)$. The $Q_{inject} = 15$ ncoulomb pulse causes a much larger conductance increase, sufficient to partially discharge the membrane (Figs. 16.2($b$) and 3($b$)), i.e. to cause incomplete REB. The $Q_{inject} = 20$ ncoulomb and 25 ncoulomb pulses both cause still larger conductance increases (each approximately eight orders of magnitude), and this proves sufficient rapidly and completely to discharge the membrane, i.e. to cause REB. It is emphasized that these plots of $G(t)$ are theoretical, and were obtained from the same model which generates the curves of Figs. 16.2($b$) and 3($b$). The reasonable agreement of experiment and theory shown in Figs. 16.2 and 16.3 suggests that these plots of $G(t)$ are reasonable representations of the conductance changes that actually occur as a result of electroporation.

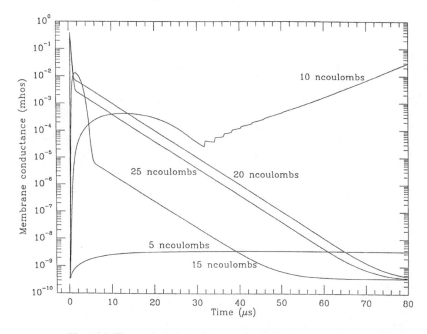

Fig. 16.5. Theoretical plots of the conductance, $G(t)$, in an artificial planar bilayer membrane as in Fig. 16.4, but for the expanded time-scale of 0 to 80 $\mu$s. All four fates are shown. The smallest pulse ($Q_{inject} = 5$ ncoulomb) results in only slight electroporation. This causes a slight rise in $G(t)$, which then persists on this time-scale, but will eventually relax to the initial value as pores are destroyed. The next largest pulse ($Q_{inject} = 10$) ncoulomb causes prompt rupture. Initially, this pulse results in a five order of magnitude, rapid increase in $G(t)$, which begins to decay, but at $t \approx 30$ $\mu$s begins to increase again as first one, and then several other, supracritical pores appear and begin their expansion that eventually (in less than $10^{-3}$ s) destroy the membrane. The $Q_{inject} = 15$ ncoulomb pulse causes a more rapid and larger increase in conductance, which is enough incompletely to discharge the membrane to a transmembrane potential, $U \approx 50$ mV (Fig. 16.3($b$)). This is an example of incomplete REB. Finally, the $Q_{inject} = 20$ ncoulomb and 25 ncoulomb pulses cause still larger conductance increases, and more rapidly, which allow the membrane to fully discharge (Fig. 16.2($b$)), and therefore represents REB.

one, and then several other, supracritical pores emerge and begin their expansion that destroys the membrane. In contrast, larger pulses result in either incomplete REB or in REB, and cause a much larger increase in $G(t)$, which allows the membrane to discharge sufficiently rapidly that rupture is avoided. Thus, a comparison of experiment and theory in artificial planar bilayer membrane is useful in providing some idea of how a dynamic pore population with many pore sizes can account for several fates, including prompt rupture. In short, prompt rupture is due to one or a small number of very large pores, while REB is due to a large number of smaller pores.

### Electrical behaviour associated with reversible electrical breakdown

Given the existence of rupture at moderate $U$, the existence of REB is tantalizing, as REB occurs at higher $U$ and rupture is usually avoided. Further, the behaviour of $U(t)$ during reversible electrical breakdown (REB) is even more dramatic than that during rupture. Essentially by definition, REB is a rapid membrane discharge, followed by complete recovery without rupture[12,14,16,17,19,48,49]. The ability of a membrane to support REB can be understood qualitatively to be the result of larger numbers of pores appearing, with the result that their ionic conductance allows the membrane to discharge (relieving the electrical pressure) before even one pore can expand to supracritical size (which would cause rupture). A quantitative description is consistent with this view, and rests on a physical model which explicitly (1) treats a rapidly changing population of pores with a distribution of sizes, (2) includes the local transmembrane potential decreases near conducting pores, and (3) incorporates a circuit equation to describe both the charging and discharging of the membrane[25-27]. Although our understanding of electroporation of artificial planar bilayer membranes is still incomplete, the success of this theory in describing several different electrical consequences of electroporation suggests that many features of the model are essentially correct.

REB has several characteristic features. (1) It appears immediately to precede the longer-lasting high permeability state observed in cell membranes. (2) During REB the membrane conductance, $G(t)$, of planar membranes rapidly increases to large values, and then recovers. (3) There are characteristic combinations of magnitude and time which result in REB: typical square pulse characteristics which result in REB are a pulse width, $\Delta t$, in the range $10^{-7} < \Delta t < 10^{-4}$ second, and transmembrane potential magnitudes in the range $500 < U < 1500$ mV. (4) Experiments using these short pulses show that the recovery process occurs within microseconds[16]. (5) An incomplete discharge (incomplete REB) can also occur, if the increase in $U(t)$ does not result in quite enough pores (size and number) to completely discharge the membrane. This has been observed experimentally in the same membrane preparations which exhibit complete REB[12], and is described quantitatively by a theory which also correctly describes rupture and REB occurrence[27].

If a series of charge pulse experiments is carried out, REB is found to occur with an increasingly rapid discharge as the pulse amplitude, $\Delta U_i$, is increased for fixed pulse width, $\Delta t$, or as $\Delta t$ is increased at constant $\Delta U_i$. In early studies, $U_o$ was defined to be the transmembrane potential at the end of a pulse. An approximate threshold potential for REB, $U_{o,c}$ was then identified as the maximum value of $U_o$, which decreases as $\Delta t$ increases[12]. Finally, another significant attribute of electroporation in artificial planar bilayer membranes is the observation that rupture, REB or even incomplete REB followed by rupture all can be caused to occur by varying only the magnitude and duration of the applied pulse[12]. This interrelated behaviour places significant constraints on the mechanism of rupture, incomplete REB and REB.

### Electroporation is chemically mild

The energetics of electroporation are particularly interesting, because electroporation is biochemically mild. Specifically, although REB has sometimes been termed 'dielectric breakdown', this is misleading terminology because of the previously well established usage of 'dielectric breakdown' for ion-pair avalanche phenomena, a very different phenomenon which involves significantly larger energy, viz. about 10 electron volts ($1.6 \times 10^{-18}$ joule) per monovalent ion[50]. The transmembrane potential associated with REB (500 to 1500 mV) corresponds to only 0.5 to 1.5 electron volts per monovalent ion, about an order of magnitude less energy, and this smaller energy is insufficient for ion-pair formation. In contrast, pore formation and expansion can occur at the lower energies.

### Electrical behaviour: comparison of experiment and theory

Although molecular transport associated with electroporation is of greater biological importance, electrical behaviour is usually more readily measured. For this reason, it is worthwhile to present several illustrations of electrical behaviour, particularly at early times after a pulse. A recent

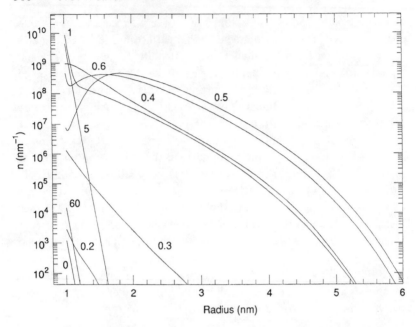

Fig. 16.6. Plots of the computed pore population distribution at different times for REB (the 20 ncoulomb case of Fig. 16.2(*b*)) in an artificial planar bilayer membrane[27]. A wide range of pore sizes is involved. This is displayed by computing the number of pores, $n(r,t)\Delta r$ with radii between $r$ and $r + \Delta r$ which is shown as a function of $r$ for different times. Initially, only a small number of pores are present (the short slanting curve labeled with '0' at the lower left corner). Then, as $U(t)$ rises because of the 0.4 $\mu$s pulse (not instantaneously experienced by the membrane), pores increase in number and size. The pore population thus first expands (curves labelled 0.2, 0.3, 0.4 and 0.5 $\mu$s), and then collapses as $U(t)$ decays (curves labelled 0.6, 5 and 60 $\mu$s). A large number of pores with diameters exceeding 6 nm are transiently present. If a cell membrane can trap, or otherwise create metastability, a single large pore, a high permeability state can exist.

theoretical model of electroporation of artificial planar bilayer membranes provides a unified, quantitative description of several aspects of electrical behaviour following electroporation, and therefore allows some insight into pore behaviour which cannot be directly measured[27]. The results shown in Figs 16.2–16.7 are in good agreement with experimental behaviour[12]. The theory is based on a number of simplifying hypotheses and approximations in the physical description of pores. One major weakness is that a detailed description of the dynamic process of pore formation and pore disappearance does not exist yet. Instead, pores are assumed to be created and destroyed by a process dependent on $U(t)$, with

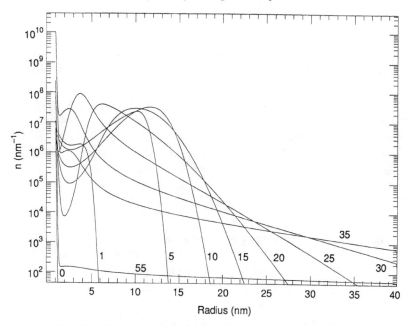

Fig. 16.7. Corresponding plots of $n(r,t)\Delta r$ for the case of rupture, i.e. the curve of Fig. 16.2 with $Q_{\text{inject}} = 10$ ncoulomb[27]. As in Fig. 16.4, the membrane initially (prior to a moderate 0.4 $\mu$s pulse) contains a small number of pores. The times labelling the curves are in $\mu$s from the time the pulse begins. As time progresses, there is a build-up of larger pores, until one or more pores becomes supracritical, and expands to rupture the membrane. In summary form, prompt rupture is due to one or a small number of very large pores, while REB is the result of a large number of smaller pores.

an assumed form for creation and destruction. Once formed, however, the response of the pores to thermal fluctuations, mechanical forces and electric fields is described by a first principles' physical theory.

### Electroporation involves pores of many sizes

An important implication results from the success of this theoretical model: a large number of pores with a significant distribution in sizes is required. Different subpopulations of the total pore population are responsible for different aspects of the electrical behaviour. Briefly, a small number of large pores are responsible for rupture, while a much larger number of smaller pores are responsible for REB. The complexity of the pore population is illustrated in Figs 16.6 and 16.7, where the number of pores, $n(r,t)\Delta r$ with radii between $r$ and $r + \Delta r$ is shown as a function of time during a REB curve. For the theoretical results of Fig. 16.6, initially fewer than ten pores are present for the macroscopic planar bilayer membrane modeled. As time progresses, the rapidly increasing $U(t)$ results in both more and larger pores, and then a recovery as the pore population collapses upon discharge of the membrane. In a cell membrane, any mechanism that 'captures' one or a small number of the larger pores could provide a persistent high permeability that allows transport of fairly large molecules. Figure 16.7 illustrates the corresponding behaviour in the case of membrane rupture for the same membrane; only the applied pulse is different.

### Molecular transport associated with electroporation

Transport of molecules, not electrical behaviour, has generated most of the recent interest in electroporation. Of particular interest is the empirical evidence that almost any macromolecule can be transported across cell membranes[1-3]. The introduction of genetic material into cells by electroporation has already become important, but the large transient molecular fluxes are likely to have much wider applications. For example, it has been shown recently that very large numbers of molecules can be introduced into cells by a single pulse[51]. The transport of very large numbers of small molecules, large numbers of macromolecules, and at least some of DNA, RNA and even small particles, is impressive. Presently, however, there is very little quantitative understanding of molecular transport due to electroporation. Qualitatively, there is evidence that a transient high permeability state is believed to occur immediately following REB[4,33,52,53]. However, the nature of the openings (pores, or coalesced pores which may form cracks[54]) remains to be elucidated.

During the relatively short interval when $U(t)$ is large, and many rapidly changing pores are present, significant electric fields exist across the membrane. After taking into account the spreading resistance[55], which results in significant potential drops within the electrolyte outside but near the pore's mouths, a field still exists within the pores. Electrokinetic transport of molecules is therefore possible[53], and is suspected of occurring in addition to hindered diffusion[28,29]. After $U(t)$ has decayed, significant molecular transport can still occur. Calculation shows that hindered diffusion is sufficient to transport large numbers of molecules across a cell membrane, even if only one large pore (e.g. $r \approx 5$ nm) has a long lifetime. For example, with an initial concentration difference of $\Delta C = C_{ext} - C_{int} = C_{ext} = 100$ $\mu$m, this size pore can transport of order $10^6$ macromolecules of diffusion constant of $D_s \approx 10^{-7}$ cm$^2$/s across a 5 nm membrane in 100 s. Although qualitatively plausible, there is presently no detailed understanding of how the long lifetime, high permeability state actually occurs, and what conditions subsequently affect its disappearance.

In partial summary, it is presently unknown how large metastable pores are formed, and what governs their rate of decay. A number of candidate interactions between pores and different aspects of a cell membrane have been identified, and can be considered for their significance in explaining persistent large pores. An example is a 'foot-in-the-door' mechanism, in which the presence of a partially inserted macromolecule repels the pore edge, preventing pore shrinkage until the macromolecule has diffused back out or across the membrane (Weaver & Barnett, unpublished observations). It remains to incorporate such hypotheses into theoretical models, and thereby to determine whether the dramatic behaviour of a persistent but metastable high permeability can be explained by such a pore mechanism.

### Membrane recovery after electroporation

Membrane recovery can be described by a progressively smaller molecular weight cut-off as pores shrink and/or disappear. Electrical measurements can reveal changes due to the conduction of small ions, while molecular transport measurements can probe a larger range of pores. The rapid time response and relative ease of electrical measurements mean that recovery probed by small ions can be readily carried out on a continuous basis. However, the more difficult molecular transport measurements have not usually been reported. Early studies reported that in an artificial planar bilayer membrane, the conductance, $G(t)$, decays approximately exponentially with a time constant, $\tau_{RC}$, of several microseconds[16], while more recent studies, using a different experiment arrangement, report considerably longer recovery times, of the order of seconds[17]. Further, in terms of overall reversibility, it has been shown that an oxidized cholesterol planar membrane can undergo REB and recover many times[12]. Similar behaviour has been demonstrated in a tissue[10]. Complete membrane recovery must also occur in many electroporated cells, as application of electroporation to gene transfer first causes uptake of DNA, and the subsequent obtaining of viable, transformed cells[1-3]. In the case of artificial planar bilayer membranes it is likely that membrane recovery takes place in two stages: (1) a rapid shrinkage of most pores as $U(t)$ is in its decreasing phase, and (2) a reduction in pore number, as small pores are somehow destroyed[27]. Any metastable pores presumably present additional complication, as it is likely that both the shrinkage and disappearance stages will be different from those of transient aqueous pores in an artificial membrane or the bilayer portion of a cell membrane.

### Recovery from cell stress: death or survival

The temporary disruption of the cell membrane's ability to restrict transport of all but selected molecules creates the possibility of cell stress. A number of possible mechanisms have been identified (see Table 16.2):

### Tissue electroporation

Only a few studies, to date, have considered tissue electroporation explicitly, i.e. application of fields or currents which cause electroporation in some or all of the cells of the exposed tissue. As noted earlier, the sparsity of direct studies on tissue means that studies of electroporation in isolated cells must be relied on, and then estimates made. As with the more thoroughly studied isolated cell preparations, both reversible and irreversible effects can be anticipated. From the perspective of electrical injury, the degree of tissue damage, rather than reversibility or irreversibility of electroporation phenomena themselves, is probably more relevant[11].

With this in mind, the studies on skeletal muscle are particularly interesting, as they provide evidence that some of the tissue injury associated with electrocution is nonthermal, and is due to electroporation[7-9]. Specifically, these studies show that skeletal muscle cells are lysed under conditions for which the temperature rise is negligible (less than 1 °C). The field strength, pulse width and number of pulses were important. Changes in the membranes of the cells comprising the tissue were determined by electrical impedance measurements, with a large, permanent decrease after 100 pulses of duration 10 ms and separation 10 s for an applied field of 120 V/cm. Overall, these studies provide strong evidence that electroporation is an important damage mechanism.

Another study demonstrates that completely reversible tissue electroporation behaviour can occur, without any evidence of damage[10]. In this study, the evidence for the occurrence of electroporation is also compelling. Isolated, viable frog skin was used in order to provide a tissue preparation which had well-defined electrical conditions, and which allowed direct electrical measurements that could be interpreted at the cellular level. The frog skin preparation presents a barrier to transport which is essentially

Table 16.2. *Candidate stress mechanisms*

- Loss of essential intracellular molecules
- Admission of molecules normally excluded
- Loading/shunting of transmembrane pumps
- Denaturation of intracellular proteins by altered intracellular conditions
- Nonrecovery of a portion of the membrane (equivalent to rupture of that portion)

that of a monolayer of cells which are connected laterally by tight junctions[56]. Thus, if this tissue is placed in a conventional tissue chamber, with electrodes on both sides, the resulting configuration is essentially a macroscopic monolayer of cells, and therefore similar to an artificial planar bilayer experiment. This allowed direct measurements of the transtissue potential and transtissue resistance, due mainly to a monolayer of cells. Results similar to REB in an artificial bilayer membrane were obtained, but with somewhat smoothed curves, which is not surprising because cells of the order of $10^6$ were involved. Specifically, the characteristic behaviour of increasingly rapid decays, and of curve crossing was observed as (1) the pulse amplitude was increased for fixed pulse width, and (2) the pulse width was increased for fixed pulse amplitude. This behaviour is the characteristic electrical signature of electroporation, as has been observed previously in artificial planar bilayer[12,14], and in isolated cells[19] under charge injection conditions[27].

Reversibility was also observed directly, by monitoring the transtissue resistance after a pulse on a time-scale of several minutes. The resistance recovered most of its original value within 20 seconds, and returned completely within 2 to 3 minutes ($25 \pm 2$ °C). Further, there was no measurable evidence of tissue damage, as could be estimated from either transtissue resistance or open circuit potential measurements. By considering the measurement error and the resistance change that should have been caused by the complete lysis of one cell (creating a hole in the tissue), it was estimated that a single pulse causing electroporation resulted in fewer than four cells being lysed. The corresponding cell lysis rate was therefore less than about $10^{-6}$ per cell. Finally, because some preparations were subjected to 20 or more pulses without finding measurable damage, it was estimated that the cell lysis rate per pulse was even lower, having an upper bound of about $10^{-7}$ per cell per pulse.

The potential importance of tissue electroporation to tissue damage suggests the need for additional studies. Presently, there is strong evidence that both reversible and irreversible phenomena can occur, and that tissue damage can be undetectable or pronounced[11]. However, the electrical conditions which separate nondamaging from damaging electroporation behaviour in a particular tissue have not been established yet. In considering the potential contribution of electroporation to tissue damage, it is essential to estimate the transmembrane potential of the cells of the tissue correctly. Generally, this will involve estimating local electric field, $E_e$, which is experienced by the cells of the tissue, and then carrying out computations that take into account the geometry of the cells within the tissue. As part of this procedure, it may often be difficult to estimate $E_e$ directly. In this case, the local current density, $\vec{J_e}$, and the corresponding electrical conductivity, $\sigma_e$, must be estimated. By combining these parameters with knowledge of the geometry (size and shape) of the cells in the tissue, generally it should be possible to estimate whether or not electroporation occurs in various parts of the tissue. Generally it will require another step, however, to determine whether any occurrence of electroporation causes acceptable levels of tissue damage. Usually, this can be expected to depend on the type of tissue (essentially no studies to date), and the composition of the extracellular medium at the time of electrical exposure.

### Summary

Electroporation occurs universally in cell membranes if the transmembrane potential reaches values greater than about 200 mV, but also depends on the duration of this increase. In order to estimate whether or not electroporation occurs in a particular tissue, it is essential to estimate the extent and duration of changes in the transmembrane potential of the cells of the tissue. Whether or not significant tissue damage occurs requires further information, as electroporation itself can be reversible or irreversible. Cellular damage may occur through membrane rupture, and be prompt, or may occur as a consequence of a high permeability state which follows REB, and be delayed. Further, whether delayed rupture occurs can depend significantly on the composition of the extracellular medium relative to the intracellular medium. Presently, electroporation is understood incompletely, and what knowledge there is comes mostly from studies on artificial planar bilayer membranes or on isolated cells. Significantly more studies on mechanisms of cell damage following electroporation are needed, as are further explicit investigations of tissue electroporation.

### Acknowledgements

The author thanks Tian Y. Tsong, Kevin T. Powell, Raphael C. Lee, Gail I. Harrison, Stephen H. Grund, Jonathan G. Bliss, and, particularly, Alan Barnett for stimulating discussions. Supported by the Office of Naval Research through Contract N00014–87–K–0479.

### References

1 Zimmermann, U. (1986). Electrical breakdown, electropermeabilization and electrofusion. *Review of Physiological and Biochemical Pharmacology*, **105**, 175–256.
2 Neumann, E., Sowers, A. & Jordan, C. (eds). (1989). *Electroporation and Electrofusion in Cell Biology*, New York: Plenum.
3 Potter, H. (1988). Electroporation in biology: methods, applications, and instrumentation. *Analytical Biochemistry*, **174**, 361–73.
4 Zimmermann, U., Riemann, F. & Pilwat, G. (1976). Enzyme loading of electrically homogeneous human red blood cell ghosts prepared by dielectric breakdown. *Biochimica et Biophysica Acta*, **436**, 460–74.
5 Uno, I., Fukami, K., Kato, H., Takenwa, T. & Ishikawa, T. (1988). Essential role for phosphatidylinositol 4,5-bisphosphate in yeast cell proliferation. *Nature*, **333**, 188–90.
6 Sale, A.J.H. & Hamilton, W.A. (1967). Effects of high electric fields on microorganisms: I. Killing of bacteria and yeasts. *Biochimica et Biophysica Acta*, **148**, 781–8.
7 Lee, R.C. & Kolodney, M.S. (1987). Electrical injury mechanisms: electrical breakdown of cell membranes. *Plastic and Reconstructive Surgery*, **80**, 672–9.
8 Lee, R.C., Gaylor, D.C., Bhatt, D. & Israel, D.A. (1988). Role of cell membrane rupture in the pathogenesis of electrical trauma. *Journal of Surgical Research*, **47**, 709–19.
9 Bhatt, D.L., Gaylor, D.C. & Lee, R.C. (1990). Rhabdomyolysis due to pulsed electric fields. *Plastic and Reconstructive Surgery*, **86**, 1–11.
10 Powell, K.T., Morgenthaler, A.W. & Weaver, J.C. (1989). Tissue electroporation: observation of reversible electrical breakdown in viable frog skin. *Biophysical Journal*, **56**, 1163–71.
11 Weaver, J.C. (1990). Electroporation: a new phenomenon to consider in medical technology. In *Emerging Electromagnetic Medical Technology*, O'Connor, Bentall and Monahan (eds), pp. 81–102, Springer-Verlag.
12 Benz, R., Beckers, F. & Zimmermann, U. (1979). Reversible electrical breakdown of lipid bilayer membranes: a charge-pulse relaxation study. *Journal of Membrane Biology*, **48**, 181–204.
13 Abidor, I.G., Arakelyan, V.B., Chernomordik, L.V., Chizmadzhev, Yu. A., Pastushenko, V.F. & Tarasevich, M.R. (1979). Electric breakdown of bilayer membranes: I. The main experimental facts and their qualitative discussion. *Bioelectrochemistry and Bioenergetics*, **6**, 37–52.
14 Benz, R. & Zimmermann, U. (1980). Pulse-length dependence of the electrical breakdown in lipid bilayer membranes, *Biochimica et Biophysica Acta*, **597**, 637–42.

15  Chernomordik, L.V. & Abidor, I.G. (1980). The voltage-induced local defects in unmodified BLM, *Bioelectrochemistry and Bioenergenetics*, 7, 617–23.

16  Benz, R. & Zimmermann, U. (1981). The resealing process of lipid bilayers after reversible electrical breakdown, *Biochimica et Biophysica Acta*, **640**, 169–78.

17  Chernomordik, L.V., Sukharev, S.I., Popov, S.V., Pastushenko, V.F., Sokirko, A.V., Abidor, I.G. & Chizmadzhev, Y.A. (1987). The electrical breakdown of cell and lipid membranes: The similarity of phenomenologies, *Biochimica et Biophysica Acta*, **902**, 360–73.

18  Chernomordik, L.V. & Chizmadzhev, Y.A. (1989). Electrical breakdown of lipid bilayer membranes: phenomenology and mechanism. In *Electroporation and Electrofusion in Cell Biology*, Neumann, E., Sowers, A.E. & Jordan, C.A. eds, pp. 83–95, New York: Plenum.

19  Benz, R. & Zimmermann, U. (1980). Relaxation studies on cell membranes and lipid bilayers in the high electric field range, *Bioelectrochemistry and Bioenergenetics*, 7, 723–39.

20  Farkas, D.L. (1989). External electrical field-induced transmembrane potentials in biological systems: features, effects and optical monitoring. In *Electroporation and Electrofusion in Cell Biology*, Neumann, E., Sowers, A.E. & Jordan, C.A. pp. 409–31, New York: Plenum.

21  Bliss, J.G., Harrison, G.I., Mourant, J.R., Powell, K.T. & Weaver, J.C. (1988). Electroporation: the distribution of macromolecular uptake and shape changes in red blood cells following a single 50 $\mu$second square wave pulse. *Bioelectrochemistry and Bioenergetics*, **19**, 57–71.

22  Hofmann, G.A. (1989). Cells in electric fields: physical and practical electronic aspects of electro cell fusion and electroporation. In *Electroporation and Electrofusion in Cell Biology*, Neumann, E., Sowers, A.E. & Jordan, C.A. eds, pp. 389–407, New York: Plenum.

23  Geddes, L.A. (1972). *Electrodes and the Measurement of Bioelectric Events*, New York: Wiley.

24  Foster, K.R. & Schwann, H.P. (1986). Dielectric properties of tissues. In *CRC Handbook of Biological Effects of Electromagnetic Fields*, Polk, C. & Postow, E. eds, pp. 27–96, Boca Raton: CRC Press.

25  Powell, K.T., Derrick, E.G. & Weaver, J.C. (1986). A quantitative theory of reversible electrical breakdown, *Bioelectrochemistry and Bioenergenetics*, **15**, 243–55.

26  Weaver, J.C. & Powell, K.T. (1989). Theory of electroporation. In *Electroporation and Electrofusion in Cell Biology*, Neumann, E., Sowers, A. & Jordan, C. eds, pp. 111–126, New York: Plenum.

27  Barnett, A.S. & Weaver, J.C. (1991). Electroporation: a unified, quantitative theory of reversible electrical breakdown and rupture. *Bioelectrochemistry and Bioenergetics*, **25**, 163–82.

28  Wang, H. & Skalak, R. (1969). Viscous flow in a cylindrical tube containing a line of spherical particles, *Journal of Fluid Mechanics*, **83**, 75–96.

29  Weaver, J.C., Powell, K.T., Mintzer, R.A., Sloan, S.R. & Ling, H. (1984). The diffusive permeability of bilayer membranes: the contribution of transient aqueous pores, *Bioelectrochemistry and Bioenergetics*, **12**, 405–12.

30 Konosita, K. Jr. & Tsong, T.Y. (1977). Hemolysis of human erythrocytes by a transient electric field, *Proceedings of the National Academy of Sciences*, **74**, 1923–7. 1977.

31 Weaver, J.C., Harrison, G.I., Bliss, J.G., Mourant, J.R. & Powell, K.T. (1988). Electroporation: high frequency of occurrence of the transient high permeability state in red blood cells and intact yeast, *FEBS Letters*, **229**, 30–4.

32 Michel, M.R., Eligizoli, M., Koblet, H. & Kempf, Ch. (1988). Diffusion loading conditions determine recovery of protein synthesis in electroporated P3X63 Ag8 cells, *Experientia*, **44**, 199–203.

33 Kinosita, K. Jr. & Tsong, T.Y. (1977). Formation and resealing of pores of controlled sizes in human erythrocyte membrane, *Nature*, **268**, 438–41.

34 Neumann, E., Schaefer-Ridder, M., Wang, Y. & Hofschneider, P.H. (1982). Gene transfer into mouse lyoma cells by electroporation in high electric fields, *EMBO Journal*, **1**, 841–5.

35 Zimmermann, U., Schultz, J. & Pilwat, G. (1973). Transcellular ion flow in *Escherichia coli B* and electrical sizing of bacterias, *Biophysical Journal*, **13**, 1005–13.

36 El-Mashak, E.M. & Tsong, T.Y. (1985). Ion selectivity of temperature-induced and electric field induced pores in dipalmitoylphosphatidylcholine vesicles, *Biochemistry*, **24**, 2884–8.

37 Rechsteiner, A.C. (1982). Transfer of macromolecules using erythrocyte ghosts. In *Techniques in Somatic Cell Genetics*, Shay, J.W. (ed.) pp. 385–398, New York: Plenum.

38 Chizmadzhev, Yu. A. & Abidor, I.G. (1980). Bilayer lipid membranes in strong electric fields. *Bioelectrochemistry and Bioenergetics*, **7**, 83–100.

39 Glaser, R.W., Leikin, S.L., Chernomordik, L.V., Pastushenko, V.F. & Sokirko, A.I. (1988). Reversible electrical breakdown of lipid bilayers: formation and evolution of pores, *Biochimica et Biophysica Acta*, **940**, 275–87.

40 Szabo, G. & Waldbillig, R.C. (1982). Lipid model membranes. In *Methods of Experimental Physics: Biophysics*, ed. Ehrenstein, G. & Lecar, H. eds, vol. 20, pp. 513–43, New York: Academic Press.

41 Weaver, J.C. & Mintzer, R.A. (1981). Decreased bilayer stability due to transmembrane potentials, *Physics Letters*, **86A**, 57–9.

42 Sugar, I.P. (1981). The effects of external fields on the structure of lipid bilayers, *Journal of Physiology (Paris)*, **77**, 1035–42.

43 Powell, K.T. & Weaver, J.C. (1986). Transient aqueous pores in bilayer membranes: a statistical theory, *Bioelectrochemistry and energetics*, **15**, 211–27.

44 Sugar, I.P. & Neumann, E. (1984). Stochastic model for electric field-induced membrane pores: electroporation, *Biophysical Chemistry*, **19**, 211–25.

45 Crowley, J.M. (1973). Electrical breakdown of bimolecular lipid membranes as an electromechanical instability, *Biophysical Journal*, **13**, 711–24.

46 Dimitrov, D.S. (1984). Electric field-induced breakdown of lipid bilayers and cell membranes: a thin viscoelastic film model, *Journal of Membrane Biology*, **78**, 53–60.

47 Dimitrov, D.S. & Jain, R.K. (1984). Membrane stability, *Biochimica et*

*Biophysica Acta*, **779**, 437–68.

48  Stämpfi, R. (1958). Reversible electrical breakdown of the excitable membrane of a ranvier node, *An. Acad. Brasil. Ciens*, **30**, 57–63.

49  Benz, R. & Conti, F. (1981). Reversible electrical breakdown of squid giant axon membrane. *Biochimica et Biophysica Acta*, **645**, 115–23.

50  Condon, E.U. & Odishaw, H. (1958). *Handbook of Physics*, New York: McGraw-Hill.

51  Bartoletti, D.C., Harrison, G.I. & Weaver, J.C. (1989). The number of molecules taken up by electroporated cells: quantitative determination. *FEBS Letters*, **256**, 4–10.

52  Neumann, E. & Rosenheck, K. (1972). Permeability changes induced by electric impulses in vesicular membranes. *Journal of Membrane Biology*, **10**, 279–90.

53  Sowers, A.E. & Lieber, M.R. (1986). Electropore diameters, lifetimes, numbers, and locations in individual erythrocyte ghosts. *FEBS Letters*, **205**, 179–84.

54  Sugar, I.P., Förster, W. & Neumann, E. (1987). Model of cell electrofusion: membrane electroporation, pore coalescence and percolation. *Biophysical Chemistry*, **26**, 321–35.

55  Newman, J. (1966). Resistance for flow of current to a disk. *Journal of the Electrochemical Society*, **113**, 501–2.

56  Berridge, M.J. & Oschman, J.L. (1972). *Transporting Epithelia*, New York: Academic Press.

# 17

# An anisotropic, elastomechanical instability theory for electropermeabilization of bilayer–lipid membranes

CHARLES MALDARELLI
KATHLEEN STEBE

## Introduction

The application of short, intense, electric fields across the bilayer–lipid membranes of natural or artificial cells can create transient, self-resealing holes in the bilayer lamellae. This hole-forming or electroporative effect was first identified from the collective results of early studies which applied transverse fields to lipid membranes in an effort to probe their ultrastructure[1-4]. The phenomenology of electroporation was established and systematized in later studies by Zimmermann et al.[5-14], Tsong et al.[15-22], and Abidor, Chizmadzhev and co-workers[23-29]. (Cf. also the review articles by Zimmermann[30,31], and the monograph by Neumann, Sowers and Jordan[32]). As identified in these experimental studies, the usual methodology for electroporating cells is to apply a direct current field of a few kV/cm to a cell or vesicle suspension in the form of a pulse (or pulses) of the order of 10 $\mu$s in duration. The pulse waveform is usually rectangular or of exponential decay (cf. Potter[33] for a summary of methods), although recent studies have demonstrated that a pulse of a dc shifted radio-frequency field can efficiently electroporate cells[34,35]. Resealment of the holes takes place approximately 10–100 s after application of the pulse. The holes which are created have been estimated to be of the order of 5–10 nm in diameter and cover the cell surface with a density of $10^7$ pores/cm[2,36,37]. A critical field strength appears necessary to cause the electroporation; however, if the field strength is too high, or the duration or number of pulses too great, this prompt, reversible response is replaced by an irreversible breakdown of the membrane[23,28].

Since electroporation creates self-resealing holes in the membrane, it has the potential to be used as a technology for producing functioning cells loaded with macromolecules which would otherwise have been unable to penetrate the membrane. Indeed, recent studies have shown that electropermeabilization can be used to introduce genes into mammalian[50-55] and plant cells[56,57] and bacteria[58] (see also the review article by Zimmermann[59]).

The physicochemical basis of electropermeabilization is as yet unresolved, although many theoretical investigations as to its origin have been undertaken. The starting point for understanding the electroporative mechanism is the transmembrane potential ($V$) developed across the membrane by the application of the field. Because the conductivity of the membrane is so much less than that of the surrounding medium, very high potential differences develop across the membrane when the external field is applied. These differences, in turn, create large electric fields in the membrane interior because the membrane thickness is usually of the order of 10 nm or less.

Crowley[39] (see also White[40] and Dimitrov[41,42]) first examined the effect of a high, transverse, electric field on the mechanical equilibrium of a flat, isotropic, elastic membrane sheet. Through a linear stability analysis, he demonstrated that, when the interfaces of the membrane are perturbed by disturbance waves, the transverse electric field gives rise to electric (Maxwell) surface stresses which destabilize the system, and cause squeezing deformations of the bilayer, as depicted in Fig. 17.1, to grow. The growth is resisted by elastic tensions caused by straining in the membrane, and Crowley showed that below a critical transmembrane potential $V_c$ all disturbance wavelengths are stable, while above this value waves which are unstable exist. This critical potential is given for an incompressible membrane (in Gaussian electrostatic units) by:

$$\epsilon_m V_c^2 / (4\pi h^2) = 2G \tag{1}$$

In this expression, $\epsilon_m$ and $G$ denote, respectively, the membrane dielectric constant and elastic shear modulus, and $h$ is the unperturbed membrane thickness in the presence of the electric field. This base state thickness is smaller than the membrane thickness in the absence of the field because the high electric fields in the membrane compress the lipid bilayer. Crowley obtained the following expression for this compression by equating the squeezing Maxwell tension to the elastic stress due to the transverse strain:

$$ln(h/h_0) = -\epsilon_m V^2 / (24\pi G h^2) \tag{2}$$

In Equation (2), $h_0$ is the thickness in the absence of the field.

Crowley conjectured that pore formation results when the membrane potential exceeds the threshold value, and growth of squeezing disturbances eventually cause the membrane to snap, locally creating a hole. He

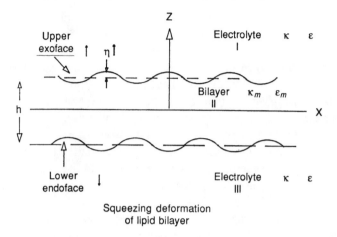

Fig. 17.1. The Crowley hypothesis: electric surface stresses destablize the squeezing mode of bilayer vibration and cause the membrane to snap thereby creating pores.

compared the value for $V_c$ predicted by Equation (1) and Equation (2) with early electroporative experiments and found that Equation (1) gave the correct order of magnitude for $V_c$, but underpredicted the critical potential by approximately a factor of 2. Several other comparisons of Equation (1) with data have been made in the literature, and the results show somewhat better agreement (for example, Zimmermann *et al.*[5]).

The explanation of electroporation as a linear, electromechanical instability has been criticized in the literature primarily because of Equation (2) which predicts an inordinately large value (a factor of $e^{-1/3}$) for the compression of the bilayer at the critical potential. Most experimental evidence and other lines of theoretical study[47] indicate that this compression is no more than a few per cent. As a result of this discrepancy, other mechanisms for electroporation have been proposed. Needham and Hochmuth[47] disregard the stability framework, and more simply propose that, because the bilayer is incompressible, the electrocompression causes the membrane area to be stretched to a critical value at which permeabilization commences. Other lines of research have focused on statistical pore theories: among them, Weaver *et al.*[43–46] have suggested a theory in which the distribution of pore sizes is skewed towards larger diameters as the transmembrane potential is increased. (Other statistical pore theories are those of Chizmadzhev *et al.*[24] and Sugar and Neumann[48].) Still other theories have focused on defects in the membrane[26] and electric-field induced redistribution of proteins[49].

In this study, the instability mechanism for electroporation is reconsidered in light of the mechanical anisotropy of the lipid bilayer. The underlying reason for the unacceptably large electrocompression at the critical potential, which is predicted by the Crowley theory, can be traced to the incorrect assumption that the lipid bilayer is isotropic in its elastic response. This is clearly not the case: for example, mechanical studies of red cell membrane bilayers[60-63] have shown conclusively that material deformations which increase the bilayer area require much larger force resultants than those necessary to shear the bilayer in the lateral plane. The mechanics of deformations in planes *perpendicular* to the membrane sheet have not been as well studied because such deformations are difficult to impose mechanically on a cell. It would be expected, however, that the modulus for shearing the bilayer in the transverse plane should, in analogy with the lateral case, be smaller than either the modulus for deformations which increase the membrane thickness or the area. Note that the material deformations involved in the bilayer squeezing of Fig. 17.1 require shearing the bilayer in its transverse plane as well as changing its thickness and area. By assuming an isotropic model, the elastic resistance to the squeezing deformation is overestimated because it does not take into account the ease of the transverse shearing deformation. Since the elastic resistance is overaccounted for, the critical transmembrane potential ($V_c$) is too high and the electrocompression is too large.

The aim of this study is to correct this deficiency of the Crowley model by developing a more complete electromechanical linear instability theory for electroporation which incorporates the effects of mechanical anisotropy. This study is divided into four sections. In the next section, the base state which forms the starting point of the linear stability analysis is described in detail. The stability analysis is described next, followed by the results. In the final section, some of the predictions of the model are compared to the recent data of Needham and Hochmuth[47] on the electroporation of reconstituted cholesterol-containing bilayers.

### The base state

The base state from which the instability develops is steady (time independent) and consists of an unperturbed, planar, laterally infinite membrane sheet bounded by motionless, semi-infinite, media (Fig. 17.1). The semi-infinite media represent the extra- and intracellular fluids, and, in this study, they are considered as identical aqueous electrolytes. The application, to these electrolytes, of a constant (positive) electric field perpendicular to the membrane lamellae causes migration of positive ions in the positive $z$ direction, and negative ions in the opposite direction. Since the membrane phase is hydrophobic, charged species reaching the membrane faces are repelled from its interior and either accumulate at the faces or pass through via small channels. In this development, this channel pathway for electrical conduction is accounted for by an overall isotropic conductivity, $\kappa_m$, which is assumed orders of magnitude smaller than the conductivity $\kappa$ of the electrolyte media. Within the context of this approximation, upon application of the field, current flows only in the $z$ direction. When the field is applied, the initial current in the membrane is much less than that in the surrounding phases, and negative charge accumulates at the exoface and positive charge at the endoface. This accumulation continues until the field in the membrane, raised by the interfacial charges, increases to the extent that the migration fluxes become equal at the interface boundary. The steady fields which so develop are given by the following balances of current densities at the unperturbed interfaces ($z = h/2$ and $z = -h/2$):

$$\kappa E^{I}_{z(o)} = \kappa_m E^{II}_{z(o)} \ (z = h/2) \text{ and}$$
$$\kappa_m E^{II}_{z(o)} = \kappa E^{III}_{z(o)} = \kappa E^{I}_{z(o)} \ (z = -h/2) \tag{1}$$

In Equation (1), $E^{\alpha}_{z(o)}$ denotes the base state electric field of phase $\alpha$ ($\alpha = $ I, II and III demarcate the upper, film and lower regions, cf. Fig. 17.1 and the subscripts denote that this vector quantity is a base state variable in the $z$-direction). As noted in the second equality of Equation (1), because the conductivities of the surrounding phases are equal, the electric fields in these regions are the same.

The steady, interfacial charges which develop at each of the membrane faces are equal in magnitude and opposite in sign, and are given in terms of the membrane ($\epsilon_m$) and surrounding phase ($\epsilon$) dielectric constants by:

$$\epsilon E^{I}_{z(o)} - \epsilon_m E^{II}_{z(o)} = \epsilon E^{I}_{z(o)} \ (1 - (\epsilon_m/\epsilon)(\kappa/\kappa_m)) = 4\pi \sigma^{\uparrow}_{(o)} \ (z = h/2)$$
$$\epsilon_m E^{II}_{z(o)} - \epsilon E^{III}_{z(o)} = 4\pi \sigma^{\downarrow}_{(o)} = -4\pi \sigma^{\uparrow}_{(o)} \qquad\qquad (z = -h/2) \tag{2}$$

where $\sigma$ denotes the interfacial charge, and the superscripted arrows denote the upper ($\uparrow$) and lower ($\downarrow$) interfaces.

The quiescent base state is in a mechanical equilibrium in which pressures and electromechanical stresses balance. To describe this equilibrium, consider first the electrical forces which act per unit volume on a polarizable medium in the presence of an electric field. For the purposes here, these may be divided into two effects: the first is the force exerted by the field on the ions carrying the current; the resultant of this interaction per unit volume is the local volume charge density ($\rho_e$) multiplied by the electric field. The second force derives from the polarization of the medium. An applied field creates a separation of charge in an otherwise neutral medium described by a dipole moment vector (per unit volume)$P_j$. (Here, and in what follows, the subscript ($j$, for example) attached to a vector quantity indicates the component of the vector in the $j^{th}$ Cartesian direction where $j = 1$, 2 and 3 denote respectively the $x$, $y$ and $z$ directions.) In the absence of orientation effects, the direction of this moment aligns itself with the field, and the magnitude of the moment is proportional to the field. Thus $P_j$ is given by $\chi_e E_j$, where $\chi_e$ is the susceptibility ($\chi_e = (\epsilon - 1)/4\pi$). The interaction of the field with the dipole creates a force in the Cartesian $j^{th}$ direction on the medium which is equal to $P_i \dfrac{\partial E_j}{\partial x_i}$; thus the total force in that direction is $\rho_e E_j + P_i \dfrac{\partial E_j}{\partial x_i}$, where a sum on $i$ is indicated by the repeated index. (For a complete treatment of the incorporation of electrical stresses in continuum theory, see the text by Melcher[66].)

In the base state of this study, current is conducted steadily and unidirectionally through the membrane and the surrounding electrolyte regions, with the electric field constant within each region and the volume charge density equal to zero. Hence, no electrical forces are exerted on the bulk continua by the application of the field. The bounding phases are incompressible fluids and therefore, with no flow, the only mechanical force which can be exerted is the isotropic pressure. In the case of the membrane phase, it is also regarded as incompressible but elastic. Consequently, the membrane can sustain a state of stress with no media motion by straining the body from some reference state in which elastic stresses are zero. However, in this study, it is assumed that *the membrane is unstrained in the base state and therefore only pressure forces are present*. Mechanical equilibrium within each phase under isotropic pressure simply requires:

$$\frac{\partial p^a_{(0)}}{\partial z} = 0 \tag{3}$$

i.e. the base state pressure ($p^a_{(0)}$) in region $a$ ($a = $ I, II or III) is uniform.

Owing to the discontinuity in the electric field across the membrane faces, and the presence of a surface charge density, electrical stresses are exerted on the membrane faces. To evaluate this action, the membrane interfaces must be examined on the microscale of the transition region between the electrolyte and membrane phase: in this region, the field change is not abrupt but continuous, and the charge density is not singular along a surface but distributed. Consider this transition region to have thickness $\Delta$, and locate a surface within this region equidistant from the edges of the transition region. (This construction can be done for any dynamic state of the membrane phase, not just the spatially invariant base state. Here the general case is presented so as to derive expressions for electrical forces on interfaces applicable as well to the linear dynamic states.)

As reasoned above, the volume force acting on the region interior to the transition region is equal to $\rho_e E_j + P_i \dfrac{\partial E_j}{\partial x_i}$. Since from Gauss's Law, $\rho_e = \dfrac{1}{4\pi} \dfrac{\partial}{\partial x_i} (\epsilon E_i)$, the volume force may be rewritten as $\dfrac{\partial T_{ij}}{\partial x_i}$, where $T_{ij}$ denotes the components of the Maxwell stress tensor. These are given by:

$$T_{ij} = \frac{\epsilon}{4\pi} E_i E_j - \frac{1}{8\pi} (E_m E_m)\delta_{ij} \tag{4a}$$

where $\delta_{ij}$ denotes the Kronecker $\delta$ symbol ($\delta_{ij} = 1$ if $i = j$, otherwise $\delta_{ij} = 0$) and $E_m E_m$ (sum on m) is the square magnitude of the field. The total force exerted on the transition region is obtained by integrating the force density $(\dfrac{\partial T_{ij}}{\partial x_i})$ over the volume. Consider a patch of surface *da* embedded in the transition region, and with local normal $n_j$ pointing in the direction of the adjoining semi-infinite phase and local tangent vector $t_j$ pointing outward from the demarcated area. Assuming the patch *da* to be small enough so that the electric field does not vary in directions lateral to the membrane along the patch, the electrical force exerted on the differential volume of transition region fluid enclosed by sides parallel to $n_j$ is given by $da \cdot F_{ej}$ where

$$F_{ej} = \int_{-\Delta/2}^{\Delta/2} (\rho_e E_j + P_i \frac{\partial E_j}{\partial x_i})\mathrm{d}\xi =$$

$$\int_{-\Delta/2}^{\Delta/2} (\frac{\partial T_{ij}}{\partial x_i})\mathrm{d}\xi \tag{4b}$$

The latter volume integral may be converted to an area integral by the divergence theorem: thus $\int_{-\Delta/2}^{\Delta/2} (\dfrac{\partial T_{ij}}{\partial x_i})\mathrm{d}\xi = n_i(T_{ij}^{\mathrm{I}} - T_{ij}^{\mathrm{II}}) + \int_{-\Delta/2}^{\Delta/2} t_i T_{ij}\mathrm{d}\xi$, where $T_{ij}^{\mathrm{I}}$ and $T_{ij}^{\mathrm{II}}$ are the values of the Maxwell stresses of the bulk phases at the border of the transition region. In the limit in which $\Delta \to 0$ and the interface is treated as a surface of charge at which the electric field changes discontinuously, the contributions to the area integral of the sides perpendicular to the embedded surface become negligible and the electrical force on the patch *da* becomes

$$F_{ej} = m_i(T_{ij}^{\mathrm{I}}|_s - T_{ij}^{\mathrm{II}}|_s) \tag{5}$$

where the subscripted variable '$s$' is a reminder that electric fields in the definitions of the components of the Maxwell stress tensor are to be evaluated at the surface. The electrical force given in Equation (5) may be resolved into a component normal to the surface $\Omega = F_{ej}n_j$ and one tangent to the surface $\Gamma = F_{ej}t_j$.

In the base state, the membrane interfaces are flat and the electric field is unidirectional; thus $n_3 = 1$ ($n_1 = n_2 = 0$), and the Maxwell stresses are normal $(T^a_{zz(o)} = (2\epsilon^a - 1)(E^a_{z(o)})^2/8\pi$, $T^a_{xx(o)} = T^a_{yy(o)} = -(E^a_{z(o)})^2/8\pi$ and $T^a_{ij(o)} = 0, i \neq j)$. The electrical force on the interfaces is only in the normal or $z$ direction and is given by $\Omega^\dagger_{(o)} = ((2\epsilon - 1) - (2\epsilon_m - 1)(\frac{\kappa}{\kappa_m})^2)(E^1_{z(o)})^2/8\pi$ for the upper interface and $-\Omega^\dagger_{(o)}$ for the lower interface. $\Omega^\dagger_{(o)}$ is clearly negative: characteristic values for $\epsilon$ and $\epsilon_m$ are 80 and 2, respectively, and the ratio of conductivities (under normal electroporative conditions) is of the order of $10^4 - 10^5$.[5] Thus, the action of the electrical stresses is to compress the membrane phase. At mechanical equilibrium, the electrical surface forces are balanced by the difference in pressures between the phases; thus

$$-p^1_{(o)} + p^{11}_{(o)} + \Omega^\dagger_{(o)} = 0 \ (z = h/2)$$
$$-p^{11}_{(o)} + p^{111}_{(o)} - \Omega^\dagger_{(o)} = 0 \ (z = -h/2) \tag{6a}$$

The above two equations indicate that the base state pressures of the bounding phases are equal and that the pressure in the membrane is necessarily larger than that of the surrounding phases in order to balance the electrical compression. It is important to emphasize here that as it is assumed that the membrane is unstrained in the base state, only the membrane pressure, arising from the incompressibility constraint, can balance the electrical compression exerted by the electrical forces on the interfaces.

Electrocompression without membrane elastic straining may be understood in physical terms through the following conceptualization: consider the flat membrane sheet to be enclosed by two parallel walls. The force (per unit area) which must be exerted on these walls to keep them from moving apart is denoted by $-T$, and is given by the expression:

$$p^{11}_{(o)} - T^{11}_{xx(o)} = -T \tag{6b}$$

Neglecting the electric field in the surrounding phases, $p^1_{(o)} = p^{11}_{(o)} - T^{11}_{zz(o)}$, and therefore since $T^{11}_{zz(o)} - T^{11}_{xx(o)} = \epsilon_m(E^{11}_{z(o)})^2/4\pi$,

$$\epsilon_m(E^{11}_{z(o)})^2/4\pi = -T - p^1_{(o)} \tag{6c}$$

From Equation (6c) it is clear that a (negative) stress of size $\epsilon_m(E^{11}_{z(o)})^2/4\pi$

has to be applied (in excess of $p_{(o)}^{\perp}$) to the walls to keep the membrane from straining. Thus, the requirement that the membrane be unstrained in the base state means that it is not relaxed laterally, but maintains a lateral tension transmitted from a constraining surface. For the case in which no such surface exists, the membrane is free and laterally relaxed, and $-T = P_{(o)}^{\perp}$. For this case, Equation (6c) is not satisfied, and the membrane would have to expand its area and contract its thickness. This point is discussed in more detail later.

## Linear stability analysis

Consider small, one-dimensional disturbances $\eta^{\uparrow}(x,t)$ and $\eta^{\downarrow}(x,t)$ from planarity of the membrane exo- and endofaces. These disturbances, as will be shown below, create electromechanical forces on the interfaces which can drive the system unstably away from the base state. The deformations also give rise to purely mechanical restoring forces – membrane elastic stresses and interfacial tensions – which can resist the destabilizing interfacial electromechanical stresses. The aim of this study is to understand this competition of interfacial electromechanical destabilization and stabilization due to membrane elastic stresses and interfacial tension in the regime of linear dynamics. To do so, the following initial condition-boundary value problem is posed: the base state is perturbed at time ($t$) equal to zero by interfacial deformations ordered with a small parameter $\delta$: thus $\eta^{\uparrow}(x,t=0) = \delta f^{\uparrow}(x)$ and $\eta^{\downarrow}(x,t=0) = \delta f^{\downarrow}(x)$. The initial surface and bulk phase velocities are assumed to be equal to zero. The surface deflections create stresses which cause the interfaces, the membrane phase and the surrounding electrolytes to move. The dynamic evolution is described by (a) Maxwell's equations in electroquasistatic approximation which account for charge conservation and which determine the electric field in terms of the polarization and charge density, and (b) the equations of motion and continuity expressing, respectively, momentum and mass conservation of the membrane and surrounding phase media. The equations which prescribe the dynamics are formulated in terms of the kinematic fields $u_i(x,z,t)$ (the Eulerian membrane displacement vector measured from the unstrained base state), $v_i^a(x,z,t)$ (the fluid velocity vectors), $p^a(x,z,t)$, $\eta^{\uparrow}(x,t)$ and $\eta^{\downarrow}(x,t)$ and the electrostatic field $E_i^a(x,z,t)$. Solutions for the kinematic and electrostatic fields of the initial condition-boundary value problem posed above are functions of $\delta$ as well as the indicated spatial coordinates and time. The functional dependence on $\delta$ may be expressed by an asymptotic expansion; thus,

$$\eta^\uparrow(x,t) = \delta\eta^\uparrow_{(1)}(x,t) + 0(\delta^2)$$
$$\eta^\downarrow(x,t) = \delta\eta^\downarrow_{(1)}(x,t) + 0(\delta^2)$$
$$u_j(x,z,t) = \delta u_{j(1)}(x,z,t) + 0(\delta^2)$$
$$v_j^a(x,z,t) = \delta v_{j(1)}^a(x,z,t) + 0(\delta^2)$$
$$E_i^a(x,z,t) = E_{z(0)}^a(z) + \delta E_{i(1)}^a(x,z,t) + 0(\delta^2)$$
$$p^a(x,z,t) = p_{(0)}^a(z) + \delta p_{(1)}^a(x,z,t) + 0(\delta^2) \tag{7}$$

Linear dynamics is described by the order $\delta$ terms, i.e. those subscripted by a '1'. To obtain the governing equations for the first-order variables, the asymptotic expansions are substituted into the governing equations, and only those terms of order $\delta$ are retained. The resulting equations are linear in the order one variables. Since the problem is unbounded in the $x$ direction, the dependence of the first-order variables on $x$ may be expressed by a Fourier integral. This is equivalent to assuming that the dynamics of the system may be decomposed into a set of normal modes of vibration in which the $x$ dependence of a system variable (for example, $\Theta_{(1)}(x,z,t)$) in each mode is of the form $e^{ikx}$, where $k$ is the disturbance wavenumber ($0 < k < \infty$). (The disturbance wavelength, $\lambda$, is equal to $2\pi/k$.) In order to evaluate the stability of each mode, time may be expressed in terms of a complex exponential growth parameter $\omega$ which is a function of the mode wavenumber $k$. Thus $\Theta_{(1)}(x,z,t) = \overline{\Theta}(z)\exp(ikx + \omega(k)t)$, and the system is stable to mode $k$ as long as $Re(\omega(k)) \leqslant 0$.

Wavenumbers, for which $\omega(k)$ are zero, identify neutral modes since these modes neither grow nor decay. These modes also demarcate the transition from unstable to stable modes, and they are therefore marginal modes. Since the aim of this study is to determine how large an applied field is necessary to destabilize the membrane system, this study will focus on the marginal state. The requirement that $\omega$ be equal to zero identifies the neutral modes as a function of the physical parameters of the problem: the applied field, the elastic moduli and the interfacial tensions. This functional dependence may be expressed in terms of neutral stability curves in which nondimensional ratios of the physical parameters are plotted against the neutral wavenumbers corresponding to these ratios. From these curves, one can deduce, for a given fixed value of the nondimensional ratio, which wavenumbers are unstable and which are not, and, finally, the value of the parameter ratio for which unstable waves first appear. It is this critical value which is the aim of the construction of the neutral curves, and which can be compared most readily with experiments.

For a symmetrical system, two fundamental system vibration modes exist. In the first, the film interfaces vibrate in phase, and the film thickness is preserved. This system mode is termed a stretching or bending vibration (abbreviated ST). It can be shown that this mode is not destabilized strongly by the electric field. In the second fundamental system vibration mode, the film interfaces vibrate $\pi$ radians out of phase, and the film thickness therefore alternately necks and thickens. This is the squeezing mode (abbreviated SQ and also pictured in Fig. 17.1), and it plays a crucial role in this study because, as explained in the Introduction, it may lead to the formation of pores. Thus, in the analysis detailed below, only the squeezing mode is considered. From the illustration in Fig. 17.1, it is clear that, for the squeezing mode, the $z$ component of the membrane displacement and surrounding phase velocity are antisymmetric functions of $z$. The reflectional symmetry about $z$ of the linear perturbation of the electrostatic potential follows from the form of the jump in this potential at the interfaces. From the first-order equations developed in the next section, it will become clear that for the SQ mode this jump requires antisymmetry in $z$. (Correspondingly, the $z$ and $x$ components of the first-order electric field are even and odd, respectively, with $z$.)

The neutral curves of the SQ mode are determined by solving the linear dynamic equations using the normal mode decomposition. This task is undertaken here in the following order. The electrodynamic equations are solved first in order to obtain expressions for the first-order electric force exerted on the interfaces as well as the first-order electric polarization force exerted on the bulk continua. Second, the first-order elastic stresses in the membrane are described. Third, the mass and momentum conservation equations are solved to yield the marginal functional dependence.

### The first-order electric field and Maxwell stresses

The electrodynamic equations are formulated in electroquasistatic form because the magnitude of magnetic fields induced by the current flow is small. Thus, induction effects related to time variations of these induced fields are negligible in Faraday's Law, and hence the electric field remains irrotational.[66] In electroquasistatic form, the electrodynamic equations are the conservation of charge $\dfrac{\partial \rho_e^a}{\partial t} = -\dfrac{\partial(\kappa^a E_i^a)}{\partial x_i}$ and Gauss's Law $(\dfrac{\partial}{\partial x_i}(\epsilon^a E_i^a) = 4\pi\rho_e^a)$ along with the fact that the electric field is irrotational $(\dfrac{\partial E_i^a}{\partial x_j} = \dfrac{\partial E_j^a}{\partial x_i})$. The condition of irrotationality allows the field to be expressed as the gradient of a scalar $\phi^a$ such that $E_i^a = -\dfrac{\partial \phi^a}{\partial x_i}$. The first-order equations for the electric field are obtained by substituting the asymptotic expansions (Equation (7)) into Gauss's Law, and the charge conservation equations, and collecting terms of order $\delta$. After decomposing the first-order variables into normal modes, and finally setting $\omega = 0$, it can easily be shown that the first-order volume charge density is equal to zero, and that the first-order potential field satisfies Laplace's equation:

$$D^2 \bar{\phi}^a - k^2 \bar{\phi}^a = 0 \tag{8}$$

where the operator '$D\bar{\Theta}$' indicates differentiation with respect to $z$. Equation (8) possesses, with respect to $z$, linearly independent symmetric and antisymmetric solution sets. In this problem, the electrostatic interfacial boundary conditions determine which solution set is applicable to the SQ mode. The boundary conditions on the electric field are the conservation of surface charge at the membrane faces, and the continuity of the tangential component of the electric field. The conservation of surface charge is expressed exactly by the condition $\dfrac{\partial \sigma^\uparrow}{\partial t} = -n_i^\uparrow(\kappa E_i^{\mathrm{I}} - \kappa_m E_i^{\mathrm{II}})\mid_s$, where $n_i^\uparrow$ is the unit normal vector to the exoface ($n_x^\uparrow = -\dfrac{\partial \eta^\uparrow}{\partial x}(1 + (\dfrac{\partial \eta^\uparrow}{\partial x})^2)^{-1/2}$ and $n_z^\uparrow = (1 + (\dfrac{\partial \eta^\uparrow}{\partial x})^2)^{-1/2}$). To first order, conservation of surface charge at marginal stability becomes:

$$\kappa\, D\bar{\phi}^{\mathrm{I}}\mid_{z=h/2} - \kappa_m D\bar{\phi}^{\mathrm{II}}\mid_{z=h/2} = 0 \tag{9}$$

Continuity of the tangential component of the electric field follows from integration of the irrotationality constraint on the electric field over a volume spanning the transition region of the interface in a manner as was done in the derivation of Equation (5). This condition is expressed exactly as $t_i^\uparrow(E_i^{\mathrm{I}} - E_i^{\mathrm{II}})\mid_s = 0$, where $t_i^\uparrow$ is the unit tangent vector to the exoface ($t_x^\uparrow = (1 + (\dfrac{\partial \eta^\uparrow}{\partial x})^2)^{-1/2}$ and $t_z^\uparrow = \dfrac{\partial \eta^\uparrow}{\partial x}(1 + (\dfrac{\partial \eta^\uparrow}{\partial x})^2)^{-1/2}$). To first order, continuity of the tangential component of the electric field becomes the following condition on the jump in the first-order potential:

$$\bar{\phi}^{\mathrm{I}}\mid_{z=h/2} - \bar{\phi}^{\mathrm{II}}\mid_{z=h/2} = \bar{\eta}^\uparrow(E_{z(o)}^{\mathrm{I}} - E_{z(o)}^{\mathrm{II}}) \tag{10}$$

In order that conditions similar to Equation (9) and Equation (10) be satisfied at $z = -h/2$, it is clear that the potential field must be antisymmetric. The antisymmetric solution set to Equation (8) which remains bounded as $z \to \pm \infty$ may be expressed as:

$$\bar{\phi}^{\mathrm{I}}(z) = a \cdot e^{-kz},\ \bar{\phi}^{\mathrm{II}}(z) = b \cdot \sinh(kz) \text{ and } \bar{\phi}^{\mathrm{III}}(z) = -a \cdot e^{kz} \tag{11}$$

where $a$ and $b$ are unknown constants. The constants $a$ and $b$ in the solution set may be expressed in terms of $\bar{\eta}^{\uparrow}$ from Equations (9) and (10); thus

$$\bar{\phi}^{\mathrm{I}}(z) = (-\cdot\bar{\eta}^{\uparrow}(E^{\mathrm{I}}_{z(\mathrm{o})} - E^{\mathrm{II}}_{z(\mathrm{o})})\mathrm{e}^{k(h/2-z)})K/(K+\tanh(kh/2))$$
$$\bar{\phi}^{\mathrm{II}}(z) = (-\cdot\bar{\eta}^{\uparrow}(E^{\mathrm{I}}_{z(\mathrm{o})} - E^{\mathrm{II}}_{z(\mathrm{o})})\sinh(kz))/\sinh(kh/2)+K\cosh(kh/2))$$
$$(12)$$

where $K$ is the ratio of the membrane to electrolyte conductivity ($K = \kappa_{\mathrm{m}}/\kappa$). The first-order charge density can be computed directly from the electrostatic fields of Equation (12) from the condition $-4\pi\bar{\sigma}^{\uparrow} = \epsilon\mathrm{D}\bar{\phi}^{\mathrm{I}}|_{z=h/2}$ $-\epsilon_{\mathrm{m}}\mathrm{D}\bar{\phi}|^{\mathrm{II}}_{z=h/2}$. Note also that it follows, from the antisymmetry of the solution set for $\bar{\phi}(z)$, that the first-order charge density at the lower face is equal to that of the upper face ($\bar{\sigma}^{\uparrow} = \bar{\sigma}^{\downarrow}$).

As noted above, at marginal stability, the first-order volume charge density is equal to zero. Hence, to this order, the only force the electric field can exert on the electrolyte and membrane phases is the polarization force $P^{\alpha}_{z(\mathrm{o})} \cdot \dfrac{\partial E_{i(1)}{}^{\alpha}}{\partial z} = \dfrac{1}{4\pi} (\epsilon^{\alpha}-1) \cdot \dfrac{\partial}{\partial x_i} (E^{\alpha}_{z(1)}E^{\alpha}_{z(\mathrm{o})})$. The later equality, which follows from the irrotationality of the first-order electric field, states that the electric force density can be represented as the gradient of the scalar field $\Xi^{\alpha}_{(1)} = \dfrac{1}{4\pi}$ $(\epsilon^{\alpha}-1)E^{\alpha}_{z(1)}E^{\alpha}_{z(\mathrm{o})}$ and is therefore also irrotational. As will become clear below, the representation of the polarization force as the gradient of a scalar field proves useful in solving the first-order equations of motion expressing the balance of linear momentum.

At the interfaces, the force exerted by the electric field is given exactly by $\Omega^{\uparrow} = n_i^{\uparrow}(T^{\mathrm{I}}_{ij} - T^{\mathrm{II}}_{ij})\,|_s n_j^{\uparrow}$ for the force normal to the interface, and $\Gamma^{\uparrow} = n_i^{\uparrow}(T^{\mathrm{I}}_{ij} - T^{\mathrm{II}}_{ij})\,|_s t_j^{\uparrow}$ for the force tangent to the interface. To first order, these tractions become:

$$\bar{\Omega}^{\uparrow} = (\bar{T}^{\mathrm{I}}_{zz} - \bar{T}^{\mathrm{II}}_{zz})\,|_{z=h/2}$$
$$= ((2\epsilon-1)/4\pi)(\bar{E}^{\mathrm{I}}_{z(1)|z=h/2}E^{\mathrm{I}}_{z(\mathrm{o})}) - ((2\epsilon_{\mathrm{m}}-1)/4\pi)(\bar{E}^{\mathrm{II}}_{z(1)|z=h/2}E^{\mathrm{II}}_{z(\mathrm{o})})$$
$$\bar{\Gamma}^{\uparrow} = (\bar{T}^{\mathrm{I}}_{zx} - \bar{T}^{\mathrm{II}}_{zx})\,|_{z=h/2} + \mathrm{i}k\bar{\eta}^{\uparrow}(T^{\mathrm{I}}_{zz(\mathrm{o})} - T^{\mathrm{II}}_{zz(\mathrm{o})})$$
$$(13)$$

Using the integrated solutions of the first-order state (Equation 12)), these tractions may be expressed entirely in terms of $\bar{\eta}^{\uparrow}$. From the antisymmetry of the potential field, it can be shown easily that the normal interfacial electromechanical stresses exerted on the endoface are equal in magnitude but opposite in sign $(n_i^{\downarrow}(T^{\mathrm{II}}_{ij} - T^{\mathrm{III}}_{ij})\,|_s n_j^{\downarrow})_{(1)} = \Omega^{\downarrow}_{(1)} = -\Omega^{\uparrow}_{(1)}$, while the tangential shears are equal: $(n_i^{\downarrow}(T^{\mathrm{II}}_{ij} - {}^{\mathrm{III}}_{ij})\,|_s t_j^{\downarrow})_{(1)} = \Gamma^{\downarrow}_{(1)} = \Gamma^{\uparrow}_{(1)}$.

## Membrane elasticity

The electromechanical interfacial tractions and volume polarization forces cause material motion of the membrane and electrolyte phases. The electrolytes are assumed to be incompressible Newtonian fluids. To first order, the electrolyte motion can be described by an equation of continuity $(ik\bar{v}_x^a + D\bar{v}_z^a = 0)$ expressing mass conservation of an incompressible medium, and Navier–Stokes equations augmented with the polarization force $(\rho\omega\bar{v}_x^a = -ik(\bar{p}^a - \bar{\Xi}^a) + \mu(D^2\bar{v}_x^a - k^2\bar{v}_x^a)$ and $\rho\omega\bar{v}_z^a = -D(\bar{p}^a - \bar{\Xi}^a) + \mu(D^2\bar{v}_z - k^2\bar{v}_z^a)$ expressing momentum conservation of a Newtonian fluid. (Here $\mu$ and $\rho$ represent the electrolyte fluid viscosity and density, respectively.) After elimination of $\bar{p}^a$, $\bar{\Xi}^a$ and $\bar{v}_x^a$, and setting $\omega = 0$, an Orr–Sommerfield equation for the $z$-component of the first order velocity field results:

$$(D^2 - k^2)^2 \; \bar{v}_z^a = 0 \tag{14}$$

Describing the mechanics of the membrane bilayer is a more complicated task. The only cell membrane whose mechanics has been studied in detail is that of the red blood cell (RBC) membrane. Experimental deformation studies of this membrane, particularly those using micropipette aspiration techniques, together with the associated modelling, have demonstrated that the RBC membrane strongly resists changes in its area, but, more readily, shears and stretches (at constant area) in its own plane. This in-plane response has also been shown to be visco-elastic. Constitutive equations describing in-plane membrane stresses as a function of in-plane shears and stretches have been developed, and are applicable to plate and shell-type calculations of membrane shapes[65].

Unlike the deformations which the membrane undergoes when subject to the stresses of micropipette aspiration, the interfacial electromechanical stresses ($\Omega$ and $\Gamma$) subject the membrane to strong forces tending to stretch and shear the membrane in planes perpendicular to the bilayer plane. To incorporate these responses in a three-dimensional mechanical picture, the membrane is modelled here as a transversely isotropic visco-elastic body. Stresses caused by small-strain deformations from an unstrained state can be described generally by a convolution integral of the linear strain rate history. Thus, the value of the first-order membrane stress tensor $\sigma_{ij(1)}$ at time $t$ and position $x,y,z$ is given by:

$$\sigma_{ij(1)} = \int_0^t G_{ijkl}(t - \tau)\dot{e}_{kl}(\tau)\mathrm{d}\tau \tag{15}$$

where the overdot indicated partial differentiation with respect to $\tau$, and where $G_{ijkl}(\tau)$ is a stress relaxation tensor, and $e_{kl}$ is the (linear) strain tensor

$(e_{kl} = \frac{1}{2}(\frac{\partial u_{k(1)}}{\partial x_l} + \frac{\partial u_{l(1)}}{\partial x_k}))$. For a transversely isotropic body, the convolution integral takes the forms:

$$\sigma_{xx(1)} = \int_o^t (2G_1(t-\tau)\dot{e}_{xx}(\tau) + (E_1(t-\tau) - G_1(t-\tau))(\dot{e}_{xx} + \dot{e}_{yy}))d\tau$$

$$\sigma_{xy(1)} = \int_o^t (2G_1(t-\tau)\dot{e}_{xy}(\tau)d\tau$$

$$\sigma_{yy(1)} = \int_o^t (2G_1(t-\tau)\dot{e}_{yy}(\tau) + (E_1(t-\tau) - G_1(t-\tau))(\dot{e}_{xx} + \dot{e}_{yy}))d\tau$$

$$\sigma_{xz(1)} = \int_o^t (2G_2(t-\tau)\dot{e}_{xz}(\tau)d\tau$$

$$\sigma_{yz(1)} = \int_o^t (2G_2(t-\tau)\dot{e}_{yz}(\tau)d\tau$$

$$\sigma_{zz(1)} = \int_o^t (2E_2(t-\tau)\dot{e}_{zz}(\tau)d\tau \tag{16}$$

where $G_1(\tau)$ and $G_2(\tau)$ are stress relaxations for, respectively, $xy$ shear deformations in the plane of the bilayer, and $xz$ and $yz$ shears in the plane perpendicular to the bilayer. $E_1(\tau)$ is a relaxation corresponding to changes in membrane area ($e_{xx} + e_{yy}$ defines the change in the membrane area), and $E_2(\tau)$ is a relaxation for stretching in the $z$ direction in the plane perpendicular to the bilayer plane.

The fact that the $G_i(\tau)$ and $E_i(\tau)$ are stress relaxations to applied deformations may be demonstrated as follows. Consider suddenly stretching the membrane in the $z$ direction by the applied deformation $u_{z(1)}(z)U(t)$, where $U(t)$ is the step function and $u_{z(1)}(z)$ is time independent. Thus $e_{zz} = U(t) \cdot \frac{\partial u_{z(1)}}{\partial_z}$ and $\sigma_{zz}(t) = E_2(t) \cdot \frac{u_{z(1)}}{\partial z}$. Note, finally, that the elastic response corresponds to the stress after the relaxation is completed and is given by $\sigma_{zz}(\infty) = E_2(\infty)\frac{\partial u_{z(1)}}{\partial z}$. Therefore, the elastic moduli are $\bar{G}_i = \lim\limits_{t\to\infty} G_i(t)$ and $\bar{E}_i = \lim\limits_{t\to\infty} E_i(t)$.

Linear membrane mechanics in normal mode form is described by an equation of continuity for the incompressible membrane phase ($D\bar{u}_z + ik\bar{u}_x = 0$) and linear momentum balances ($\rho_m\omega^2\bar{u}_x = -ik(\bar{p}^{II} - \bar{\Xi}^{II}) + ik\bar{\sigma}_{xx} + D\bar{\sigma}_{xz}$ and $\rho_m\omega^2\bar{u}_z = -D(\bar{p}^{II} - \bar{\Xi}^{II}) + ik\bar{\sigma}_{xz} + D\bar{\sigma}_{zz}$) augmented with the polarization force. After elimination of the in-plane displacement $\bar{u}_x$, the pressure and the polarization force fields, and upon taking the limit as $\omega \to 0$, the following analogue of Equation (14) is derived:

$$(D^4 - 2k^2 YD^2 + k^4)\bar{u}_z = 0, \tag{17}$$

where $Y = \lim\limits_{\omega\to 0} ((\omega E_1(\omega) + \omega G_1(\omega) + \omega E_2(\omega) - 2\omega G_2(\omega))/2\omega G_2(\omega))$ and $G_i(\omega)$ and $E_i(\omega)$ denote the Laplace transforms of the stress relaxation functions. Since, from the final value theorem of the Laplace transformation, $\bar{E}_i = \lim\limits_{\omega\to 0} \omega E_i(\omega)$ and $\bar{G}_i = \lim\limits_{\omega\to 0} \omega G_i(\omega)$, the marginal state (and, in particular, $\Upsilon$) is only a function of the elastic moduli. Note that, when the membrane is isotropic, $G_1(\omega) = E_1(\omega) = G_2(\omega)$ and $E_2(\omega) = 2G_2(\omega)$; with these relations, $\Upsilon$ becomes equal to one, and Equation (17) becomes of the same form as (14).

The solution set to Equations (14) and (17) which describes squeezing vibrations of the membrane system is antisymmetric with respect to $z$ and is given by:

$$
\begin{aligned}
\bar{v}_z^{\mathrm{I}}(z) &= c_1 \cdot e^{-kz} + c_2 \cdot z \cdot e^{-kz} \\
\bar{u}_z(z) &= c_3 \cdot \sinh(ka_1 z) + c_4 \cdot \sinh(ka_2 z) \\
\bar{v}_z^{\mathrm{III}}(z) &= -c_1 \cdot e^{+kz} + c_2 \cdot z \cdot e^{+kz}
\end{aligned}
\tag{18}
$$

where the additional constraint of boundedness at $z \to \pm\infty$ has been imposed and where $a_1 = (\Upsilon + (\Upsilon^2 - 1)^{1/2})^{1/2}$ and $a_2 = (\Upsilon - (\Upsilon^2 - 1)^{1/2})^{1/2}$ The constants are determined from the kinematic and stress boundary conditions at the interfaces. Consider first the kinematic conditions. These are (i) continuity of the normal and tangential components of the velocity field at the interfaces and (ii) an equation relating the movement of the boundary surface defining the interface (i.e., $\eta^{\uparrow}(x,t)$ and $\eta^{\downarrow}(x,t)$). Since the displacement field in the membrane is Eulerian, the velocity field is given implicitly by the equation $v_i^{\mathrm{II}} = \dfrac{\partial u_i^{\mathrm{II}}}{\partial t} + v_{\mathrm{m}}^{\mathrm{II}} \cdot \dfrac{\partial u_i^{\mathrm{II}}}{\partial x_{\mathrm{m}}}$. To first order in $\delta$, however, the displacement and velocity fields are related simply by $\dfrac{\partial u_{\mathrm{m}(1)}^{\mathrm{II}}}{\partial t} = v_{\mathrm{m}(1)}^{\mathrm{II}}$.

Continuity of the normal and tangential components of the velocity field at the upper surface is given exactly by $(m_i^{\mathrm{I}}(v_i^{\mathrm{I}} - v_i^{\mathrm{II}})) = 0$ and $(t_i^{\mathrm{I}}(v_i^{\mathrm{I}} - v_i^{\mathrm{II}})) = 0$, and to first order in normal mode form by:

$$
\bar{v}_z^{\mathrm{I}}|_{z=h/2} = \omega \cdot \bar{u}_z|_{z=h/2}; \quad D\bar{v}_z^{\mathrm{I}}|_{z=h/2} = \omega \cdot D\bar{u}_z|_{z=h/2}
\tag{19}
$$

Similar equations exist at $z = -h/2$, and are satisfied by the antisymmetric solution set (18). At marginal stability ($\omega = 0$), continuity requires that $\bar{v}_z^{\mathrm{I}}|_{z=h/2} = D\bar{v}_z^{\mathrm{I}}|_{z=h/2} = 0$, and hence that $c_1 = c_2 = 0$. Thus, in the marginal state, the interfaces are deformed ($\bar{\eta}^{\uparrow}$ is nonzero) and the membrane is strained ($c_3$ and $c_4$ are nonzero) but the fluid media are motionless.

The motion of the interfaces is defined in the following way. The interfaces are conceptualized as being composed of particles which remain on the surface for all time, and which move at the velocity of the media which adjoin them. (These are sufficient, though not necessary, conditions for the interfaces to act as bounding surfaces for the bulk media, i.e. surfaces which do not allow transfer of bulk fluid.) If a surface is defined by the relation $F(z,x,t) = z - \eta(x,t)$, and the particle trajectories by $z_p(t)$ and

$x_p(t)$, then for a particle to remain on the surface the trajectory functions must satisfy $F(z_p(t),x_p(t))=0$. Differentiating the latter expression with respect to time, and noting that $\dot{z}_p$ and $\dot{x}_p$ define the particle velocity (and therefore the instantaneous fluid velocity), the following equation is obtained:

$$\frac{\partial \eta^\uparrow}{\partial t} = v_z^{\text{II}}|_s - v_x^{\text{II}}|_s \cdot \frac{\partial \eta^\uparrow}{\partial x} \tag{20}$$

To first order in the normal mode domain, Equation (20) becomes $\bar{u}_z|_{z=h/2} = \eta^\uparrow$.

The final conditions are the normal and tangential stress balances at the interfaces. The normal stress balance at the upper interface is expressed exactly by the relation:

$$-p^{\text{I}}|_s + p^{\text{II}}|_s + \Omega\uparrow + (n_i^\uparrow(\tau_{ij}^{\text{I}} - \sigma_{ij})\,|_s n_j^\uparrow) +$$
$$\gamma \cdot \frac{\partial^2 \eta^\uparrow}{\partial x^2} \cdot (1 + (\frac{\partial \eta^\uparrow}{\partial x})^2)^{-3/2} = 0 \tag{21}$$

where $\gamma$ denotes the interfacial tension and $\tau_{ij}^{\text{I}}$ the viscous stress tensor of the Newtonian upper phase. The last term in the above balance is equal to twice the mean curvature of the interface, and represents the restoring action of the interfacial tension. To first order, at marginal stability, this equation may be written:

$$(k^4\gamma - k^3\Phi(k)\epsilon_{\text{m}}(E_{z(0)}^{\text{II}})^2/4\pi)\,\bar{u}\,|_{z=h/2} - \bar{G}_2 D^3\bar{u}_z|\,_{z=h/2} +$$
$$(2\Upsilon + 1)k^2\,\bar{G}_2 D\bar{u}_z|_{z=h/2} = 0 \tag{22}$$

where $k\Phi(k)$ is given explicitly by:

$$\Phi(k) = (1-K)(1-\chi K^2)/(K+\tanh{(kh/2)}) \tag{23}$$

where $\chi$ is the ratio of the electrolyte to membrane dielectric constant.

For the tangential balance, two limiting conditions are formulated. The first condition requires that the interface is constrained from the relative displacement of its material particles. To first order, this condition requires (for the upper interface) that $\bar{u}_x|_{z=h/2} = 0$ (or, equivalently, $D\bar{u}_z|_{z=h/2} = 0$). The second limiting form assumes that the interfaces are unconstrained in their lateral motion, and, therefore, the dynamics is determined by a tangential stress balance. Balance of tangential stresses exerted on the upper interface is given exactly by:

$$\Gamma^\uparrow + n_i^\uparrow(\tau_{ij}^{\text{I}} - \sigma_{ij})\,|_s t_j^\uparrow = 0 \tag{24}$$

and, to first order, in normal mode form at marginal stability, by:

$$\bar{G}_2(D^2\bar{u}_z|_{z=h/2} + k^2\bar{u}_z|_{z=h/2}) + k^2\beta(\frac{E^{II^2}_{z(0)}}{4\pi})\bar{u}_z|_{z=h/2} = 0 \tag{25}$$

where

$$\beta = (1 - \chi K)K(1 + \tanh(kh/2))/(K + \tanh(kh/2)) \tag{25}$$

Substituting the integrated solution set into Equation (22) and either Equation (25) or the surface immobility constraint $D\bar{u}|_{z=h/2} = 0$, yields the following two marginal stability conditions:

$$\varLambda = \varPhi(k)\psi_i/(1 + kh \cdot S \cdot \psi_i) \quad \text{(immobile neutral curve)} \tag{26a}$$

$$\varLambda = \varPhi(k)\psi_m/(1 + kh \cdot S \cdot \psi_m) - \beta\phi_m/(1 + kh \cdot S \cdot \psi_m)$$
$$\text{(mobile neutral curve)} \tag{26b}$$

where:

$$\varLambda = \bar{G}_2/(\epsilon_m(E^{II}_{z(0)})^2/4\pi)$$
$$S = \gamma/(\bar{G}_2 h)$$
$$\psi_i = (\tanh(kha_2/2)/a_2 - \tanh(kha_1/2)/a_1)/(a_1^2 - a_2^2)$$
$$\psi_m = (a_1 - a_2)/((a_1 + a_2)(\coth(kha_2/2)/a_2 - \coth(kha_1/2)/a_1))$$
$$\phi_m = ((\coth(kha_2/2) - \coth(kha_1/2))/(\coth(kha_2/2)/$$
$$a_2 - \coth(kha_1/2)/a_1)) \times (1/(a_1 + a_2))$$

Note, finally, the limiting forms for $\psi_i$ and $\psi_m$ under isotropic conditions ($\varUpsilon \to 1$):

$$\lim_{\varUpsilon \to 1} (\psi_i) = (\sinh(kh) - kh)/(2(\cosh(kh) + 1))$$

$$\lim_{\varUpsilon \to 1} (\psi_m) = (\cosh(kh) - 1)/(2(\sinh(kh) + kh))$$

$$\lim_{\varUpsilon \to 1} (\phi_m) = kh/(2(\sinh(kh) + kh))$$

## Marginal curves and stability maps

Consider first the properties of the neutral stability curves (Equations (26a) and (26b)) in the absence of membrane surface tension ($S = 0$). It can be shown easily analytically that, for both neutral curves, when $S$ is equal to zero, $\varLambda$ is a monotonically increasing function of kh which asymptotes for both surface conditions to the same positive constant value as $kh \to \infty$. This value is denoted by $\varLambda_\infty$ and is given by

$$\varLambda_\infty = \frac{(1 - \chi K^2)(1 - K)}{(a_1 + a_2)} \tag{26}$$

While the asymptotic behaviour of the marginal curves for very short waves is identical for both surface conditions, the behaviour for long waves $(kh \to 0)$ is different. The value of $\Lambda$ for immobile conditions tends to zero while that for a mobile interface tends to a negative value. The intersection of the mobile marginal curve with the abscissa is at values of $kh$ of $O(K)$, and therefore negative values of $\Lambda$ occur only for extremely long disturbance waves.

Illustrations of the zero surface tension neutral curves for different values of $Y(1, 10, 10^2$ and $10^3)$ are given in Figs. 17.2(a) and (b) for, respectively, immobile and mobile surface conditions. In these, and in all subsequent simulations, the ratio $K$ of the membrane conductivity to that of the surrounding phase is taken to be equal to $10^{-5}$, and the ratio $\chi$ of the surrounding phase dielectric constant to that of the membrane is set equal to 80/2.2; these are typical values (cf. Zimmermann *et al.*[5] and Needham and Hockmuth[47]). Also, note that the values used for the anisotropic parameter $Y$ are equal to, and larger than, one. This choice reflects the fact that, as explained in the Introduction, the modulus for shearing deformations in the transverse plane of the membrane $(\bar{G}_2)$ is presumed to be much less than the moduli for area enlargement $(\bar{E}_1)$ or thickness expansion $(\bar{E}_2)$. Experimental support of this assumption is presented on p. 352–6.

Recall that the neutral curves locate waves of marginal stability, i.e. those which do not grow or decay $(\omega = 0)$. To resolve the stability of waves larger or smaller than the critical one, a normal mode analysis including the unsteady terms must be done, and then the sign of $\dfrac{d\omega_r}{dk}$ must be computed at the marginal point. These details are not given here, but it can be shown that for constant $\Lambda$, waves shorter than the critical one are unstable, while those larger are stable. Thus, Figs. 17.2(a) and (b) are marginal stability curves, and the regions underneath the curve are labelled with a 'U'. The membrane is stable when all waves are stable; thus, in the absence of surface tension, a necessary and sufficient condition for instability is that $\Lambda < \Lambda_\infty$. When this condition is fulfilled, a band of unstable short waves exists.

The necessary and sufficient condition $\Lambda < \Lambda_\infty$ is a new result, and describes the influence of finite electrolyte conductivity (through the parameter $K$) and anisotropic membrane elasticity (through the parameter $Y$). The dependence on the anisotropic parameter is significant, and is illustrated by the different curves in Fig. 17.2 representing $Y = 1, 10, 10^2$ and $10^3$. As is clear from the figure, as $Y$ increases from one, the curves lie successively beneath one another, the region of instability is reduced, and larger transmembrane potentials are necessary to destabilize the system. This behaviour is in accordance with the fact that, as $Y$ increases from one,

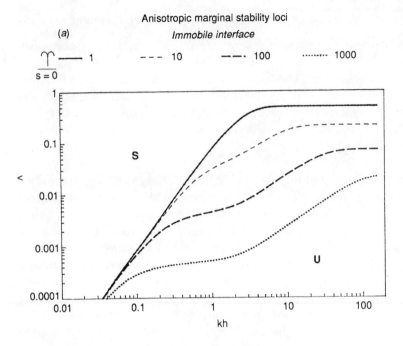

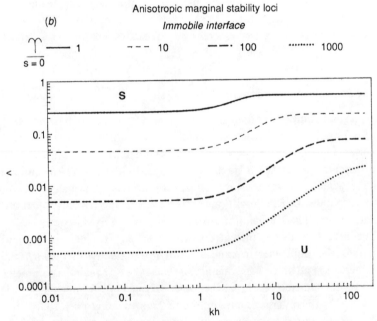

Fig. 17.2. Marginal stability curves of $\Lambda$ as a function of $kh$ for $Y=1, 10$ $10^2$ and $10^3$, $K=10^{-5}$ and $X=80/2.2$: (a) immobile surface conditions; and (b) mobile surface conditions.

the moduli for increases in membrane area ($\bar{E}_1$), thickness ($\bar{E}_2$) or strain in the $x$ direction ($\bar{G}_1$) must increase over their isotropic values, and this will necessarily restrain the disjoining action of the interfacial electromechanical stresses. In the limit of infinite electrolyte conductance ($K \to 0$) and isotropic membrane elasticity ($\Upsilon = 1$), $\Lambda_\infty$ reduces to $1/2$ and Crowley's stability criterion for an incompressible body, as given in the Introduction, Equation (1), is recovered. Note, finally, that as remarked above, in the limit of very short waves ($kh \to \infty$), both surface conditions approach the same asymptote. This behaviour is a consequence of the fact that, for short waves, the elastic forces *throughout* the membrane volume are great, and dominate the restoring action, with the lateral extensibility of the surface playing a less important role.

The presence of a membrane surface tension ($S \neq 0$) stabilizes short waves ($kh >> 1$), and this influence is shown in Fig. 17.3 for an isotropic membrane ($\Upsilon = 1$) under immobile (3a) and mobile (3b) surface conditions $S = 0.1, 1$ and $10$. When $S$ is nonzero, $\Lambda$ achieves a maximum ($\Lambda^*$) at a value of $kh = k^*h$, and then descends towards, and asymptotically approaches zero as $kh \to \infty$. Note that $\Lambda^* < \Lambda_\infty$, and therefore the condition $\Lambda < \Lambda_\infty$ is necessary but no longer sufficient for instability. Instead, the new sufficient condition for instability is that $\Lambda < \Lambda^*$; when this inequality is fulfilled, the system is unstable to a finite band of wavelengths. Marginal curves for anisotropic membranes with nonzero surface tension are shown in Figs. 17.4(a) for $\Upsilon = 10^2$ and immobile conditions and Fig. 17.4(b) for $\Upsilon = 10^2$ and mobile conditions. The stabilizing effect of surface tension is again evident in this series of figures, but, for the same value of $S$, the values of $k^*h$, for which the maximum in $\Lambda$ occurs, become progressively larger as $\Upsilon$ increases. The physical reason for this shift is that, as $\Upsilon$ increases at fixed $S$, resistance to area and thicknesses changes in the membrane interior become great and dominate the restoring response, causing the marginal curves to asymptote as $kh$ increases (Fig. 17.3). It, therefore, requires very short waves for the surface tension forces to become controlling and cause the marginal curves to turn towards zero.

Marginal stability loci which provide sufficient conditions for membrane stability as a function of $S$ can be constructed in the following implicit manner: The function $\Lambda(S,kh,\Upsilon)$ is differentiated with respect to $kh$, and the result is set equal to zero providing an implicit equation for $k^*h$ as a function of $S$. In this equation, $S$ may be expressed directly as a function of $k^*h$, and, by varying $k^*h$, the surface tensions which give these critical wavelengths may be computed. For a particular pair ($k^*h,S$), the value of $\Lambda$ is then obtained from the equation $\Lambda = \Lambda(S,k^*h)$. In this way, the $\Lambda$

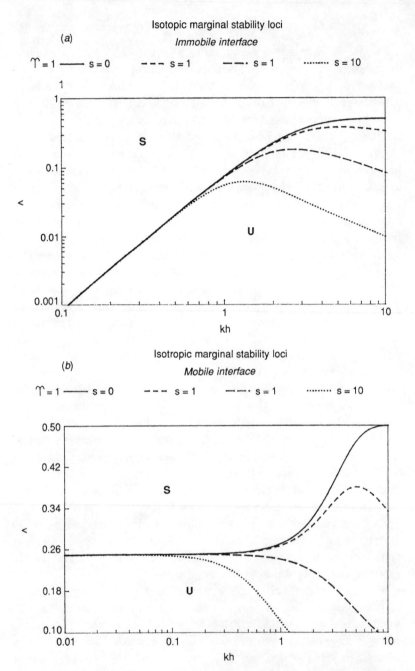

Fig. 17.3. Marginal stability curves of $\Lambda$ as a function of $kh$ for an isotropic membrane ($Y=1$) demonstrating the influence of surface tension ($K=10^{-5}$ and $\chi=80/2.2$.; $S=0.1$, 1 and 10): (a) immobile surface conditions; and (b) mobile surface conditions.

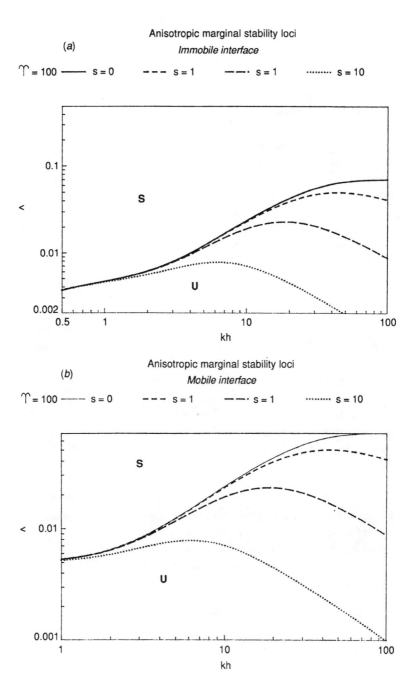

Fig. 17.4. Marginal stability curves of $\Lambda$ as a function of $kh$ for an anisotropic membrane ($Y = 10^2$) demonstrating the influence of surface tension ($K = 10^{-5}$ and $\chi = 80/2.2$.; $S = 0.1$, 1 and 10): (a) immobile surface conditions; and (b) mobile surface conditions.

corresponding to different values of $S$ may be computed. The results are presented for $Y=1$, 10 and $10^2$ in Figs. 17.5($a$) and ($b$), respectively, immobile and mobile surface conditions. Note, from Figs. 17.5($a$) and ($b$), that at fixed $S$, increasing $\Lambda$ across a marginal boundary corresponds to moving from an unstable to a stable physical parameter set. Therefore, the space underneath the marginal curves of these figures represents unstable conditions, and the space above represents stable conditions.

Consider first the stability map for immobile conditions (Fig. 17.5($a$)). As $S\rightarrow0$, $k^*h\rightarrow\infty$, and $\Lambda$ asymptotes to $\Lambda_\infty$. As $S\rightarrow\infty$, it can be shown analytically that $(k^*h)^4=(9/2)S^{-1}+O(1)$. This reflects the physical fact that as the magnitude of the surface tension coefficient increases, longer and longer waves are stabilized. Since, in the limit, as $S\rightarrow\infty$, $k^*h\rightarrow0$, $\Lambda=\Lambda(k^*h,S)$ must also tend to zero. For $K<<S^{-1/4}<<1$, the asymptotic approach of $\Lambda$ to zero is given by $\Lambda=(1/2)(6S)^{-1/2}+O(1)$ as $S\rightarrow\infty$. Denoting $E^{II}_{(0)z}$ by $\dfrac{V_c}{h}$ in the expression for $\Lambda$, where $V_c$ is the critical transmembrane potential difference and $h$ the base state membrane thickness, this asymptotic formula for the marginal curve as $S\rightarrow\infty$ may be written as $V_c^2=((24G\sigma h^3)/(\epsilon_m/4\pi)^2)^{1/2}$. This expression for the critical potential was first derived by Dimitrov[41] using a lubrication analysis in which the disturbance waves were assumed to be much longer than the membrane thickness ($kh\rightarrow0$). Dimitrov's result agrees with this study's exact analysis only in the large surface tension limit ($S\rightarrow\infty$) because it is only in this limit that the critical wave $k^*h$ which yields a maximum for $\Lambda$ becomes much larger than the membrane thickness (i.e. $(k^*h)<<1$). The lubrication result is plotted also in Fig. 17.5($a$), and it is seen that, for intermediate or low surface tensions, the Dimitrov result overpredicts $\Lambda_c$ and therefore underpredicts the critical membrane potential necessary and sufficient for instability. For even larger $S$, i.e. $K>>S^{-1/4}$, it can be shown that the asymptotic approach to zero shifts to the expression $\Lambda=(9/2S)^{3/4}/12K$. This latter asymptote is probably not physically relevant for small values of $K$ because it requires excessively high values of $S$ (e.g. for $K=10^{-5}$, $S>10^{20}$).

The stability map for mobile surface conditions is given in Fig. 17.5($b$). Once again, as $S\rightarrow0$ the curves demarcating stable and unstable parameter spaces asymptote to $\Lambda_\infty$. In the limit of large surface tension, however, the curves all appear to asymptote towards plateau values. This type of behaviour is only strictly true for an infinitely conducting electrolyte ($K=0$). For that case, the plateau values of $\Lambda$ are given by $(a_1+a_2)^{-2}$, and the curves smoothly reach this plateau for $S=(1/6)(a_1+a_2)^2$. For nonzero

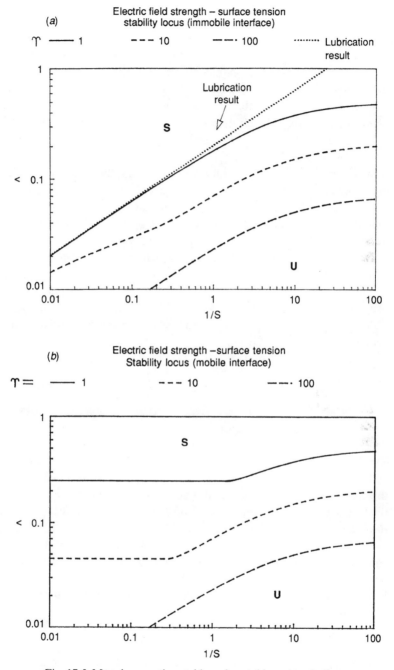

Fig. 17.5. Map demarcating stable and unstable regions in the parameter space of $\Lambda$ and $S$ for $Y = 1$, 10 and $10^2$ ($K = 10^{-5}$ and $\chi = 80/2.2$.): (a) immobile surface conditions; and (b) mobile surface conditions.

but very small $K$ (e.g. the simulation value of $10^{-5}$), the curves eventually tend towards zero for extremely large values of $S$. However, this additional stabilization is probably not physically relevant because of the excessively high values of $S$ it requires. Finally, it should be noted that, for small but finite $K$, the near plateau value and the value of $S$ at which the near plateau behaviour commences are given to a very good approximation by the $K=0$ values (i.e. the plateau in $\Lambda$ is equal to $(a_1 + a_2)^{-2}$, and the plateau begins at $S = (1/6)(a_1 + a_2)^2$).

As observed earlier in the discussion of Fig. 17.3, the values of $k^*h$, for which maxima in $\Lambda$ exist, shift to larger values of $k^*h$ as $Y$ increases from the isotropic value of one. Note further that the maxima in $\Lambda$ (i.e. $\Lambda^*$) for the two surface conditions approach each other in the limit of large $Y$ since the surface extensibility does not play a significant role for short wavelength disturbances. Therefore, for a fixed range of values of $S$ (starting at zero), as $Y$ increases, the $\Lambda - (1/S)$ stability maps should approach one another. This is, indeed, the case as can be seen from examination of the $Y = 10^2$ boundaries on Figs. 17.5(a) and (b) for the fixed surface tension parameter interval $0.1 < S < 10$. This result is extremely important because it means that, for the values of $S < 10$ and $Y > 10^2$, the stability maps are independent of the mobility of the interface.

### Comparisons of the anisotropic model results with experiments and concluding remarks

The first issue in comparing the marginal curves of the anisotropic model with electroporative experiments is to verify that the electrocompression of the membrane at $V_c$ is small. For this purpose, the pressure $-T$ applied in the lateral direction to keep the lamellae from compressing (cf. Equation (6b)) is set equal to $P_{(o)}^l$. The relaxed bilayer then compresses in the $z$ direction and expands in the $x$ direction. It is assumed here that this elastic strain is small and that, therefore, the linear constitutive equations of pp. 340–4 are valid. In that case, because the membrane is now unconstrained in the lateral direction, rather than (6b), the balance of forces in that direction becomes:

$$p_{(o)}^{ll} - T_{xx(o)}^{ll} - (\bar{G}_1 + \bar{E}_1)\, e_{xx(o)} = -T \tag{27a}$$

where $e_{xx(o)}$, a constant, represents the (one-dimensional) strain in the membrane area of the base state. In the $z$ direction, the balance of forces becomes (neglecting the electric field in the surrounding phase):

$$p^{II}_{(o)} - T^{II}_{zz(o)} - \bar{E}_2 \, e_{zz(o)} = P^I_{(o)} \tag{27b}$$

where $e_{zz(o)}$ is the elastic compression in the $z$ direction, and is equal to $-e_{xx(o)}$ as a consequence of incompressibility. Combining the above two expressions to eliminate the pressure in the bilayer results in an expression for the small strain change in the membrane area with the Maxwell compressive force:

$$T + p^I_{(o)} + \frac{\epsilon_m}{4\pi}(E^{II}_{z(o)})^2 = (\bar{E}_1 + \bar{E}_2 + \bar{G}_1)e_{xx(o)} \tag{28}$$

or simply $\dfrac{\epsilon_m}{4\pi} (E^{II}_{z(o)})^2 = (\bar{E}_1 + \bar{E}_2 + \bar{G}_1)e_{xx(o)}$ since $-T = p^I_{(o)}$. The critical potential is given by the stability maps of Fig. 17.5. Neglecting surface tension, it is clear that, for either surface condition, at the critical potential sufficient for instability, $\Lambda = \Lambda_\infty$, or

$$\frac{\epsilon_m}{4\pi} \left(\frac{V_c}{h}\right)^2 = \bar{G}_2(a_1 + a_2) \tag{29}$$

From Equations (28) and (29), the change in area of the base state at the critical potential is given by:

$$\bar{G}_2(a_1 + a_2) = (\bar{E}_1 + \bar{E}_2 + \bar{G}_1)e_{xx(o)} \tag{30}$$

Assuming that $\bar{G}_1 << \bar{E}_1$, $\bar{G}_2 << \bar{E}_2$ and $\bar{G}_2 << \bar{E}_1$, $\tau >> 1$ and $(a_1 + a_2) \approx ((\bar{E}_1 + \bar{E}_2)/\bar{G}_2)^{1/2}$. (Note that an ordering of $\bar{E}_1$ and $\bar{E}_2$ is not specified, and is not needed since it is their sum which is measured; cf. the discussion below.) With these approximations, the base state area stretch becomes:

$$e_{xx(o)} \approx (\bar{G}_2/(\bar{E}_1 + \bar{E}_2))^{1/2} << 1 \tag{31}$$

Thus, as long as the moduli inequalities are met, the base state increase in membrane area, and the constriction in the membrane thickness, are both small.

In order to use the stability maps presented in the previous section to predict critical potentials, it is clear that at least $\tau$, $\bar{G}_2$ and $S$ must be known. In micropipette aspiration experiments[65], the area of lipid bilayer membranes is increased through an imposed, measurable lateral tension $T(>0)$, and the area expansion $e_{xx(o)}$ is measured. By using Equation (28) (with the electrocompression term equal to zero) it is clear, from these studies, that $\bar{E}_1 + \bar{E}_2 + \bar{G}_1$ can be deduced. Other aspiration experiments, at constant membrane area, have been undertaken on RBCs to measure $\bar{G}_1$ [65], and it is found that $\bar{G}_1 < < (\bar{E}_1 + \bar{E}_2)$. However, the transverse moduli and the surface tension $\gamma$ are unknown. Nevertheless, the anisotropic model at least may be checked qualitatively by predicting $\bar{G}_2$ and $S$ from critical potential data. In this regard, consider the recent data of Needham and Hochmuth[47] on the electropermeabilization of three different reconstituted bilayers with increasing amounts of cholesterol: stearoyloleoylphosphatidyl choline (SOPC), red blood cell (RBC) lipid extract and SOPC cholesterol (CHOL), 1:1. Micropipette aspiration techniques were used to measure $\bar{E}_1 + \bar{E}_2$ of these membranes, and it was found that the presence of increasing amounts of cholesterol enhanced the membrane cohesiveness, and thereby increased $\bar{E}_1 + \bar{E}_2$. Neglecting for the moment the influence of surface tension, the critical potential may be obtained by equating $\Lambda = (a_1 + a_2)^{-1}$. Assuming $\bar{G}_1 < < \bar{E}_1$ and $\bar{G}_2 < < \bar{E}_1, (a_1 + a_2) \approx ((\bar{E}_1 + \bar{E}_2)/\bar{G}_2)^{1/2}$, and the following approximate equation for $\bar{G}_2$ in terms of $V_c$ may be derived:

$$\bar{G}_2 h \approx (\epsilon_m/4\pi)^2 (V_c^4/h^2)/((\bar{E}_1 + \bar{E}_2)h) \tag{32}$$

The above corresponds to a value for $\bar{G}_2$ for $S=0$. For $S>0$, $\bar{G}_2$ must decrease from Equation (32) in order that the membrane destabilize for the same value of $V_c$. These lower values of $\bar{G}_2$ at finite $S$ may be obtained from the simulations of Fig. 17.5. The values of the surface tension $\gamma$ and transverse shear modulus $\bar{G}_2$, consistent with the critical potential, are given in Fig. 17.6 for each of the reconstituted bilayers of Needham and Hochmuth's study. (Although these curves were constructed using the mobile interface condition map, Fig. 17.5, the immobile map can be shown to yield identical results because the values of $\Upsilon$ are large enough that $k^*h > > 1$. Finally, in obtaining these curves, the values used for $\bar{E}_1 + \bar{E}_2$, $V_c$ and $h$ are obtained from the Needham and Hochmuth study and are listed for each of the reconstituted cell types in Table 17.1. The tabulated values for $V_c$ are those for a laterally relaxed membrane, and are obtained from the extrapolated values as presented in Fig. 3 of Needham and Hochmuth.)

Consider Fig. 17.6, and note first that the upper bound values for $\bar{G}_2 h$ corresponding to $\gamma = 0$ and given by Equation (32) lie in the range $3 \times 10^{-1}$–$9 \times 10^{-1}$ dyne/cm, and these values are, as anticipated, approximately three orders of magnitude smaller than $(\bar{E}_1 + \bar{E}_2)h$. The upper bound for the transverse shear modulus is also two orders of magnitude larger than the value of the lateral shear modulus $(\bar{G}_1 h)$ which has been measured for red blood cells[64,65], indicating a stiffening for shear in the transverse direction. However, smaller values of $\bar{G}_2 h$ consistent with the critical potential data at finite $\gamma$ exist all the way down to $\bar{G}_2 h = 0$, with the corresponding of $\gamma$

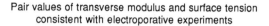

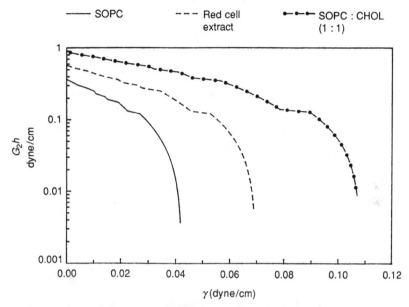

Fig. 17.6. Plot of values of $G_2h$ and $\gamma$ which are consistent with the measured values of $V_c$ necessary for electroporation for the three bilayers of Needham and Hochmuth's study. The values of the elastic moduli, critical voltages and bilayer thicknesses used to construct these plots are given in Table 17.1, and $K = 10^{-5}$ and $\chi = 80/2.2$.

increasing monotonically to an asymptotic value in the range of $0.04 - 0.1$ dyne/cm. Thus, the data also appears to establish an upper bound for the surface tension of the bilayer. Note, finally, that for fixed $\gamma$, the calculated values for $\bar{G}_2h$ increase with increasing cholesterol content, again (as with $(\bar{E}_1 + \bar{E}_2)h$) reflecting increased cohesiveness with elevated cholesterol content in the lipid bilayer.

As the above example demonstrates, the predictive capabilities of the anisoptropic theory, which has been presented in this study, rest on the knowledge of the transverse shear elastic modulus $\bar{G}_2$. Although plausible and self-consistent values for this modulus may be predicted from electroporative data, it would be much more satisfying to deduce $\bar{G}_2$ from an imposed deformation of a bilayer, and then predict $V_c$. Studies of the mechanics of lipid bilayers have not focused on transverse shear deformations, but, as this study at the very least points out, these are the very

Table 17.1. *Parameters for the determination of the transverse shear modulus*

| Bilayer | Hydrocarbon core thickness $h$ (nm) | Elastic modulus $(\bar{E}_1 + \bar{E}_2)h$ (dyne/cm) | Critical voltage (volts) |
|---|---|---|---|
| SOPC | 3.9 | 193 | 1.1 |
| RBC lipid extract | 4.0 | 420 | 1.6 |
| SOPC:CHOL | 4.0 | 594 | 2.0 |

deformations which are important in understanding the mechanics of electroporation.

### References

1 Hanai, T., Haydon, D. & Taylor, J. (1964). An investigation by electrical methods of lecithin in hydrocarbon films in aqueous solutions. *Proceedings of the Royal Society of London Series B. Biological Sciences*, **281**, 377–91.

2 Rosen, D. & Sutton, A. (1968). *Biochimica et Biophysica Acta*, **163**, 226.

3 Sale, A. & Hamilton, W. (1968). *Biochimica et Biophysica Acta*, **163**, 37–41.

4 Alvarez, O. & Latorre, R. (1978). Voltage dependent capacitance in lipid bilayers made from monolayers. *Biophysical Journal*, **21**, 1–17.

5 Zimmermann, U., Pilwat, G. & Riemann, F. (1974). Dielectric breakdown of cell membranes. *Biophysical Journal*, **14**, 881–9.

6 Riemann, F., Zimmermann, U. & Pilwat, G. (1975). *Biochimica et Biophysica Acta*, **394**, 449–62.

7 Coster, H. & Zimmermann, U. (1975). *Journal of Membrane Biology*, **22**, 73–90.

8 Zimmermann, U., Beckers, F. & Coster, H. (1977). The effects of pressure on the electrical breakdown in the membranes of *Valonia utricularis*. *Biochimica et Biophysica Acta*, **464**, 399–416.

9 Zimmermann, U., Pilwat, G., Pequeux, A. & Gilles, R. (1980). Electromechanical properties of human erythrocyte membranes: the pressure dependence of potassium permeability. *Journal of Membrane Biology*, **54**, 103–13.

10 Zimmermann, U., Vienken, J. & Pilwat, G. (1980). Development of drug carrier systems: electric field induced effects in cell membranes. *Journal of Electroanalytical Chemistry*, **116**, 553–74.

11 Benz, R. & Zimmermann, U. (1980). Pulse length dependence of the electrical breakdown in lipid bilayer membranes. *Biochimica et Biophysica Acta*, **597**, 637–42.

12 Benz, R. & Zimmermann, U. (1980). Relaxation studies on cell membranes and lipid bilayers in the high electric field range. *Bioelectrochemistry and Bioengineering*, **7**, 723–39.

13 Benz, R. & Zimmermann, U. (1981). The resealing process of lipid

bilayers after reversible electric breakdown. *Biochimica et Biophysica Acta*, **640**, 169–78.

14 Buschl, R., Ringsdorf, H. & Zimmermann, U. (1982). Electric field induced fusion of large liposomes from natural and polymerizable lipids. *Federation of European Biochemical Society & Letters*, **150**, 38–42.

15 Tsong, T. & Kingsley, E. (1975). Hemolysis of human erythrocyte induced by a rapid temperature jump. *Journal of Biological Chemistry*, **250**, 786–9.

16 Tsong, T. Y., Tsong, T., Kingsley, E. & Siliciano, R. (1976). Relaxation phenomena in human erythrocyte suspensions. *Biophysical Journal*, **16**, 1091–104.

17 Kinosita, K. & Tsong, T. (1977). Formation and resealing of pores of controlled size in human erythrocyte membrane. *Nature (London)*, **268**, 438–41.

18 Kinosita, K. & Tsong, T. (1977). Voltage-induced pore formation and hemolysis of human erythrocytes. *Biochimica et Biophysica Acta*, **471**, 227–42.

19 Kinosita, K. & Tsong, T. (1979). Voltage-induced conductance in human erythrocyte membranes. *Biochimica et Biophysica Acta*, **554**, 479–97.

20 Tessie, J. & Tsong, T. (1981). Electric field induced transient pores in phospholipid bilayer vesicles. *Biochemistry*, **20**, 1548–54.

21 Tsong, T. (1983). Voltage modulation of membrane permeability and energy utilization in cells. *Bioscience Reports*, **3**, 487–505.

22 Kinosita, K., Ashikawa, I., Saita, N., Yoshimura, H., Itoh, H., Nagayama, K. & Ikegami, A. (1988). Electroporation of cell membrane visualized under a pulsed-laser fluorescence microscope. *Biophysical Journal*, **53**, 1015–19.

23 Abidor, I.G., Arakelyan, V., Chernomordik, L., Yu, Chizmadzhev, A., Pastushenko, V. & Tarasevich, M. (1979). Electric breakdown of bilayer lipid membranes. I. The main experimental facts and their qualitative discussion. *Bioelectrochemistry and Bioenergetics*, **6**, 37–52.

24 Pastushenko, V., Chizmadzhev, Y. & Arakelyan, V. (1979). Electrical breakdown of bilayer lipid membranes: II. Calculation of the membrane lifetime in the steady-state diffusion approximation. *Bioelectrochemistry and Bioenergetics*, **6**, 53–62.

25 Chizmadzhev, Y., Arakelyan, V. & Pastushenko, V. (1979). Electrical breakdown of bilayer lipid membranes: III. Analysis of possible mechanisms of defect origination. *Bioelectrochemistry and Bioenergetics*, **6**, 63–70.

26 Chernomordik, L., Shkharev, S., Abidor, I. & Chizmadzhev, Y. (1983). Breakdown of lipid bilayer membranes in an electric field. *Biochimica et Biophysica Acta*, **736**, 203–13.

27 Patushenko, V. & Petrov, A. (1984). Electromechanical mechanism of pore formation in bilayer lipid membranes. In *7th School on Biophysics of Membrane Transport. School Proceedings* (Poland).

28 Chernomordik, L., Shkharev, S., Popov, S., Pastushenko, V., Sokirko, A., Abidor, I. & Chizmadzhev, Y. (1987). The electrical breakdown of cell and lipid membranes, the similarity of phenomenologies. *Biochimica et Biophysica Acta*, **902**, 360–73.

29 Glazer, R., Leikin, S., Chernomordik, L., Pastushenko, V. & Sokirko,

A. (1988). Reversible electrical breakdown of lipid bilayers: Formation and evolution of pores. *Biochimica et Biophysica Acta*, **940**, 275–87.

30 Zimmermann, U. (1982). Electric field-mediated fusion and related electrical phenomena. *Biochimica and Biophysica Acta*, **694**, 227–77.

31 Zimmermann, U. (1986). Electric breakdown, electropermeabilization, and electrofusion. *Reviews of Physiology, Biochemistry and Pharmacology*, **105**; 175–256.

32 Neumann, E., Sowers, A.E. & Jordan, C. (1988). *Electroporation and Electrofusion in Cell Biology*. Plenum Publishing Corp., New York.

33 Potter, H. (1988). Electroporation in biology; methods, applications and instrumentation. *Analytical Biochemistry*, **174**, 361–73.

34 Chang, D.C. (1989). Cell poration and cell fusion using an oscillating electric field. *Biophysical Journal*, **56**, 641–52.

35 Chang, D. (1988). Cell poration and cell fusion using an oscillating electric field. In *Electroporation and Electrofusion in Cell Biology*, Neumann, E., Sowers, A.E. & Jordan, C., eds, New York: Plenum Publishing Corp.

36 Sowers, A.E. & Lieber, M. (1986). Electropore diameters, lifetimes, numbers, and locations in individual erythrocyte ghosts. *FEBS Letters*, **205**, 179–84.

37 Chang, D. & Reese, T. (1989). Structure of electric field-induced membrane pores revealed by rapid-freezing electron microscopy. *Biophysical Journal*, **55**, 136a. (Abstr.)

38 Zimmermann, U. & Vienken, J. (1982). Dielectric field induced cell-to-cell fusion. *Journal of Membrane Biology*, **67**, 165–82.

39 Crowley, J. (1972). Electrical breakdown of bimolecular lipid membranes as an electromechanical instability. *Biophysical Journal*, **13**, 711–24.

40 White, S. (1974). Comments on 'Electrical breakdown of bimolecular lipid membranes as an electromechanical instability'. *Biophysical Journal*, **14**, 155–8.

41 Dimitrov, D. (1984). Electric field-induced breakdown of lipid bilayers and cell membranes: a thin viscoelastic film model. *Journal of Membrane Biology*, **78**, 53–60.

42 Dimitrov, D. & Jain, R.K. (1984). Membrane stability. *Biochimica et Biophysica Acta*, **779**, 437–68.

43 Weaver, J.C. & Mintzer, R. (1981). Decreased bilayer stability due to transmembrane potentials. *Physics Letters*, **86A**, 57–9.

44 Powell, K.T. & Weaver, J.C. (1986). Transient aqueous pores in bilayer membranes: a statistical theory. *Bioelectrochemistry and Bioenergetics*, **15**, 211–27.

45 Weaver, J.C. & Mintzer, R.A. (1986). Conduction onset criteria for transient aqueous pores and reversible electrical breakdown in bilayer membranes. *Bioelectrochemistry and Bioelectoenergetics*, **15**, 229–42.

46 Powell, K.T. Derrick, E.G. & Weaver, J.C. (1986). A quantitative theory of reversible electrical breakdown in bilayer membranes. *Bioelectrochemistry and Bioenergetics*, **15**, 243–55.

47 Needham, D. and Hochmuth, R.M. (1989). Electro-mechanical permeabilization of lipid vesicles: role of membrane tension and compressibility. *Biophysical Journal*, **55**, 1001–9.

48 Sugar, I. & Neumann, E. (1984). Stochastic model for electric-field

induced membrane pores, electroporation. *Biophysical Chemistry*, **19**, 211–25.

49  Schwister, K. & Deutike, B. (1985). Formation and properties of aqueous leaks induced in human erythrocytes by electrical breakdown. *Biochimica et Biophysica Acta*, **816**, 332–48.

50  Neumann, E., Schafer-Ridder, M., Wang, Y. & Hofschneider, P. (1982). Gene transfer into mouse myelyoma cells by electroporation in high electric fields. *European Molecular Biological Organ Journal*, **1**, 841–5.

51  Wong, T.K. & Neumann, E. (1982). Electric field-induced gene transfer. *Biochemical and Biophysical Research Communications*, **107**, 584–7.

52  Potter, H., Weir, L. & Leder P. (1984). Enhancer-dependent expression of human immunoglobin genes introduced into mouse pre-B lymphocytes by electroporation. *Proceedings of the National Academy of Sciences, USA*, **81**, 7161–5.

53  Smithies, O., Gregg, R., Boggs, S., Koralewski, A. & Kucherlapati, R. (1985). Insertion of DNA sequences into the human chromosomal β-globin locus by homologous recombination. *Nature (London)*, **317**, 230–3.

54  Knutsen, J. & Yee, D. (1987). Electroporation: parameters affecting transfer of DNA into mammalian cells. *Analytical Biochemistry*, **164**, 44–52.

55  Chu, G., Hayakawa, H. & Bert, P. (1987). Electroporation for the efficient transfection of mammalian cells with DNA. *Nucleic Acids Research*, **15**; 1311–26.

56  Yang, N. (1985). Transient gene expression in electroporated plant cells. *Trends in Biotechnology*, **3**, 191–2.

57  Fromm, M., Taylor, P. & Walbot, V. (1986). Stable transformation of maize after gene transfer by electroporation. *Nature (London)*, **319**, 791–3.

58  Miller, J., Dower, W. & Tomkins, L. (1988). High voltage electroporation of bacteria: genetic transformation of *Camphylobacter jejuni* with plasmid DNA. *Proceedings of the National Academy of Sciences, USA*, **85**, 856–60.

59  Zimmermann, U. (1988). Electrofusion and electrotransfection of cells. In *Molecular Mechanisms of Membrane Fusion*, Ohki, S., Doyle, D., Flanagan, T., Hui, S. & Mayhew, E., eds, pp. 209–22, New York: Plenum Publishing Corp.

60  Skalak, R., Tozeren, A., Zarda, R. & Chien, S. (1973). Strain energy function of red cell membranes. *Biophysical Journal*, **13**, 245–64.

61  Chien, S., Kuo-Li, P., Skalak, R., Usami, S. & Tozeren, A. (1978). Theoretical and experimental studies on viscoelastic properties of erythrocyte membrane. *Biophysical Journal*, **24**, 463–87.

62  Evans, E. (1973). A new material concept for the red cell membrane. *Biophysical Journal*, **13**, 926–40.

63  Evans, E., Waugh, R. & Melnick, L. (1976). Elastic area compressibility modulus of red cell membrane. *Biophysical Journal*, **16**, 585–95.

64  Engelhardt, H. & Sackmann, E. (1988). On the measurement of shear elastic moduli and viscosities of erythrocyte plasma membranes by

transient deformation in high frequency electric fields. *Biophysical Journal*, **54**, 495–508.

65  Evans, E. & Skalak, R. (1980). *Mechanics and Thermodynamics of Biomembranes*, Boca Rotan, Florida: CRC Press.

66  Melcher, J. (1981). *Continuum Electromechanics*, Cambridge, Massachusetts: The MIT Press.

# 18

## Electrical injury to heart muscle cells

LESLIE TUNG

### Introduction

High intensity, pulsed d.c. electric fields are applied deliberately to the heart in the clinical setting for electrical *countershock* of cardiac arrhythmia[1-5], using electrodes placed on the body surface, heart surface, or heart cavity. This chapter discusses those conditions of *defibrillation* under which cardiac tissue may be injured directly by the electric shock. Countershock is also used for *cardioversion* of cardiac arrhythmia, other than fibrillation, but is less likely to cause injury because of the lower energies used[3]. The injury effect of high-energy d.c. shocks has been utilized for tissue *ablation*[6] of some types of tachyarrhythmia, using endocardial catheters[7].

When the level of shock delivered to the heart is just at the threshold for defibrillation, electrical injury of the myocardium is absent or transient[8-10]. However, defibrillation success rates are probabilistic in nature[11]. There-fore, to assure a high probability of success with a minimal delivery of shock pulses in life-threatening situations, high suprathreshold levels of shock often are used[12]. In animal studies, depending to some extent on waveform shape, if the shock level reaches three to five times the level of current, or 20–30 times the level of energy at the threshold of defibrillation, cardiac function is depressed significantly[10,13-17]. In clinical human studies, myocardial injury has been documented following defibrillatory shocks[18-20], although not in every case, even with multiple shocks[8,21,22].

The experimental observations cited in this chapter are drawn primarily from animal studies on *internal* defibrillation in which electrodes are applied directly on, or within, the heart, since the myocardial injury is more clearly related to the shock site and shock level. It appears that cardiac electrical injury is nonthermal in nature[4,23,24], although, in cases of excessive shock levels or poor electrode contact, thermogenic injury can occur[25,26]. The shock currents and voltage gradients are not distributed uniformly throughout the heart[27 30] and are maximal in the regions directly adjacent to the electrodes[31-34]. At high suprathreshold shock levels, local current densities may reach several tenths to 1 amp/cm$^2$ and potential gradients may reach 100 volts/cm[30,35]. Myocardial damage is greatest at the shock electrodes[19,23,24,36,37], and, depending on shock strength, may extend well into the ventricular wall. Injury effects are *functional* (altered electrophysiology[23,24,38], arrhythmia[24,36,39], coronary artery dilation[38], impaired contractile force[14,15,17,24,40], *morphological* (ultrastructural changes[23-25,41], necrosis[23,24,36,37,42,43]), haemorrhage[38]) and *biochemical* (depletion of essential enzymes[18,24,25,44]) in nature. Even in the case of external defibrillation, in which electrodes are applied to the chest and much of the applied current is shunted around the heart[45-47], similar injury can occur to the myocardium[10,13,44,48-55].

Considering the shock as an entity delivered to the heart, the degree of myocardial injury is determined by the shock current, waveshape, size of the electrodes, number of shocks applied, and time between shock pulses[19,25,38,48]. Therefore, one way to minimize myocardial injury is to limit the peak level of current. Since the strength required for a successful defibrillation pulse is inversely related to the pulse duration[40,56 58], longer pulse durations should be used. This necessitates, however, a greater charge usage[59] and therefore larger storage capacitors and batteries for implantable defibrillators[5]. Peak current levels also may be reduced by distributing the shock current more evenly and effectively through the heart volume. Such strategies are undergoing active investigation, and include: improvements in electrode design and placement[5,31-33,48,60-64], waveforms with multiphasic shapes[60,65-71], and multiple electrodes and sequential shock[27,72-74].

Further improvements towards the reduction of electrical injury may be possible with an understanding of the parameters which govern injury at the tissue and cellular levels. Of the various measures of shock intensity which have been studied (energy, potential, charge, current, current density and potential gradient), the magnitude of the tissue injury is correlated best with local current density or with local potential gradient. These observations are reviewed on pp. 363–7. Recent experiments on single heart cells in our laboratory, also reviewed on pp. 368–76, suggest that breakdown of the cell membrane occurs with sufficiently large changes in transmembrane potential, as proposed recently to explain injury in skeletal muscle[75,76]. Such an event can account for many of the injury effects observed in whole heart and in *in vitro* strips of heart muscle.

Therefore, myocardial injury appears to be related to tissue potential gradient on the one hand and to cellular membrane potential on the other. Theoretical models are needed to describe the linkage between these two parameters. Unlike other excitable tissue such as skeletal muscle, heart cells are coupled electrically. This has major implications in the types of models needed to predict the effect of external electric fields on cardiac cellular membrane potential. The prevailing theoretical approaches, as well as the concept of electroporation of cell membranes, are described on pp. 376–85.

The term injury is generally reserved to describe long-lasting conditions which can be corroborated by histological evidence. In this discussion, the term injury will be defined more broadly to include transient and reversible conditions. Under this concept, the most immediate and sensitive index of myocardial injury in whole heart may be *electrophysiological* (e.g. ECG or rhythm abnormality), compared, for example, with biochemical (e.g. enzyme release) or mechanical (e.g. left ventricular rate of rise of systolic pressure, or diastolic stiffness) indices[8,24,38]. Given this viewpoint, the goal of this chapter is to review the chain of experimental and theoretical evidence which suggests that the *electro-pathological effects* of high intensity electric shock on cardiac muscle originate from *electroporation of the cell membrane*. Experimental observations obtained at four organizational levels of the heart (Fig. 18.1): whole heart, muscle strips, cell aggregates and single cells, and cell membrane, are summarized below. Next, a number of theoretical models and their supporting data which relate the four organizational levels and which may help to explain the steps involved in the electrical injury of heart muscle cells, are summarized. The final section discusses the interpretation of the experimental observations in light of the theoretical models. Together, this information may be helpful in evaluating new approaches which minimize injury in heart muscle cells owing to high-intensity electric shock.

### Experimental observations

#### Whole heart

Following high-intensity electric shock, alterations in cardiac electrophysiology occur and include: increased arrhythmia[24,50,52], changes in QRS complex, ST segment and T wave[44,52], and cellular depolarization with decreased tissue excitability or temporary arrest[24,28,77]. These alterations are accompanied by loss of tissue potassium[24,78,79], metabolic abnormalities[18,24,25,54], haemodynamic changes[80], uptake of markers of myocardial necrosis[25,81], reduced contractility[15,17,24,42,82], and a variety of histologi-

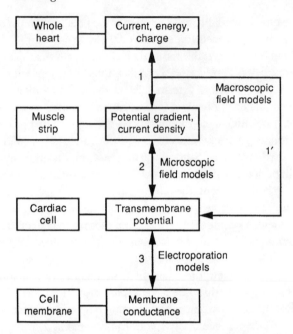

Fig. 18.1 System diagram for cardiac muscle for electric shock. Different physical parameters (charge, energy, potential, potential gradient, current and current density) are of interest at the various organizational levels of the heart. Theoretical models have been developed to interrelate the parameters at the various levels.

cal and ultrastructural changes[23-25,36,37,41,43]. In general, these effects are minimal at defibrillation threshold and are found mainly in tissue adjacent to the electrodes, but increase in severity throughout the heart with multiple suprathreshold current shocks[19,25,48]. The threshold for arrhythmia is also dependent on the phase of the cardiac cycle when the shock is delivered[50,83]. Shock may also initiate fibrillation[84]; low levels result in reversible fibrillation while high levels result in intractable fibrillation[50,85].

One difficulty with interpreting many of these studies is that the output of the defibrillator or cardioverter is expressed usually in total energy delivered, calibrated for a 50 ohm load. Since the impedance of the tissue is an uncontrolled parameter, neither the actual energy delivered, current density, or electric field distribution throughout the heart, can be determined without independent measurements. Recently, there have been efforts to adjust the output of external defibrillators to the tissue impedance or to a constant current mode to deliver a more consistent dose of energy to the heart[86-88].

Another difficulty in whole heart studies is the separation of direct effects of shock on myocardial tissue from effects on the nervous system[89], as well as from haemodynamic reflexes of the autonomic nervous system in response to myocardial depression caused by the shock[1,3,4]. These ambiguities may be avoided, in part, by the excised perfused heart preparation[14,17,24,40,79,89] and especially by the *in vitro* preparations described in the following sections.

Measurements of potential gradients during defibrillation are few[46,90,91] and come primarily from the laboratory of Ideker and co-workers, who have quantified the spatial distribution and magnitude of potential gradients during excitation and defibrillation. Potential gradients associated with electrical stimulation depend on fibre orientation and are of the order of 1–3 V/cm for 3 ms pulses[92], whereas the minimum field strength required for defibrillation is of the order of 6 V/cm for 5 ms pulses[30]. On the other hand, potential gradients distributed across the heart are highly nonuniform and highest adjacent to the shock electrodes[28,29]. Shocks with higher intensities directly depolarize a larger area of epicardium[28]. During high defibrillation level shocks, significant regions of myocardium may experience potential gradients in excess of 60 V/cm[30] and suffer conduction block, the duration of which is a function of shock intensity.

### In vitro *muscle strip*

To quantify better the effect of electric shock on cardiac cell excitability, rectangular electric field pulses with graded intensities were applied to frog ventricular muscle strips using a three pair, electrode system as diagrammed in Fig. 18.2(*a*)[93]. A graded increase in shock intensity (measured as current density) reduces the post-shock action potential amplitude, action potential duration, resting potential, excitability and conduction velocity, and prolongs the refractory period[93], as seen in other *in vitro* preparations[94–97]. Fig. 18.3 shows the effect of a 1.0 A/cm² (in bath, lower value in muscle strip), 10 ms duration shock pulse on the excitation strength–duration curve (ESD). At 5 s following the shock, the strip is unexcitable for most durations tested (not shown). At 30 s following the shock, excitability is restored over all durations, but the ESD is shifted upward uniformly to higher current levels. Thus, a transient refractory period, as observed in studies using constant amplitude stimulation[93,97], is expected as long as the ESD is positive to the stimulus pulse, represented by point S. By 60 s post-shock, the ESD has returned close to its pre-shock levels, and excitation can be obtained once again with the stimulus S.

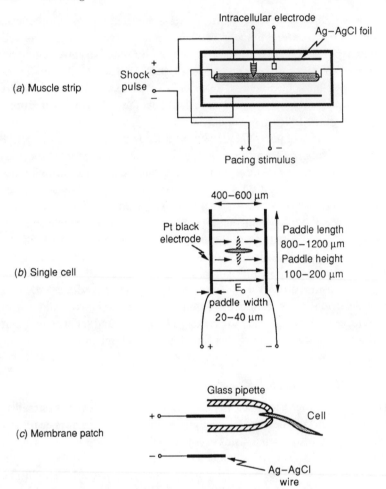

Fig. 18.2. Arrangement of electrodes used for studying cardiac muscle strips, single heart cells, and membrane patches. (*a*) Three pairs of electrodes are used for muscle strip experiments. The first electrode pair delivers constant amplitude pacing stimuli, the second pair delivers a rectangular current shock pulse orthogonal to the muscle strip, and the third pair includes a suction electrode for monitoring monophasic action potential as a measure of intracellular potential.[180] (*b*) A pair of micropaddle electrodes is placed around a single heart cell. Each electrode is constructed by compressing the exposed end of a teflon coated 0.010″ diameter platinum wire in a vice. The paddles are coated with platinum black to increase the effective surface area to minimize electrode polarization and bubble formation. (*c*) The end of a single heart cell is drawn by suction into the mouth of a glass micropipette. The pipette is connected to a custom-built, whole cell voltage clamp unit. Rectangular

### Cultured cell aggregates

The pioneering work of the laboratory of Jones, Jones and co-workers[35,68,69,98-103] has contributed much to the knowledge of the pathological effects of electric shock on cardiac muscle, and the reader is directed to the series of papers summarized below. The studies were performed on monolayer sheets of cultured chick heart cells which were subjected to spatially uniform and controlled electric fields. Ultrastructural changes were observed and included cell contracture, intracellular oedema, and swelling of intracellular organelles[103], as well as formation of microlesions on the cell surface membrane[101].

The observation that high-intensity electric fields produced a rapid membrane depolarization to around 0 mV without an action potential overshoot prompted Jones[102] to suggest that electrical breakdown of the cell membrane is the underlying basis for the shock effects observed experimentally in the whole heart. Consistent with this hypothesis was the result that sodium and calcium channel blockers did not inhibit the shock-induced depolarization[100], which has also been observed[104]. While cellular depolarization, standstill, and loss of excitability were seen at high field levels of about 100 V/cm, lower levels produced tachyarrhythmia, which correlated well with the electrophysiological changes observed on the whole heart level[35]. Various waveform shapes were studied[99], and multiphasic waveforms were shown to be less likely to produce arrhythmia compared with monophasic waveforms[68,69]. This finding has been confirmed in whole heart studies[60,67,70,71] and underscores the utility of heart cell models for studies of cardiac function.

### Enzymatically isolated single cell

The experimental preparation of choice for many present-day studies of the heart is, increasingly, the single heart cell[105,106]. Enzymatic techniques for dissociating intact tissue and isolating single cells are now well established[107]. For electrophysiological studies which utilize the voltage clamp technique, the single cell provides superior time resolution, voltage uniformity, control of the ionic and metabolic environment inside and outside the cell, and membrane patches containing single ion channels[108].

*Caption for Fig. 18.2 (Cont.)*
or ramp pulses having variable amplitude (0–4 V) and duration (4–20 ms) are applied to the pipette, and the pipette current is monitored. From[93,112,124] respectively. Typical dimension of muscle strip: $1 \times 1 \times 15$ mm; of frog cardiac cell: $10 \times 3 \times 300$ $\mu$m. See text for further description.

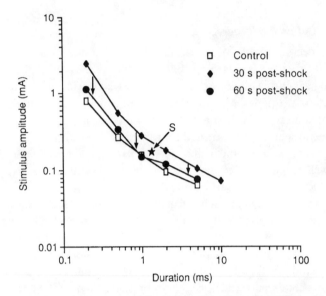

Fig. 18.3. Shift in excitation stimulus-duration curve (ESD) with electric shock. A frog ventricular muscle strip was subjected to a 10 ms duration rectangular current pulse having a current density of 1.0 A/cm². Following the shock, the excitation threshold was determined by applying a brief train of stimuli lasting less than 2 s, with each stimulus pulse in the train having constant duration but monotonically increasing amplitude up to the maximum amplitude of the stimulator. The train of shocks was applied at 5, 30, and 60 s postshock. At 5 s postshock, the strip was inexcitable for most durations tested (not shown). At 30 s postshock, the strip regained excitability at current levels higher than in control. The stimulus–duration curve was uniformly shifted towards higher current levels. By 60 s postshock, the stimulus–duration curve nearly returned to its preshock level. A pacing test pulse (point S) is shown to illustrate the dependence of relative refractory period on pacing pulse parameters and time course of recovery of the ESD. From (L. Fogelson & L. Tung, unpublished observations).

For mechanical studies, the complex three-dimensional structure and mixture of connective fibres and muscle cells found in intact tissue are eliminated at the single cell level[109]. Furthermore, cell shape and ultrastructural parameters such as sarcomere length can be observed directly, and cell length and force of contraction can be measured now in real time[110].

Single ventricular heart cells from frog and guinea pig were used in the laboratory for studies of electric shock. It has been found that the electrophysiological and contractile properties of the frog cells are comparable in most respects with those of intact muscle strips[109,111]. The

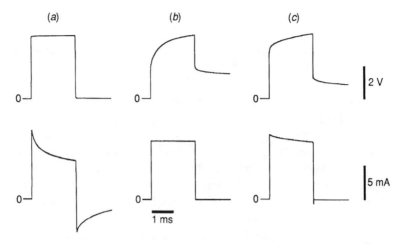

Fig. 18.4. Voltage and current waveforms measured from micro-paddle, platinum/platinum black electrodes. The left hand panels (*a*) were obtained under voltage-controlled conditions; the centre panels (*b*) under current-controlled conditions; the right-hand panels (*c*) with a commercial stimulator (model SD9, Grass Instruments, Quincy, MA) with its output terminals isolated from ground and output voltage range at maximum setting (10–100 V). The upper row is voltage measured across the electrodes; the lower row is total current injected between the electrodes.

parallel plate shock electrodes used (Fig. 18.2(*b*)) are miniaturized[104,112] to take advantage of the small cell size, which is typically $10 \times 3 \times 300$ $\mu$m (frog) or $30 \times 10 \times 100$ $\mu$m (guinea pig). Typical dimensions for the paddles are 800–1200 $\mu$m in length, 20–40 $\mu$m in width, 100–200 $\mu$m in height, and 400–600 $\mu$m separation. The small size of the paddles provides several significant advantages. First, the large volume of the bath surrounding the paddles serves as a heat sink and minimizes joule heating effects. Secondly, the geometric leverage gained in the small size permits high-intensity electric fields to be produced with relatively small currents and voltages. Consequently, conventional analogue circuits can be used to construct the waveform generator.

Monophasic, rectangular constant current pulses were applied through the electrodes by a custom-built stimulator. Rectangular pulses were used for the reasons that: 1) they are effective at lower peak currents compared to the exponential, damped sinusoidal or trapezoidal waveform shapes[56,58,99], and 2) they simplify the analysis by electrical models[58,59,113]. The difference in using *current*-controlled waveforms rather than *voltage*-controlled waveforms is shown in Fig. 18.4, which shows the interelectrode current and voltage measured simultaneously from the micro-paddles under both controlled conditions. Panel A was obtained for a rectangular voltage pulse. In this case, the current response, and therefore the electric field (Equation 1), is *not* rectangular and surges at the beginning of the pulse due to electrode capacitance. A substantial current continues to flow after the cessation of the pulse. Panel B was obtained for reciprocal current-controlled conditions. The voltage response is nonlinear and shows a very slow decay (90% decay time was 2.3 s) following the cessation of the current pulse. However, the current (and hence electric field) *is* rectangular. Panel C was obtained using a commercial stimulator, with its output terminals isolated from ground. Under these conditions with these electrodes, the stimulator is a close approximation to a constant current source. The time-dependent effects seen in all three panels can be attributed to the time-varying impedance and polarization of the platinum electrodes, which contribute significant artefacts at the low voltages (but high current densities) used with the micro-paddle system. Nonpolarizable electrodes such as silver/silver chloride could not be used since free silver ion is apparently toxic to these single cell preparations[109]. Therefore, current-controlled waveforms are essential for these types of studies. Current-based shock delivery has also been proposed for clinical use, in part for similar reasons to minimize electrical instability and nonlinearity due to the electrode/tissue interface, and, in part, to eliminate the dependence of the shock pulse on the geometry and impedance of the medium[86 88].

Pulse duration of the stimulator varied from 20 $\mu$s–10 ms, and pulse amplitude could be varied between 0–70 mA. This corresponded to a peak current density of 13 A/cm$^2$. The micro-paddle electrode voltage divided by the intra-electrode distance could not be used as a measure of the electric field, since, as noted already, distortion due to electrode impedance and polarization was significant at the low voltages used by these electrodes (Fig. 18.4). In principle, the electric field also can be derived from the current density (Equation 1), but two factors must be known with precision: the surface area of the paddle electrodes and the conductivity of the bath solution. Instead, the system was calibrated directly by an exploring electrode. The voltage gradient at the floor of the chamber between the paddles had a peak value of about 800 V/cm at the highest current setting.

### Stimulus threshold and effect of cell orientation

Since cardiac cells are thought to be stimulated to contract when a constant voltage threshold is reached[59,113], measurement of the stimulus–duration curve for excitation (ESD) with applied fields yields information on the coupling between the applied field and the induced change in membrane potential. The micro-paddle electrodes were placed as a unit to straddle single cells for the purpose of field stimulation (Fig. 18.2(*b*)). The orientation of the cell could be adjusted as desired with respect to the electric field, and cells were tested with their long axis aligned either parallel to, or perpendicular to, the applied electric field as shown[112,114,115]. Figure. 18.5 compares on a log–log scale the ESD of a frog ventricular cell (panel A) or guinea pig cell (panel B) with its long axis aligned perpendicular to the applied electric field, then to the ESD obtained for the same cell after it was rotated to be parallel (Fig. 18.2(*b*)) to the electric field. The first point to be noted is that both curves for the frog cell (Fig. 18.5(*a*)) deviate from the expected straight line hyperbolic relation[59,116]. The 'notch' in the ESD seen at a pulse duration around 1 ms was observed in many of the frog heart cells[104,112] but never in the guinea pig cells. The notch is not usually observed in multicellular preparations (although see [116]), but this may be because stimulus durations are tested rarely below 1 ms. The notch may reflect two modes of stimulation of the cell membrane or perhaps local peaks of transmembrane potential owing to the convoluted cell shape[104]. The second point is that even ultrashort duration pulses (20–40 $\mu$s) are sufficient to stimulate the cell, as observed previously for dog and turtle heart[51,116], although the potential gradient needed may reach 100 V/ cm, at which cell injury may occur. The third point is that there is a reduction in intensity required for stimulation when the cell is parallel as opposed to perpendicular to the electric field[112,114,117], consistent with measurements of the extracellular field required for stimulation in whole heart[92]. Since cell stimulation occurs when the membrane potential reaches a fixed threshold[59], this observation suggests that the field-induced change in membrane potential is greater when the poles of the cell are farther apart along the electric field axis, as predicted by field theoretic models (see pp. 382–4). Similar results were obtained on single guinea pig heart cells (Fig. 18.5(*b*)). These data may explain, in part, the cellular basis for the efficacy of orthogonal pulses compared with single pulse defibrillation[72,74].

### *Cell contractility and threshold for cell contracture*

At high external field strengths, heart cells undergo irreversible contracture and die. Since the cells were observed to remain quiescent in response to the same levels of field strength if calcium were absent from the bathing solution, contracture evidently is not a direct effect of electric field and, more likely, is a result of intracellular overload of calcium ions[118]. Frog

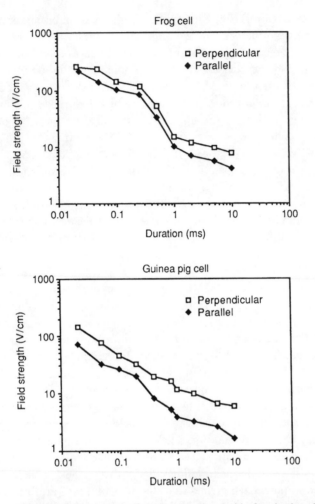

Fig. 18.5. Effect of cell orientation on threshold of excitation. Stimulus–duration curves were obtained for a single heart cell under field stimulation with rectangular current waveforms. Plotted on the abscissa is the waveform duration and on the ordinate the field strength corresponding to the current magnitude. For both frog and guinea pig heart cells, the stimulus–duration curve was shifted towards higher field strengths when the cell was oriented perpendicular to, instead of parallel to, the applied electric field. From [112] © 1988 IEEE, reprinted with permission, and N. Sliz L. Tung, unpublished observations.

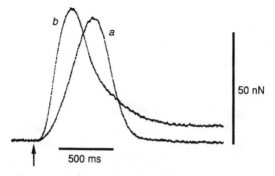

Fig. 18.6. Isometric contraction of a single frog ventricular heart cell. Trace *a* was obtained with a slightly suprathreshold 3.4 V, 2 ms stimulus pulse; trace *b* was the response to the fourth of a series of 20 V, 50 μs high intensity stimulus pulses. Arrow indicates time of the stimulus pulse. From L. Tung, unpublished observations.

heart cells were used for these studies since they, unlike avian cells, do not have significant intracellular storage compartments of calcium ion (i.e. the sarcoplasmic reticulum[119]) and do not exhibit a dose-dependent pattern of tachyarrhythmia[35,102], both of which can complicate the interpretation of the experiments in terms of membrane breakdown. Occasionally, a range of field intensities intermediate between that for stimulation and that for contracture was observed to produce no visible contraction at all, as reported for skeletal muscle cells[75] and avian cardiac cells[102]. This may be due, however, to a stimulus sufficiently great to reverse the normal electrochemical gradient for calcium ion through voltage-gated channels in the cell membrane, thereby preventing calcium influx and cell contraction[119,120].

The difference between normal cell contraction and that occurring at the threshold of contracture is shown in Fig. 18.6, recorded under isometric conditions from a single frog ventricular heart cell. The cell was mounted on an ultrasensitive force transducer[121] and field stimulated. In this study, the micro-paddle system was not used. The anode electrode was an electrolytically sharpened tungsten wire with its tip placed approximately 20 μm from the cell, and the cathode was a remote platinum electrode. Trace *a* is the normal twitch obtained with a 3.4 V, 2 ms stimulus pulse. Trace *b* is the twitch after a series of four 20 V, 50 μs suprathreshold pulses was delivered. Note the marked increase in rate of rise of force, slowed rate of relaxation, and decay of force to an elevated diastolic level. Considering the known role of calcium in the generation of force in heart cells and pathways for calcium entry into the cell[120], these observations are consistent with a rapid influx of calcium from the bathing solution by a pathway *other* than normal excitation pathways, e.g. membrane breakdown, resulting in a state of calcium overload in this cell. The cell later went on to generate a level of force much larger than that of the twitch, detached from the transducer and shortened irreversibly.

Figure 18.7 compares the stimulus–duration curve for threshold excitation ($T_e$) to a curve obtained at higher intensities which induced cell contracture ($T_c$). In these studies, force was not recorded, but contracture was observed as an abrupt and irreversible reduction of cell length[112]. It is apparent that cell contracture is a function of pulse intensity and pulse duration. $T_c$ was not affected statistically by addition of calcium channel blockers, tetrodotoxin, or KCl depolarization[104], again consistent with the notion that calcium is entering the cell by some means other than normal excitation pathways. Furthermore the curve for $T_c$ has a hyperbolic shape similar to the excitation curve, which suggests that contracture, like excitation, occurs when a given voltage threshold in membrane potential is reached. The two curves diverge slightly, however, for increasing pulse duration. Similar results obtained by Jones and Jones[99] show that the curves for excitation and injury (defined as arrhythmia) begin to converge for pulse durations exceeding 10 ms.

### Cell membrane

Figures 18.6 and 18.7 showed the combined use of calcium ion and cell contractility to assess the permeability of the cell membrane. Membrane permeability appears to increase substantially when a certain threshold level of membrane potential is reached, i.e. a breakdown effect as proposed by Jones and co-workers[102]. However, this conclusion is tentative, since the membrane potential is not known truly (although it could be estimated theoretically using appropriate field models – step 2, Fig. 18.1). A variation of the cell-attached 'loose patch clamp' technique[122] has therefore been adopted. The end of the cell is drawn by suction into the tip of a glass pipette (Fig. 18.2(c)). A voltage applied to the pipette will be divided across the portions of cell membrane inside (surface area $S_1$) and outside (surface area $S_2$) the pipette (refer to Fig. 18.11(b) for explanation). Because $S_1$ is much smaller than $S_2$ and therefore has a much higher impedance, most of the pipette voltage drop occurs across $S_1$. By monitoring the pipette current, the kinetics of change in impedance of $S_1$ can then be observed as the threshold for breakdown is exceeded[123,124].

A key element in this study was the use of voltage ramps as a test

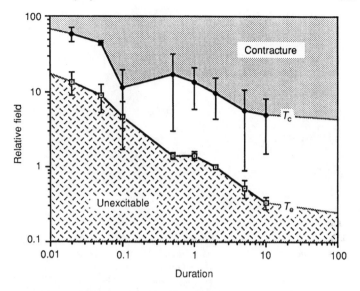

Fig. 18.7. Stimulus–duration curves for excitation and contracture thresholds for single frog ventricular heart cells. Rectangular current waveforms were used to field stimulate individual cells oriented parallel to the field axis. Eight cells were observed at each of the eight durations tested. The field intensity producing excitation and contracture for each cell at its test duration was normalized to the intensity required to excite that cell at a (standard) 2 ms duration. In this way, variations due to cell shape, orientation, and electrode placement could be minimized. From M. Mulligan and L. Tung, unpublished observations.

waveform. Unlike conventional studies of electroporation in which rectangular voltage steps are applied[125,126], the voltage ramp permits the observation of the kinetics of membrane breakdown uncomplicated by a simultaneous step change in membrane potential[124]. Because the currents involved were much smaller than those in the whole cell studies, nonpolarizable silver/silver chloride could be used for the electrodes instead of platinum (Fig. 18.2(*b*)). For low-amplitude ramps of either polarity, the current response was proportional to the applied pipette potential and, most likely, reflected the leakage of current through the seal between cell and pipette (Fig. 18.11(*b*)). However, for the test ramp with 2 V amplitude as shown in Fig. 18.8, the current response was markedly nonlinear. Typically, at potentials about 0.5 V, the current increased slope and occasionally became noisy, suggesting an instability in membrane resistance. When the membrane potential reached a critical threshold of about 0.8 V, the current exhibited a step increase over a time interval less

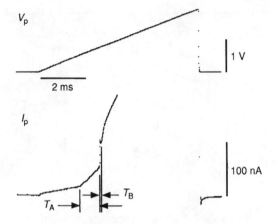

Fig. 18.8. Electrical breakdown of cardiac cell membrane. A ramp in pipette voltage ($V_p$) was applied to the end of a frog ventricular heart cell using a loose patch clamp technique. At the onset of the ramp there was an initial linear response in the pipette current ($I_p$). In this cell, an increase in membrane conductance was observed at a membrane potential of 0.56 V (onset of period $T_A$). A permanent increase in membrane conductance occurred at a membrane potential of ~0.8 V (period $T_B$), which was completed in less than 30 μs. From [123] © 1988 IEEE, reprinted with permission.

than 30 μs (the time resolution of the instrumentation system), suggesting a rapid breakdown of the membrane patch. Similar results were obtained with opposite polarity test ramps and with solutions of varying ionic compositions[124].

### Theoretical models

The overall theoretical scheme which is proposed to unify the experimental observations of pp. 363–76 is depicted in Fig. 18.1. The physical parameters of charge, energy, and current are used to characterize defibrillators and cardioverters at the level of the whole heart, and each parameter can be associated with an injury effect. Loosely speaking, charge may be associated with electrolytic decomposition at the electrode–electrolyte interface, energy with joule heating, current with potential gradient, and potential gradient with membrane depolarization[58]. Depending on which parameter is to be minimized, a different shock pulse duration is required[58,59]. The first part that follows describes the conventional class of macroscopic field models which relates these parameters to local electric fields and current density at the tissue level (step 1, Fig. 18.1), as well as a newer class of macroscopic field models which can also relate these parameters to changes in transmembrane potential (steps 1 and 1', Fig. 18.1). The second part describes, on a microscopic level, the effect of local electric field on transmembrane potential of the cardiac cell (step 2, Fig. 18.1). Finally, electroporation is described, a process by which sufficiently large transmembrane potentials can produce pores within the cell surface membrane (step 3, Fig. 18.1). These electric field-induced pores then result in the decline of cellular homeostasis through the intracellular loss of $K^+$ and essential enzymes, or gain of $Ca^{2+}$ and water, which together may account for many of the pathological effects of strong countershock.

### Distribution of electric field in the heart

#### 1. Potential gradient and current density

The stimulation and defibrillation of cardiac muscle has been related to the localized *potential gradient* (or electric field)[28,35,92,127] or to *current density*[34,128], rather than *energy, voltage, or charge* delivered[87]. At the same time, both the potential gradient $E$ and current density $J$ have been correlated to histological and electrophysiological damage[30,35]. Since Ohm's law[129] states that $J$ is directly proportional to $E$ for a conductive medium (conductivity $\sigma$) such as heart muscle:

$$J = \sigma E \tag{1}$$

the experimental evidence suggests that the potential gradient $E$ in the tissue, rather than energy or charge, is the critical parameter governing myocardial stimulation and myocardial injury (although see pp. 386–7).

The tissue parameters can, in turn, be related to the shock parameters at the electrodes. Current density integrated over the electrode surface area is equal to the applied current. The charge delivered is equal to the total current integrated over time. Energy delivered can be calculated given a measurement of the shock current and either the interelectrode potential difference or the tissue impedance.

#### 2. Monodomain, bidomain, and periodic structure models

The reader is referred to the review by Plonsey and Barr[130] for a comprehensive summary of the various types of electrical models of the heart. In brief, the two- or three-dimensional distribution of electric field and current density in the heart volume can be calculated for a given electrode geometry and placement using a conventional volume conductor model (step 1, Fig. 18.1) in which the tissue is characterized by a bulk

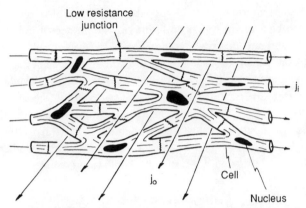

Low resistance
junction

$j_i$

$j_o$

Cell

Nucleus

Fig. 18.9. Microscopic flow of current through cardiac muscle. Intracellular ($j_i$) may flow from cell to cell via low resistance gap junctions. Extracellular current ($j_o$) flows around cells. The average (macroscopic) orientation of intracellular and extracellular currents can differ, as shown. Adapted from an illustration by A. Miller[181], reproduced with permission.

resistivity[131,132]. The tissue resistivity may be anisotropic to account for the preferential orientation of the myocardial fibres[133,134]. Such models are advantageous in that standard numerical techniques such as finite element analysis can be readily applied[33,47]; however, no distinction is made between currents which flow inside, outside, or across the cell membrane.

To address this issue, 'bidomain' volume conductor models (steps 1 and 1', Fig. 18.1) have been developed and describe electrically excitable tissues in which the cells are *electrically coupled*[130,135-138]. A microscopic view of cardiac tissue is shown in Fig. 18.9. Low-resistance gap junctions in the intercalated discs permit the flow of intracellular current between neighbouring cells[139]. Electrical currents flow in a complicated pattern through, and around, each cell and may differ in average direction, depending on whether they are intracellular (density $j_i$) or extracellular (density $j_o$). With bidomain models, current is viewed macroscopically (densities $J_o$ or $J_i$) over distances much larger than a single cell, and the small perturbations in flow at the cell boundaries are ignored. The intracellular and extracellular spaces are modelled as two interpenetrating, conductive domains which occupy the same volume but which are separated by a volume distributed boundary (the cell membrane) (Fig. 18.10($a$)). Conventional volume conductor models can then be regarded as a degenerate case of bidomain models in which the membrane impedance goes to zero. Bidomain models can predict the spatial distribution of *intracellular* and *extracellular electric fields* and, most importantly for this discussion, *transmembrane potentials*. Finite

(a)

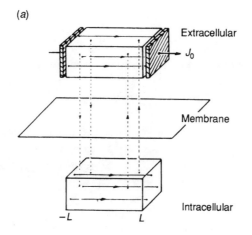

(b)

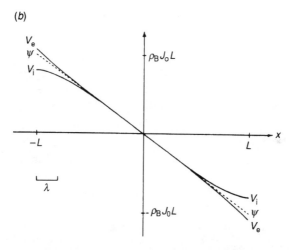

Fig. 18.10. Flow of electrical current in heart muscle using a simplified bidomain model. (*A*) A rectangular slab of cardiac muscle of length $2L$ is placed between two parallel plate electrodes. $J_o$ is the current density at the electrode. Extracellular and intracellular domains coexist in the same three-dimensional volume but are separated at every point in space by a volume-distributed membrane. Current can flow between the electrodes either through the extracellular domain or across the volume-distributed membrane and through the intracellular domain. (*B*) Plotted are the theoretical profiles for extracellular ($V_e$, and intracellular ($V_i$) potentials as a function of position. Membrane potential ($V_m$) is equal to ($V_i$-$V_e$) and is nonzero only in a region on the order of $\lambda$ from each electrode. Terms are defined in the text.

element analysis recently has been extended from monodomain to bidomain models[140].

A simple example drawn from the measurement of myocardial longitudinal resistance[141] is shown in Fig. 18.10 and serves to illustrate the different predictions made by the bidomain and conventional monodomain models. Current (with density $J_o$) can flow between the two electrodes either 1) directly through the extracellular space or 2) across the cell membrane, through the intracellular space, and back across the cell membrane (panel A). If a one-dimensional model is used, the potential profiles in the muscle strip, calculated by Weidmann[141], can be rewritten for steady-state conditions in a form used by Peskoff[142]:

$$V_e = \left(\frac{-\rho_e}{\rho_e + \rho_i}\right)\phi + \psi \tag{2a}$$

$$V_i = \left(\frac{-\rho_i}{\rho_e + \rho_i}\right)\phi + \psi \tag{2b}$$

$$V_m = V_i - V_e = \phi \tag{2c}$$

where $V_i$, $V_e$ and $V_m$ are the intracellular, extracellular and transmembrane potentials, $\phi$ and $\psi$ are auxiliary potentials, $\rho_i$ and $\rho_e$ are the effective intracellular and extracellular resistivities (which take into account the relative cross-sectional areas of the two spaces), and $\rho_b$ is the parallel combination of $\rho_i$ and $\rho_e$. The term $\phi$ is a solution to the Helmholtz equation, is unique to bidomain systems, and gives rise to domain currents which have opposite signs (and hence are 'antiparallel'). The term $\psi$ is a solution to Poisson's equation, is shared by monodomain systems, and gives rise to domain currents which have the same sign (and hence are 'parallel'). For the examples of Fig. 18.10,

$$\phi = 2\lambda\rho_e J_o \frac{\sinh L/\lambda}{\sinh 2L/\lambda} \sinh x/\lambda \tag{3a}$$

$$\psi = -\rho_b J_o x \tag{3b}$$

$$\lambda^2 = \frac{R_m}{\chi(\rho_e + \rho_i)} \tag{3c}$$

where $\lambda$ is the space constant, $\chi$ is the cell surface membrane area per unit volume of tissue, and $R_m$ is the specific membrane resistance. Longitudinal current through the cell membrane at the ends of the muscle has been neglected. For the bulk of the tissue, $V_i$ and $V_e$ (plotted in panel B, Fig. 18.10) are approximately equal to $\psi$, and therefore the interelectrode potential gradient is approximately equal to $\rho_b J_o$ in the case where $L \gg \lambda$. Thus, under these conditions, $\rho_b$ can be interpreted as the *bulk resistivity* of the tissue, treated as a monodomain volume conductor. Interestingly, the bidomain model predicts that the induced $V_m$ will be nonzero only in regions on the order of a space constant from the two electrodes, and *zero* throughout the bulk of the myocardium (since all of the current is flowing longitudinally along the muscle axis and not across the cell membrane). However, since the potentials $V_i$, $V_e$ and $V_m$ are macroscopic potentials which represent averages of the local potential distribution around each cardiac cell, this conclusion may not account correctly for the microscopic variations in transmembrane potential which can contribute to membrane breakdown.

By way of example, discontinuous bidomain[130] and periodic structure[143] models (steps 1, 1' and 2, Fig. 18.1) have been formulated, based on significant coupling resistances in the intercalated disks between cells, which then can act as secondary sources and produce microscopic gradients in membrane potential from one end of the cell to the other[144]. The continuous bidomain model predicts only the average potential in each cell under these conditions.

Since monodomain models make no distinction between intracellular and extracellular domains, the transmembrane potential is indeterminate. However, if cells are assumed to be arranged in a periodic structure, the transmembrane potential *can* be predicted from a *monodomain* model. In the 'periodic structure' model[143], the total potential is decomposed into aperiodic and periodic terms. The aperiodic term is a large-scale potential which may be derived from an equivalent monodomain model (step 1, Fig. 18.1). The periodic term is based on the geometry of a unit cell, or unit bundle of cells, and is a small-scale potential whose magnitude is a function of the spatial *gradient* of the aperiodic term (step 2, Fig. 18.1). In regions well removed from boundaries and sources, the transmembrane potential is determined primarily by the periodic term. For the example of Fig. 18.10, the aperiodic term would take the form of Equation (3b), but with $\rho_b$ replaced by an equivalent, homogenized resistivity. In the bulk of the tissue, $V_m$ is predicted by the bidomain model to be nearly zero, but is predicted by the periodic structure model to be equal to a nonzero periodic function, changing sign between hyperpolarized and depolarized values from end to end of each unit bundle similar to that observed for single cells exposed to extracellular electric fields (see next section). This oscillatory behaviour would be identical from bundle to bundle. Experimental measurements are needed to determine whether the bidomain or periodic structure model is applicable under conditions of electric shock, or whether more complex models are necessary.

The models above assume passive membrane properties for the cell membrane. The known active properties of the cell membrane[145 147] can be incorporated into tissue models[148,149] but apparently do not play a significant role in the genesis of electrical injury, as suggested by experiments with ion channel blockers[100,104].

### Effect of external electric field on cardiac cell potential

#### Electric field intensity

Lepeschkin and co-workers[35] found, in their autorhythmic cardiac cell cultures, that increasing levels of electric shock produced first, a single, premature contraction ('stimulation'), then a series of irregular contractions ('tachyarrhythmia'), a period of standstill, and, finally, fibrillation. The threshold levels for local potential gradients sufficient to produce these effects, as well as defibrillation, were estimated[35] in their own, and in other tissue preparations and animal species, to be [mean ± s.d., in V/cm and normalized to a hypothetical 2 ms, exponential waveform]: stimulation [1.45 ± 0.34], tachyarrhythmia [52.8 ± 14.3], defibrillation [96 ± 25.8], standstill [99 ± 58], and fibrillation [158 ± 92]. With whole heart preparations, electric fields are not known unless measured directly, since, in general, the tissue is anisotropic, and the electric field is three-dimensional and nonuniform over the heart volume[28–30,90,92]. On the other hand, with single cells or cell cultures, uniform electric fields of known intensity and orientation can be applied[68,69,99,102,112,114,115].

#### Cell orientation

Spherical and spheroidal cell models have been used to calculate the change in cell membrane potential in response to an externally applied electric field[150–153] (step 2, Fig. 18.1). By way of illustration, Fig. 18.11(a) shows a prolate spheroidal cell oriented with the major axis parallel to an externally applied d.c. electric field ($\mathbf{E_o}$). The change in transmembrane potential is biphasic (one end of the cell hyperpolarized and the other end depolarized), maximum at the poles of the cell closest to the two electrodes, and dependent on field intensity, pulse duration, cell length, and cell shape[150,153]. Thus, longer cells will theoretically have a greater change in transmembrane potential at their ends than shorter cells with the same shape.

(a)

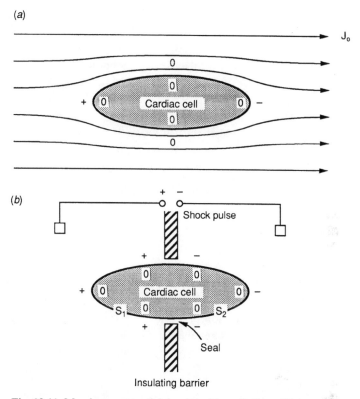

(b)

Fig. 18.11. Membrane potential developed in a cardiac cell in response to an externally applied potential gradient. The cell is described here as a prolate spheroid immersed in a conductive medium. (*a*) A spatially uniform electric field $\mathbf{E}_o$, producing a uniform density of current $\mathbf{J}_o$, is applied to the cell parallel to its long axis. Because the cell membrane has a high resistance compared to the bath, the flow of current is perturbed around the cell. The extracellular potential gradient results in a change in membrane potential which is maximal at the two poles of the cell. The polarity of potential change is indicated by +, 0, or −. The maximum induced potential is given for steady state conditions[153] by the expression $V_m = [a^2 A^2 \sin^2\theta + c^2 C^2 \cos^2\theta]^{\frac{1}{2}} E_o$, where $\theta$ is the angle between major axis of the cell and the field axis, $c$ is the semiprincipal major axis, $a$ the semiprincipal minor axis, and $C$ and $A$ are shape constants which are each functions of $c$ and $a$. (*b*) The cell is inserted into the orifice of an insulating barrier (e.g. particle volume analyser or glass pipette), across which is applied a potential difference. The potential developed in the two halves of the membrane surface ($S_1$, $S_2$) will be a function of applied potential, membrane impedance and seal resistance between cell and barrier. Given that the cell membrane has a naturally high impedance, very little current will flow across the gap if the resistance of the seal between the cell and barrier is sufficiently high. The applied potential difference will be divided across $S_1$ and $S_2$ in a manner inversely proportional to their relative areas.

If the cell is rotated by 90°, so that it is perpendicular to the electric field axis, the peak transmembrane potential still occurs at the edges of the cell closest to the two electrodes[153]. Since there is now a shorter projection of cell length along the electric field axis, the membrane depolarization will be smaller than in the case of a parallel orientation (although the shape factor also comes into play). This results in an apparently higher threshold of excitability, when the cell is perpendicular, as opposed to parallel to the electric field[112,114,117]. The effect, if any, of cell orientation on the threshold of arrhythmia or contracture has yet to be determined.

A feature common to all the models referred to above is that the cell membrane is in a spatially uniform, highly nonconductive state compared with the intracellular and extracellular fluids. Once the membrane has been electroporated, however, this may no longer be the case, and the models then will need revision.

### Restricted extracellular space

The models described in the previous section assumed a cell placed in an infinite volume conductor. The presence of neighbouring cells can perturb significantly the distribution of extracellular potential and current flow. Reduction of the cross-sectional area of the extracellular space around the cell is predicted to increase the maximum transmembrane potential developed at the poles of the cell[154]. In the limiting case in which neighbouring cells are joined tightly so that no extracellular current may flow, the change in membrane potential induced by an applied potential gradient will be maximal (Fig. 18.11(*b*)).

### Effective cell length: cell-to-cell coupling

Cardiac cells are coupled by low-resistance junctions[139] to form an electrical syncytium which permits the propagation of electrical impulses, just as in electrical cables. The coupling resistance has been studied in isolated cell pairs and is known to be nonselective, nonvarying with time, and linear in its current–voltage relation[155-158]. Therefore, although individual cardiac cells are relatively small in dimension compared to skeletal muscle fibres, they can act functionally as long muscle fibres. Since the change in transmembrane potential of a cell subjected to an applied electric field depends on the length of the cell, the results of the single cell studies described earlier should be applied with caution to the intact tissue, since the effective *electrical* length of the cardiac cell may be longer than its *anatomical* length[127].

### Electroporation

Electrical breakdown of the cell membrane ('electroporation' or 'electro-permeabilization') by high-intensity, pulsed electric fields appears to occur universally for lipid bilayers and cell membranes when the membrane potential reaches a threshold value of about 0.2–1 volt (at room temperature), depending on pulse duration (for reviews, see [125,126,160]). Electroporation has been studied in cell membranes using: 1) resistance change of cells flowing through a particle volume analyser, 2) impedance change or exchange of substances from cell suspensions in a discharge chamber, 3) microelectrode voltage clamp in large cells, and 4) voltage-sensitive fluorescent dyes[126,152,161–164]. Thus, with an applied electric field (Fig. 18.11(*a*)) membrane breakdown should occur symmetrically at the opposite poles of the cell (although asymmetric breakdown can occur primarily at one pole if the cell has a significant intrinsic membrane potential[165]). Data such as those in Fig. 18.8 are a direct confirmation of electroporation in cardiac cell membranes[124]. The event indicated by $T_A$ in Fig. 18.8 may correspond to pore growth and the event $T_B$ to membrane breakdown, as observed previously in lipid bilayers and in cell membranes[161,166]. Thus, electroporation of the cell membrane may be the last link (step 3, Fig. 18.1) in the sequence of events leading to the electropathological effects as described on pp. 363–76. It is unlikely that electroporation itself is a mechanism for electrical defibrillation as has been suggested[167], considering, first, that 6 V/cm may be sufficient for defibrillation whereas 60–100 V/cm may be required for electroporation as inferred by conduction disturbances[30], and, second, that injury effects are absent or transient at shock levels just at the defibrillation threshold [8–10].

The formation and resealing of pores are functions of pulse intensity, pulse duration, number of pulses applied, time between pulses, membrane stress and temperature[125,126,152,161–164,168,169]. The time course of membrane breakdown has been shown to occur in cell membranes on a microsecond time-scale[161,162,168]. Data are consistent with these observations and show that membrane breakdown occurs in less than 30 $\mu$s[124]. Pore size has been measured in cardiac cell membranes by Jones *et al.*[101] using fluorescent dextran molecules. It is a function of shock intensity, and is at least 44 Å in diameter following a series of six 5 ms, 200 V/cm shock pulses. Recently, electrically induced pores with diameters of 20–120 nm have been visualized in red blood cell membranes by Chang and Reese using electron microscopy[170].

## Discussion

### The potential gradient

The working hypothesis of this chapter is that electroporation of the cell membrane is responsible for electrical injury effects in heart muscle and is dependent on the level of transmembrane potential. Although the transmembrane potential can be related to local electric field (steps 1' or 2, Fig. 18.1), the cell size, cell orientation, specific pathways of current, and syncytial structure of the cardiac tissue all can influence this relationship. It is on the basis of size, for example, that electroporation in bacteria requires electric fields on the order of 10 kV/cm, whereas, in the much larger skeletal muscle cell, fields serveral orders of magnitude *smaller* may be sufficient. Furthermore, the field intensity required to porate the cell membrane depends on the pulse duration used. Therefore, it might be expected that local electric field can be used to predict the extent of electrical injury only if *all* of these other factors are accounted for. On the other hand, it is membrane potential which governs pore formation, and a threshold value of about 0.8 V is consistent with our experimental results on single cardiac cells[124]. Recently, preliminary data have been obtained suggesting that the threshold for electroporation may be as low as 0.4 V for monophasic and biphasic rectangular pulses of transmembrane potential[171].

The theoretical considerations described on pp. 376–85 may help to explain some of the observations regarding the anatomical site of myocardial damage. For the case of two plate electrodes applied to the heart surface, injury to the myocardium occurs preferentially in the neighbourhood of the electrodes[24,37]. This can be explained either by: 1) higher current density (and therefore greater induced change in transmembrane potential), or 2) bidomain model predictions of a current induced transmembrane potential which is greatest in a region about a space constant wide from the electrodes even in the case of uniform tissue current density (Fig. 18.10($b$)). In either case, cellular injury then can be accounted for by electroporation, provided that $V_m$ exceeds about 0.8 volt. Histological studies have also found severely damaged fibres immediately adjacent to normal or minimally injured fibres[1,4,23]. This might be explained on the basis that adjoining cells which are better coupled have a longer 'electrical' cell length, and hence are more prone to electroporation.

Field-induced pores form large nonselective openings through the cell surface membrane[101,170]. It is unknown at this time whether electroporation of internal membrane systems (sarcoplasmic reticulum, mitochondria, T-tubules, nucleus) occurs in cardiac cells. However, these systems may be protected by virtue of their smaller diameters compared to the cell length, and therefore would require much higher field intensities for membrane breakdown. On the other hand, swelling of these structures has been observed[103], perhaps as a result of electrolyte and consequent osmotic imbalance produced by the shock-induced depolarization (see below).

### Alterations in cellular homeostasis

With pore formation in cell membrane, the transmembrane potential will be shunted to zero, resulting in a period of standstill[102]. A reduction in resting potential may account also for the changes in excitability, conduction velocity, electrocardiogram and contractility observed experimentally in whole hearts. If the pore lifetime is long compared with the diffusion time for monovalent ions, intracellular potassium could be lost and sodium gained. Resting potential recovers with a time course which depends on the shock level[93,102]. The recovery process must involve, first, the resealing of the field-induced membrane pores, and, second, restoration of resting levels of intracellular potassium and sodium by the ATP-dependent Na/K pump, which can be inhibited by cardiac glycosides[98].

Increase in intracellular calcium through the field-induced pores may result in 'calcium overload'[118], which results in contractile oscillations and arrhythmogenic currents[172]. Use of a calcium channel blocker (verapamil) fails to prevent the electrophysiological alterations seen immediately following shock[44,100], suggesting that calcium entry is not by way of the calcium channel. Influx of calcium could occur also via Na/Ca counter-exchange[119,120], secondary to elevation of intracellular sodium by sodium influx through the field-induced pores. The rise in intracellular calcium may also account for the formation of granules in the mitochondria[25,103], loss of mitochondrial function[173], appearance of contraction bands[25,41], activation of membrane phospholipases[174], and, ultimately, development of tissue necrosis[23,24,118]. Uncoupling of cardiac cells can occur[139], reducing conduction velocity or even preventing the propagation of electrical activity[175-177].

Other effects could arise with the formation of relatively large openings in the cell membrane. The alterations in electrolyte content described above could result in osmotically driven water flow across the cell membrane[126,151,178], producing intracellular oedema and swelling of intracellular organelles[103]. Pores with large openings also could permit the loss of essential enzymes, electrolytes and metabolites to the extracellular medium, as observed in the haemolysis of red blood cells[126,151].

### *Future directions*

Many questions remain regarding electric field-mediated electroporation of the cardiac cell membrane. Although membrane breakdown appears to be a well-defined event, the membrane pores can reseal if irreversible rupture[125,159,160] has not occurred. Pore resealing is an essential step in the recovery of the cell from depolarization-induced standstill and unexcitability and in the prevention of further overload of calcium ions. Thus, further experimental work is needed to identify the parameters which control the resealing process in heart cell membranes, so that the recovery of myocardial tissue from shock can be better understood. Preliminary data have been obtained which indicate a highly variable time course for resealing, ranging from less than 1 second to more than 3 minutes[179].

The monodomain, bidomain, and periodic structure models described on pp. 377–82 can be used to describe the coupling of extracellular electric field in the myocardium to cellular membrane potential. For the example of Fig. 18.10, the bidomain model predicts a significant change in membrane potential only in regions directly adjacent to the shock electrodes, whereas the periodic structure model predicts oscillations in membrane potential in the bulk of the tissue. The validity of either model can be determined by experiments which pinpoint the locations where the membrane potential changes significantly.

The effects of high levels of current on gap junctions and cell-to-cell connections need to be explored. While single cells cannot be used for these types of studies, cell pairs can[155,158]. Studies of cell pairs thus far have limited transjunctional potentials to less than 80 mV, in which case the junctional conductance is ohmic and linear[155,156]. The characteristics of the junctional conductance at higher transjunctional potentials and current densities are, as yet, unknown. However, changes in intracellular calcium and pH can mediate the electrical coupling between heart cells[139]. If the junctional resistance between cells becomes comparable to the intracellular resistance, simulations show that the junction acts as a secondary source during the flow of externally applied current and produces microscopic potential gradients from one end of the cell to the other, which is superimposed on a background potential gradient varying slowly over many cell lengths[127,144]. This situation could result then in sites for electroporation which could be distributed over additional regions of the heart.

In summary, electrical injury to heart muscle, broadly defined to include even reversible electrophysiological changes, may occur by nonthermal, membrane breakdown in the region of the shock electrodes during the application of electric countershock for defibrillation or cardioversion, particularly for shock levels much greater than the defibrillation threshold level. By better understanding 1) the coupling between cell membrane potential and the externally applied electric field by appropriate theoretical models, and 2) the parameters which control the size, formation rate, and recovery rates of electrically induced membrane pores, it may be possible to select better waveform shapes, waveform durations and amplitudes, shock protocols, electrode configurations and electrode placement to minimize this form of myocardial injury, while preserving the therapeutic effects of countershock.

### Acknowledgements

I am indebted to Drs Nitish Thakor, Thomas Guarnieri, Janice Jones and Wanda Krassowska for their critical reading and helpful suggestions for this manuscript, to my students Rory O'Neill, Michele Mulligan, Larry Fogelson, Nicholas Sliz, and Andrew Westdorp for their contributions to the chapter material, and to Doug Price for his assistance with the preparation of the manuscript. This work was supported by a grant from the Whitaker Foundation.

### References

1 Crampton, R. (1980). Accepted, controversial, and speculative aspects of defibrillation. *Progress in Cardiovascular Diseases*, **23**, 167–86.
2 DeSilva, R.A., Graboys, T.B., Podrid, P.J. & Lown, B. (1980). Cardioversion and defibrillation. *American Heart Journal*, **100(6)**, 881–95.
3 Lerman, B.B. (1987). Electrical cardioversion and defibrillation. In *Management of Cardiac Arrhythmias*, E.V. Platia, ed. Chap. 11, pp. 236–56, Philadelphia: J.B. Lippincott Co.
4 Tacker, W.A. & Geddes, L.A. (1980). *Electrical Defibrillation*, Boca Raton, Fl. CRC Press.
5 Troup, P.J. (1989). Implantable cardioverters and defibrillators. *Current Problems in Cardiology*, **14(12)**, 675–815.
6 Bardy, G.H., Sawyer, P.L., Johnson, G.W., Ivey, T.D. & Reichenbach, D.D. (1989). Effect of voltage and charge of electrical ablation pulses on canine myocardium. *American Journal of Physiology*, **257**, H1534–42.
7 Scheinmen, M.M. (1986). Catheter ablation for patients with cardiac arrhythmias. *PACE*, **9**, 551–64.
8 Avitall, B., Port, S., Gal, R., McKinnie, J., Tchou, P., Jazayeri, M., Troup, P. & Akhtar, M. (1990). Automatic implantable cardioverter/

defibrillation: histopathology and temporal stability of defibrillation energy requirements. *Journal of the American College of Cardiology*, **9**, 631–8.

10  Tacker, W.A., Davis, J.S., Lie, J.T., Titus, J.L. & Geddes, L.A. (1978). Cardiac damage produced by transchest damped sine wave shocks. *Medical Instrumentation*, **12**, 27–30.

11  Davy, J.M., Fain, E.S., Dorian, P. & Winkle, R.A. (1987). The relationship between successful defibrillation and delivered energy in open-chest dogs: reappraisal of the 'defibrillation threshold' concept, *American Heart Journal*, **113**, 77–84.

12  Lown, B., Crampton, R.S., DeSilva, R.A. & Gascho, J. (1978). The energy for ventricular defibrillation – too little or too much?, *New England Journal of Medicine*, **298(22)**, 1252–3.

13  Babbs, C.F., Tacker, W.A., Van Fleet, J.F., Bourland, J.D. & Geddes, L.A. (1980). Therapeutic indices for transchest defibrillator shocks: effective damaging and lethal electrical doses. *American Heart Journal*, **99**, 734–8.

14  Geddes, L.A., Tacker, W.A., Rosborough, J., Cabler, J., Chapman, R. & Rivera, R. (1976). The increased efficacy of high-energy defibrillation. *Medical and Biological Engineering*, **14**, 330–3.

15  Kerber, R.E., Martins, J.B., Gascho, J.A., Marcus, M.L. & Grayzel, J. (1981). Effect of direct-current countershocks on regional myocardial contractility and perfusion. *Circulation*, **63**, 323–32.

16  Niebauer, M.J., Babbs, C.F., Geddes, L.A. & Bourland, J.D. (1983). Efficacy and safety of defibrillation with rectangular waves of 2 to 20 milliseconds duration. *Critical Care Medicine*, **11**, 95–8.

17  Niebauer, M.J., Babbs, C.F. Geddes, L.A., Carter, J.E. & Bourland, J.D. (1984). Functional cardiac depression caused by defibrillator shocks, *Japanese Heart Journal*, **25**, 773–81.

18  Ehsani, A., Ewy, G.A. & Sobel, B.E. (1976). Effects of electrical countershock on serum creatine phosphokinase (CPK) isoenzyme activity. *American Journal of Cardiology*, **37**, 12–18.

19  Singer, I., Hutchins, G.M., Mirowski, M., Mower, M.M., Veltri, E.P., Guarnieri, T., Griffith, L.S.C., Watkins, L., Juanteguy, J., Fisher, S., Reid, P.R. & Weisfeldt, M.L. (1987). Pathologic findings related to the lead system and repeated defibrillations in patients with the automatic implantable cardioverter-defibrillator. *Journal of the American College of Cardiology*, **10**, 382–8.

20  Turner, J.R.B. & Towers, J.R.H. (1965). Complications of cardioversion, *Lancet*, **ii**, 612–613.

21  Kong, T.Q. & Proudfit, W.L. (1964). Repeated direct-current countershock without myocardial injury. *Journal of the American Medical Association*, **187**, 160–61.

22  Marriott, H.J.L. & Sandler, A.I. (1964). Multiple countershocks. *New England Journal of Medicine*, **270**, 1019.

23  Anderson, H.N., Reichenbach, D., Steinmetz, G.P. & Merendino, K.A. (1964). An evaluation and comparison of effects of alternating and direct current electrical discharges on canine hearts. *Annals of Surgery*, **160**, 251–62.

24  Koning, G., Veefkind, A.H. & Schneider, H. (1980). Cardiac damage caused by direct application of defibrillator shocks to isolated Langendorff-perfused rabbit heart, *American Heart Journal*, **100**, 473–82.

25 Doherty, P.W., McLaughlin, P.R., Billingham, M., Kernoff, R., Goris, M.L. & Harrison, D.C. (1979). Cardiac damage produced by direct current countershock applied to the heart, *American Journal of Cardiology*, **43**, 225–32.

26 Rivkin, L.M. (1963). The defibrillator and cardiac burns, *Journal of Thoracic Cardiovascular Surgery*, **46**, 755–64.

27 Bourland, J.D., Tacker, W.A., Wessale, J.L., Kallok, M.J., Graf, J.E. & Geddes, L.A. (1986). Sequential pulse defibrillation for implantable defibrillators. *Medical Instrumentation*, **20**, 138–42.

28 Chen, P.S., Wolf, P.D., Claydon, F.J., Dixon, E.G., Vidaillet, H.J., Danieley, N.D., Pilkington, T.C. & Ideker, R.E. (1986). The potential gradient field created by epicardial defibrillation electrodes in dogs, *Circulation*, **74(3)**, 626–36.

29 Tang, A.S.L., Wolf, P.D., Claydon, F.J., Smith, W.M., Pilkington, T.C. & Ideker, R.E. (1988). Measurement of defibrillation shock potential distributions and activation sequences of the heart in three dimensions. *Proceedings of the IEEE*, **76**, 1176–86.

30 Yabe, S., Smith, W.M., Daubert, J.P., Wolf, P.D., Rollins, D.L. & Ideker, R.E. (1990). Conduction disturbances caused by high current density electric fields. *Circulation Research*, **66**, 1190–203.

31 Kim, Y., Fahy, J.B. & Tupper, B.J. (1986). Optimal electrode designs for electrosurgery, defibrillation, and external cardiac pacing. *IEEE Transactions on Biomedical Engineering*, **33(9)**, 845–53.

32 Koning, G., Schneider, H., Reneman, R.S. & Hoelen, A.J. (1972). An electrode system with rounded edges for direct ventricular defibrillation, *Medical and Biological Engineering*, **10**, 201–6.

33 Kothiyal, K.P., Shankar, B., Fogelson, L.J. & Thakor, N.V. (1988). Three-dimensional computer model of electric fields in internal defibrillation, *Proceedings of the IEEE*, **76(6)**, 720–30.

34 Lindemans, F.W. & Denier van der Gon, J.J. (1978). Current thresholds and liminal size in excitation of heart muscle, *Cardiovascular Research*, **12**, 477–85.

35 Lepeschkin, E., Jones, J.L., Rush, S. & Jones, R.E. (1978). Local potential gradients as a unifying measure for threshold of stimulation, standstill, tachyarrhythmia, and fibrillation appearing after strong capacitor discharges. *Advances in Cardiology*, **21**, 268–78.

36 Barker-Voelz, M.A., Van Vleet, J.F., Tacker, W.A., Bourland, J.D., Geddes, L.A. & Schollmeyer, M.P. (1983). Alterations induced by a single defibrillating shock applied through a chronically implanted catheter electrode. *Journal of Electrocardiology*, **16(2)**, 167–80.

37 Van Fleet, J.F., Tacker, W.A., Cechner, P.E., Bright, R.M., Greene, J.A., Raffee, M.R., Geddes, L.A. & Ferrans, V.J. (1978). Effect of shock strength on survival and acute cardiac damage induced by open-thorax defibrillation of dogs, *American Journal of Veterinary Research*, **39**, 981–7.

38 Knox, M.A., Hughes, H.C. Jr., Tyers, G.F.O., Seidl, D. & Demers, L.M. (1980). The induction of myocardial damage by open-chest low-energy countershock. *Medical Instrumentation*, **14**, 63–6.

39 Kouwenhoven, W.B. & Milnor, W.R. (1954). Treatment of ventricular fibrillation using a capacitor discharge. *Journal of Applied Physiology*, **7**, 253–7.

40 Geddes, L.A., Niebauer, M., Babbs, C.F. *et al.* (1985). Fundamental criteria underlying the efficacy and safety of ventricular defibrillating

current waveforms. *Medical and Biological Engineering and Computing*, **23**, 122–30.

41  Reichenbach, D. & Benditt, E.P. (1969). Myofibrillar degeneration: a common form of cardiac muscle injury. *Annals of the New York Academy of Science*, **156**, 164–76.

42  Mehta, J., Runge, W., Cohn, J.N. & Carlyle, P. (1978). Myocardial damage after repetitive direct current in the dog: correlation between left ventricular end-diastolic pressure and extent of myocardial necrosis, *Journal of Laboratory and Clinical Medicine*, **91**, 272–9.

43  Van Fleet, J.F., Ferrans, V.J., Barker, M.A., Tacker, W., Bourland, J.D. & Schollmeyer, M.P. (1982). Ultrastructural alterations in the fibrous sheath, endocardium, and myocardium of dogs shocked with chronically implanted automatic defibrillator leads. *American Journal of Veterinary Research*, **43**, 909–15.

44  Patton, N., Allen, J.D. & Pantridge, J.F. (1984). The effects of shock energy, propranolol, and verapamil on cardiac damage caused by transthoracic countershock. *Circulation*, **69(2)**, 357–68.

45  Deale, O.C. & Lerman, B.B. (1990). Intrathoracic current flow during transthoracic defibrillation in dogs. *Circulation Research*, **67**, 1405–19.

46  Hoyt, R., Grayzel, J. & Kerber, R.E. (1981). Determinants of intracardiac current in defibrillation experimental studies in dogs. *Circulation*, **64**, 818–23.

47  Nadarajan, R. & Seshadri, V. (1976). Electric field distribution in the human body using finite-element method. *Medical and Biological Engineering*, **14**, 489–93.

48  Dahl, C.F., Ewy, G.A., Warner, E.D. & Thomas, E.D. (1974). Myocardial necrosis from direct current countershock. Effect of paddle electrode size and time interval between discharges. *Circulation*, **50**, 956–61.

49  Ewy, G.A., Taren, D., Bangert, J., McClung, S. & Hellman, D.A. (1980). Comparison of myocardial damage from defibrillator discharges at various dosages. *Medical Instrumentation*, **14**, 9–12.

50  Peleska, B. (1963). Cardiac arrhythmias following condenser discharges and their dependence upon strength of current and phase of cardiac cycle, *Circulation Research*, **13**, 21–32.

51  Schuder, J.C., Rahmoeller, G.A., Nellis, S.H., Stoeckle, H. & Mackenzie, J.W. (1967). Transthoracic ventricular defibrillation with very high amplitude rectangular pulses. *Journal of Applied Physiology*, **22(6)**, 1110–14.

52  Tacker, W.A., Van Fleet, J.F. & Geddes, L.A. (1979). Electrocardiographic and serum enzyme alterations associated with cardiac alterations induced in dogs by single transthoracic damped sinusoidal defibrillator shocks of various strengths. *American Heart Journal*, **98**, 185–93.

53  Van Fleet, J.F., Tacker, W.A., Geddes, L.A. *et al.* (1980). Sequential ultrastructural alterations in ventricular myocardium of dogs given large single transthoracic damped sinusoidal waveform defibrillator shocks. *American Journal of Veterinary Research*, **41**, 493–501.

54  Warner, E.D., Dahl, C. & Ewy, G.A. (1975). Myocardial injury from transthoracic defibrillator countershock. *Archives of Pathology*, **99**, 55–9.

55  Wilson, C.M., Allen, J.D., Bridges, J.B. & Adgey, A.A.J. (1988). Death

and damage caused by multiple direct current shocks: studies in an animal model. *European Heart Journal*, **9**, 1257–65.

56 Bourland, J.D., Tacker, W.A. & Geddes, L.A. (1978). Strength–duration curves for trapezoidal waveforms of various tilts for transchest defibrillation in animals. *Medical Instrumentation*, **12(1)**, 38–41.

57 Geddes, L.A., Tacker, W.A., McFarlane, J. & Bourland, J. (1970). Strength–duration curves for ventricular defibrillation in dogs. *Circulation Research*, **27**, 551–60.

58 Koning, G., Schneider, H., Hoelen, A.J. & Reneman, R.S. (1975). Amplitude-duration relation for direct ventricular defibrillation with rectangular current pulses. *Medical and Biological Engineering*, **13**, 388–95.

59 Geddes, L.A. & Bourland, J.D. (1985). Tissue stimulation: theoretical considerations and practical applications. *Medical and Biological Engineering and Computing*, **23**, 131–7.

60 Dixon, E.G., Tang, A.S.L., Wolf, P.D., Meador, J.T., Fine, M.J., Calfee, R.V. & Ideker, R.E. (1987). Improved defibrillation thresholds with large contoured epicardial electrodes and biphasic waveforms. *Circulation*, **76(5)**, 1176–84.

61 Fahy, J.B., Kim, Y. & Ananthaswamy, A. (1987). Optimal electrode configurations for external cardiac pacing and defibrillation: an inhomogeneous study. *IEEE Transactions on Biomedical Engineering*, **34**, 743–8.

62 Langer, A., Heilman, M.S., Mower, M.M. & Mirowski, M. (1976). Considerations in the development of the automatic implantable defibrillator. *Medical Instrumentation*, **10**, 163–7.

63 Santel, D.J., Kallok, M.J. & Tacker, W.A. (1985). Implantable defibrillator electrode systems: a brief review. *PACE*, **8**, 123–31.

64 Troup, P.J., Chapman, P.D., Olinger, G.N. & Kleinman, L.H. (1985). The implanted defibrillator: relation of defibrillating lead configuration and clinical variables to defibrillation threshold. *Journal of the American College of Cardiology*, **6(6)**, 1315–21.

65 Chapman, P.D., Vetter, J.W., Souza, J.J., Troup, P.J., Wetherbee, J.N. & Hoffmann, R.G. (1988). Comparative efficacy of monophasic and biphasic truncated exponential shocks for nonthoracotomy internal defibrillation in dogs. *Journal of the American College of Cardiology*, **12(3)**, 739–45.

66 Fain, E.S., Sweeney, M.B. & Franz, M.R. (1989). Improved internal defibrillation efficacy with a biphasic waveform. *American Heart Journal*, **117(2)**, 358–64.

67 Flaker, G.C., Schuder, J.C., McDaniel, W.C., Stoeckle, H. & Dbeis, M. (1989). Superiority of biphasic shocks in the defibrillation of dogs by epicardial patches and catheter electrodes. *American Heart Journal*, **118**, 288–91.

68 Jones, J.L. & Jones, R.E. (1983). Improved defibrillator waveform safety factor with biphasic waveforms. *American Journal of Physiology*, **245**, H60–5.

69 Jones, J.L. & Jones, R.E. (1989). Improved safety factor for triphasic defibrillator waveforms. *Circulation Research*, **64(6)**, 1172–1177.

70 Tang, A.S.L., Yabe, S., Wharton, M., Dolker, M., Smith, W.M. & Ideker, R.E. (1989). Ventricular defibrillation using biphasic

waveforms: the importance of phasic duration. *Journal of the American College of Cardiology*, **13(1)**, 207–14.

71  Winkle, R.A., Mead, R.H., Ruder, M.A., Gaudiani, V., Buch, W.S., Pless, B., Sweeney, M. & Schmidt, P. (1989). Improved low energy defibrillation efficacy in man with the use of a biphasic truncated exponential waveform. *American Heart Journal*, **117(1)**, 122–6.

72  Bardou, A.L., Degonde, J., Birkui, P.J., Auger, P., Chesnais, J.M. & Duriez, M. (1988). Reduction of energy required for defibrillation by delivering shocks in orthogonal directions in the dog. *PACE*, **11**, 1990–5.

73  Chang, M.S., Inoue, H., Kallok, M.J. & Zipes, D.P. (1986). Double and triple sequential shocks reduce ventricular defibrillation threshold in dogs with and without myocardial infarcation. *Journal of the American College of Cardiology*, **8(6)**, 1393–405.

74  Jones, D.L., Klein, G.J., Guiraudon, G.M. & Sharma, A.D. (1988). Sequential pulse defibrillation in humans: orthogonal sequential pulse defibrillation with epicardial electrodes. *Journal of the American College of Cardiology*, **11(3)**, 590–6.

75  Lee, R.C., Gaylor, D.C., Bhatt, D. & Israel, D.A. (1988). Role of cell membrane rupture in the pathogenesis of electrical trauma. *Journal of Surgical Research*, **44(6)**, 709–19.

76  Lee, R.C. & Kolodney, M.S. (1987). Electrical injury mechanisms: electrical breakdown of cell membranes. *Plastic and Reconstructive Surgery*, **80(5)**, 672–9.

77  Coraboeuf, E., Suekane, K. & Breton, D. (1963). Some effects of strong stimulations on the electrical and mechanical properties of isolated heart. *International Symposium on the Electrophysiology of the Heart*, Taccardi, B. & Marchetti, G., eds, pp. 133–45, Oxford, New York: Pergamon Press.

78  Arnsdorf, M.F., Rothbaum, D.A. & Childers, R.W. (1977). Effect of direct current countershock on atrial and ventricular electrophysiological properties and myocardial potassium efflux in the thoracotomized dog. *Cardiovascular Research*, **11**, 324–33.

79  Niebauer, M.J., Geddes, L.A. & Babbs, C.F. (1986). Potassium efflux from myocardial cells induced by defibrillator shock. *Medical Instrumentation*, **20(3)**, 135–7.

80  Pansegrau, D.G. & Abboud, F.M. (1970). Hemodynamic effects of ventricular defibrillation. *Journal of Clinical Investigation*, **49**, 282–97.

81  DiCola, V.C., Freedman, G.S., Downing, S.E. & Zaret, B.L. (1976). Myocardial uptake of technetium-99m stannous pyrophosphate following direct current transthoracic countershock. *Circulation*, **54(6)**, 980–6.

82  Tacker, W.A., Geddes, L.A., McFarlane, J., Milnor, W., Gullet, J., Havens, W., Green, E. & Moore, J. (1969). Optimum current duration for capacitor-discharge defibrillation of canine ventricles. *Journal of Applied Physiology*, **27(4)**, 480–3.

83  Shibata, N., Chen, P.S., Dixon, E.G., Wolf, P.D., Danieley, N.D., Smith, W.M. & Ideker, R.E. (1988). Influence of shock strength and timing on induction of ventricular arrhythmias in dogs. *American Journal of Physiology*, **255**, H891–901.

84  Chen, P.S., Shibata, N., Dixon, E.G., Martin, R.O. & Ideker, R.E. (1986). Comparison of the defibrillation threshold and the upper limit of ventricular vulnerability. *Circulation*, **73(5)**, 1022–28.

85 Lesigne, C., Levy, B., Saumont, R., Birkui, P., Bardou, A. and Rubin, B. (1976). An energy-time analysis of ventricular fibrillation and defibrillation thresholds with internal electrodes. *Medical and Biological Engineering*, 617–622.

86 Kerber, R.E., Martins, J.B., Kienzle, M.G., Constantin, L., Olshansky, B., Hopson, R. & Charbonnier, F. (1988). Energy, current, and success in defibrillation and cardioversion: clinical studies using an automated impedance-based method of energy adjustment. *Circulation*, **77(5)**, 1038–46.

87 Lerman, B.B., Halperin, H.R., Tsitlik, J.E., Brin, K., Clark, C.W. & Deale, O.C. (1987). Relationship between canine transthoracic impedance and defibrillation threshold. Evidence for current-based defibrillation. *Journal of Clinical Investigation*, **80(3)**, 797–803.

88 Monzón, J.E. & Guillén, S.G. (1985). Current defibrillator: new instrument of programmed current for research and clinical use. *IEEE Transactions on Biomedical Engineering*, **32**, 928–34.

89 Cobb, F.R., Wallace, A.G. & Wagner, G.S. (1968). Cardiac inotropic and coronary vascular responses to countershock. *Circulation Research*, **23**, 731–42.

90 Lepeschkin, E., Herrlich, H.C., Rush, S., Jones, J.L. & Jones, R.E. (1980). Cardiac potential gradients between defibrillation electrodes. *Medical Instrumentation*, **14**, 57.

91 Witkowski, F.X., Penkoske, P.A. & Plonsey, R. (1990). Mechanism of cardiac defibrillation in open-chest dogs with unipolar DC-coupled simultaneous activation and shock potential recordings. *Circulation*, **82**, 244–60.

92 Frazier, D.W., Krassowska, W., Chen, P.S., Wolf, P.D., Dixon, E.G., Smith, W.M. & Ideker, R.E. (1988). Extracellular field required for excitation in three-dimensional anisotropic canine myocardium. *Circulation Research*, **63(1)**, 147–64.

93 Fogelson, L.J., Tung, L. & Thakor, N.V. (1988). Electrophysiologic depression in myocardium by defibrillation-level shocks. *Proceedings of the 10th Annual Conference IEEE Engineering in Medicine and Biology Society*, pp. 963–64.

94 Antoni, H. (1970). Electrophysiological studies of the mechanism of DC defibrillation of the heart. *Symposium of Cardiac Arrhythmias*, Sandoe, E., Flensted -, Jensen, E. & Olensen, K. eds, pp. 379–92, Elsinore, Denmark.

95 Knisley, S., Zhou, X., Guse, P., Wolf, P., Rollins, D., Smith, W. & Ideker, R. (1990). Shocks first prolong, then shorten, action potentials in heart muscle. *PACE*, **13**, 517.

96 Levine, J.H., Spear, J.F., Weisman, H.F., Kadish, A.H., Prood, C., Siu, C.O. & Moore, E.N. (1986). The cellular electrophysiologic changes induced by high-energy electrical ablation in canine myocardium. *Circulation*, **73(4)**, 818–29.

97 Moore, E.N. & Spear, J.F. (1985). Electrophysiologic studies on the initiation, prevention, and termination of ventricular fibrillation. In *Cardiac Electrophysiology and Arrhythmias*, Zipes, D.P. & Jalife, J. eds, Chap. 35, pp. 315–322, New York: Grune & Stratton.

98 Jones, J.L. & Jones, R.E. (1980*b*). Postcountershock fibrillation in digitized myocardial cells *in vitro*. *Critical Care Medicine*, **8(3)**, 172–6.

99 Jones, J.L. & Jones, R.E. (1982*a*). Determination of safety factor for defibrillator waveforms in cultured heart cells. *American Journal of*

*Physiology*, **242**, H662–70.
100 Jones, J.L. and Jones, R.E. (1982*b*). Effects of tetrodotoxin and verapamil on the prolonged depolarization produced by high-intensity electric field stimulation in cultured myocardial cells. *Federation Proceedings*, **41**, 1383.
101 Jones, J.L., Jones, R.E. & Balasky, G. (1987*b*). Microlesion formation in myocardial cells by high-intensity electric field stimulation. *American Journal of Physiology*, **253**, H480–6.
102 Jones, J.L., Lepeschkin, E., Jones, R.E. & Rush, S. (1978). Response of cultured myocardial cells to countershock-type electric field stimulation. *American Journal of Physiology*, **235(2)**, H214–22.
103 Jones, J.L., Proskauer, C.C., Paull, W.K., Lepeschkin, E. & Jones, R.E. (1980). Ultrastructural injury to chick myocardial cells *in vitro* following 'electric countershock'. *Circulation Research*, **46(3)**, 387–94.
104 Mulligan, M.R. (1989). The Effects of Pulsed DC Electric Fields on the Cardiac Myocyte Membrane and Threshold Levels, Master's Thesis, Dept. Biomed. Engr., Johns Hopkins University.
105 Lieberman, M., Hauschka, S.D., Hall, Z.W., Eisenberg, B.R., Horn, R., Walsh, J.V., Tsien, R.W., Jones, A.W., Walker, J.L., Poenie, M., Fay, F., Fabiato, F. & Ashley, C.C. (1987). Isolated muscle cells as a physiological model. *American Journal of Physiology*, **253**, C349–63.
106 Piper, H.M. & Isenberg, G. (1989). *Isolated Adult Cardiomyocytes, Vol. I. Structure and Metabolism, Vol. II. Electrophysiological and Contractile Function*. Boca Raton, Fl: CRC Press.
107 Jacobson, S.L. (1989). Techniques for isolation and culture of adult cardiomyocytes. In *Isolated Adult Cardiomyocytes, Vol. I. Structure and Metabolism*, H.M. Piper & G. Isenberg, eds, Chap. 2, pp. 43–80, Boca Raton, Fl: CRC Press.
108 Pelzer, D. & Trautwein, W. (1987). Currents through ionic channels in multicellular cardiac tissue and single heart cells. *Experientia*, **43**, 1153–62.
109 Tung, L. & Morad, M. (1988). Contractile force of single heart cells compared with muscle strips of frog ventricle. *American Journal of Physiology*, **255**, H111–20.
110 Capogrossi, M.C. & Lakatta, E.G. (1989). Intracellular calcium and activation of contraction as studied by optical techniques. In *Isolated Adult Cardiomyocytes, Vol. II. Electrophysiological and Contractile Function*, H.M. Piper & G. Isenberg, eds, Chap. 9, pp. 183–212, Boca Raton, Fl: CRC Press.
111 Tung, L. & Morad, M. (1985). A comparative electrophysiological study of enzymatically isolated single cells and strips of frog ventricle. *Pflugers Archives*, **405**, 274–84.
112 Mulligan, M.R., O'Neill, R.J., Zei, P. & Tung, L. (1988). Graded effects of pulsed electric fields on contractility of single heart cells. *Proceedings of the 10th Annual Conference IEEE Engineering in Medicine and Biology Society*, pp. 902–3.
113 Geddes, L.A. & Bourland, J.D. (1989). Ability of the Lapicque and Blair strength–duration curves to fit experimentally obtained data from the dog heart. *IEEE Transactions on Biomedical Engineering*, **36(9)**, 971–4.
114 Mulligan, M.R. & Tung, L. (1989). Influence of electrical axis of stimulation on excitation of cardiac myocytes. *Circulation*, **80(4)**, II–532.

115 Tung, L., Sliz, N. & Mulligan, M.R. (1991). Influence of electrical axis of stimulation on excitation of cardiac muscle cells. Circulation Research, **69**, 722–30.

116 Pearce, J.A., Bourland, J.D., Neilsen, W., Geddes, L.A. & Voelz, M. (1982). Myocardial stimulation with ultrashort duration current pulses. *PACE*, **5**, 52–8.

117 Bardou, A.L., Degonde, J., Birkui, P.J. & Chesnais, J.M. (1988). Stimulation threshold of isolated myocytes and crossed shock defibrillation. *IEEE EMBS Conference Proceedings*, **10**, 961–2.

118 Fleckenstein, A., Janke, J., Doring, H.J. & Leder, O. (1974). Myocardial fiber necrosis due to intracellular Ca overload – a new principle in cardiac pathophysiology. *Recent Advances in Cardiac Structure and Metabolism*, **4**, 563–80.

119 Chapman, R.A. (1979). Excitation-contraction coupling in cardiac muscle. *Progress in Biophysics Molecular Biology*, **35**, 1–52.

120 Isenberg, G. and Wendt-Gallitelli, M.F. (1989). Cellular mechanisms of excitation contraction coupling. In *Isolated Adult Cardiomyocytes. Vol. II. Electrophysiological and Contractile Function*, Piper, H.M. & Isenberg, G. eds, Chap. 10, pp. 213–48, Boca Raton, Fl: CRC Press.

121 Tung, L. (1986). An ultrasensitive transducer for measurement of isometric contractile force from single heart cells. *Pflugers Archives*, **407**, 109–15.

122 Stuhmer, W., Roberts, W.M. & Almers, W. (1983). The loose patch clamp. In *Single-Channel Analysis*, B. Sakmann and E. Neher, eds, Chap. 8, pp. 123–32, New York: Plenum Press.

123 O'Neill, R.J. & Tung, L. (1989). The dynamic breakdown of heart cell membranes exposed to ramp increases in transmembrane potential. *Proceedings of the IEEE 11th Annual Conference Engineering in Medicine and Biology Society*, 1731–32.

124 O'Neill, R.J. & Tung, L. (1991). A cell-attached patch clamp study of the electropermeabilization of amphibian cardiac cells. *Biophysical Journal*, **59**, 1028–39.

125 Tsong, T.Y. (1983). Voltage modulation of membrane permeability and energy utilization in cells. *Bioscience Reports*, **3**, 487–505.

126 Zimmerman, U., Pilwat, G., Beckers, F. & Riemann, F. (1976). Effects of external electrical fields on cell membranes. *Bioelectrochemistry and Bioengineering*, **3**, 58–83.

127 Krassowska, W., Frazier, D.W., Pilkington, T.C. & Ideker, R.E. (1990). Potential distribution in three-dimensional periodic myocardium–Part II: application to extracellular stimulation. *IEEE Transactions on Biomedical Engineering*, **37**, 267–84.

128 Lindemans, F.W., Heethaar, R.M., Denier van der Gon, J.J. & Zimmerman, A.N.E. (1975). Site of initial excitation and current threshold as a function of electrode radius in heart muscle. *Cardiovascular Research*, **9**, 95–104.

129 Plonsey, R. & Barr, R.C. (1988). *Bioelectricity*, Chapter 2, New York: Plenum Press.

130 Plonsey, R. & Barr, R.C. (1987). Mathematical modeling of electrical activity of the heart. *Journal of Electrocardiology*, **20(3)**, 219–26.

131 Plonsey, R. & Barr, R.C. (1982). The four-electrode resistivity technique as applied to cardiac muscle. *IEEE Transactions on Biomedical Engineering*, **29**, 541–546.

132 Rush, S., Abildskov, J.A. & McFee, R. (1963). Resistivity of body

tissues at low frequencies. *Circulation Research*, **12**, 40–50.

133  Clerc (1976). Directional differences of impulse spread in trabecular muscle from mammalian heart. *Journal of Physiology*, **255**, 335–46.

134  Roberts, D.E., Hersh, L.T. & Scher, A.M. (1979). Influence of cardiac fiber orientation on wavefront voltage, conduction velocity and tissue resistivity in the dog. *Circulation Research*, **44**, 701–12.

135  Plonsey, R. (1989). The use of the bidomain model for the study of excitable media. *Lectures on Mathematics in the Life Sciences*, **21**, 123–49.

136  Henriquez, C.S., Trayanova, N. & Plonsey, R. (1990). A Planar slab bidomain model for cardiac tissue. *Annals of Biomedical Engineering*, **18**, 367–76.

137  Roth, B.J. & Wikswo, J.P. Jr. (1986). A bidomain model for the extracellular potential and magnetic field of cardiac tissue. *IEEE Transactions on Biomedical Engineering*, **33**, 467–9.

138  Tung, L. (1978). A bidomain model for describing ischemic myocardial D-C potentials. PhD dissertation, Dept. Elec. Eng., Massachusetts Institute of Technology, Cambridge, Massachusetts.

139  De Mello, W.C. (1982). Cell-to-cell communication in heart and other tissues. *Progress in Biophysics and Molecular Biology*, **39**, 117–82.

140  Sepulveda, N.G., Roth, B.J. & Wikswo, J.P. Jr. (1988). Finite element bidomain calculations. *Proceedings of the 10th Annual International Conference IEEE Engineering in Medicine and Biology Society*, p. 950–1.

141  Weidmann, S. (1970). Electrical constants of trabecular muscle from mammalian heart. *Journal of Physiology*, **210**, 1041–54.

142  Peskoff, A. (1979). Electric potential in three-dimensional electrically syncytial tissues. *Bulletin in Mathematical Biology*, **41**, 163–81.

143  Krassowska, W., Pilkington, T.C. & Ideker, R.E. (1990). Potential distribution in three-dimensional periodic myocardium – Part I: Solution with two-scale asymptotic analysis. *IEEE Transactions on Biomedical Engineering*, **37**, 252–66.

144  Plonsey, R. & Barr, R.C. (1986). Inclusion of junction elements in a linear cardiac model through secondary sources: application to defibrillation. *Medical and Biological Engineering and Computing*, **24**, 137–44.

145  Beeler, G.W. & Reuter, H. (1977). Reconstruction of the action potential of ventricular myocardial fibers. *Journal of Physiology*, **286**, 177–210.

146  Ebihara, L. & Johnson, E.A. (1980). Fast sodium current in cardiac muscle. A quantitative description. *Biophysical Journal*, **32**, 779–90.

147  Noble, D. & DiFrancesco, D. (1985). A model of cardiac electrical activity incorporating ionic pumps and concentration changes. *Philosophical Transactions Royal Society of London Series B*, **307**, 353–98.

148  Rudy, Y. & Quan, W. (1987). A model study of the effects of the discrete cellular structure on electrical propagation in cardiac tissue. *Circulation Research*, **61**, 815–23.

149  Spach, M.S., Dolber, P.C., Heidlage, J.F., Kootsey, J.M. & Johnson, E.A. (1987). Propagating depolarization in anisotropic human and canine cardiac muscle: apparent directional differences in membrane capacitance. *Circulation Reseach*, **60**, 206–19.

150 Jeltsch, E. & Zimmermann, U. (1979). Particles in a homogeneous electrical field: a model for the electrical breakdown of living cells in a Coulter counter. *Bioelectrochemistry and Bioenergetics*, **6**, 349–84.

151 Knosita, K. Jr. & Tsong, T.Y. (1977). Voltage-induced pore formation and hemolysis of human erythrocytes. *Biochimica et Biophysica Acta*, **471**, 227–42.

152 Kinosita, K. Jr. & Tsong, T.Y. (1979). Voltage-induced conductance in human erythrocyte membranes. *Biochimica Biophysica Acta*, **554**, 479–97.

153 Klee, M. & Plonsey, R. (1976). Stimulation of spheroidal cells – the role of cell shape. *IEEE Transactions on Biomedical Engineering*, **23(4)**, 347–54.

154 Gaylor, D.C., Prakah-Asante, K. & Lee, R.C. (1988). Significance of cell size and tissue structure in electrical trauma. *Journal of Theoretical Biology*, **133**, 223–37.

155 Veenstra, R.D. & DeHaan, R.L. (1988). Cardiac gap junction channel activity in embryonic chick ventricle cells. *American Journal of Physiology*, **254(1 Pt 2)**, H170–80.

156 Weingart, R. (1986). Electrical properties of the nexal membrane studied in rat ventricular cell pairs. *Journal of Physiology*, **370**, 267–84.

157 White, R.L., Spray, D.C., Campos de Carvalho, A.C., Wittenberg, B.A. & Bennett, M.V.L. (1985). Some electrical and pharmacological properties of gap junctions between adult ventricular myocytes. *American Journal of Physiology*, **249**, C447–55.

158 Wittenberg, B.A., White, R.L., Ginzberg, R.D. & Spray, D.C. (1986). Effect of calcium on the dissociation of the mature rat heart into individual and paired myocytes: electrical properties of cell pairs. *Circulation Research*, **59(2)**, 143–50.

159 Neumann, E., Sowers, A.E. & Jordan, C.A. (1989). *Electroporation and Electrofusion in Cell Biology*, New York: Plenum Press.

160 Zimmermann, U. (1982). Electric field-mediated fusion and related electrical phenomena. *Biochimica et Biophysica Acta*, **694**, 227–77.

161 Chernomordik, L.V., Sukharev, S.I., Popov, S.V., Pastushenko, V.F., Sokirko, A.V., Abidor, I.G. & Chizmadzhev, Y.A. (1987). The electrical breakdown of cell and lipid membranes: the similarity of phenomenologies. *Biochimica et Biophysica Acta*, **902**, 360–73.

162 Kinosita, K., Ashikawa, I., Saita, N., Yoshimura, H., Itoh, H., Nagayama, K. & Ikegami, A. (1988). Electroporation of cell membrane visualized under a pulsed-laser fluoresence microscope. *Biophysical Journal*, **53**, 1015–19.

163 Weaver, J.C., Harrison, G.I., Bliss, J.G., Mourant, J.R. & Powell, K.T. (1988). Electroporation: high frequency of occurrence of a transient high-permeability state in erythrocytes and intact yeast. *FEBS Letters*, **229**, 30–4.

164 Zimmermann, U., Scheurich, P. *et al.* (1981). Cells with manipulated functions: new perspectives for cell biology, medicine and technology. *Angewandte Chemic International Edition English*, **20**, 325–44.

165 Mehrle, W., Hampp, R. & Zimmermann, U. (1989). Electric pulse induced membrane permeabilisation. Spatial orientation and kinetics of solute efflux in freely suspended and dielectrophoretically aligned plant mesophyll protoplasts. *Biochimica et Biophysica Acta*, **978**, 267–75.

166 Glaser, R.W., Leikin, S.L., Chernomordik, L.V., Pastushenko, V.F. &

Sokirko, A.I. (1988). Reversible electrical breakdown of lipid bilayers: formation and evolution of pores. *Biochimica et Biophysica Acta*, **940**, 275–87.

167 Chernysh, A.M., Tabak, V.Y. & Bogushevich, M.S. (1988). Mechanisms of electrical defibrillation of the heart. *Resuscitation*, **16**, 169–78.

168 Benz, R. & Zimmermann, U. (1980). Relaxation studies on cell membranes and lipid bilayers in the high electric field range. *Bioelectrochemistry and Bioenergetics*, **7**, 723–39.

169 Needham, D. & Hochmuth, R.M. (1989). Electro-mechanical permeabilization of lipid vesicles: role of membrane tension and compressibility. *Biophysical Journal*, **55**, 1001–9.

170 Chang, D.C. & Reese, T.S. (1990). Changes in membrane structure induced by electroporation as revealed by rapid-freezing electron microscopy. *Biophysical Journal*, **58**, 1–12.

171 Tovar, O. & Tung, L. (1991). Electropermeabilization of cardiac cell membranes with monophasic or biphasic rectangular voltage pulses. *PACE*, **14** (4, pt.2), 667.

172 Berlin, J.R., Cannell, M.B. & Lederer, W.J. (1989). Cellular origins of the transient inward current in cardiac myocytes. *Circulation Research*, **65**, 115–26.

173 Nayler, W.G. (1981). The role of calcium in the ischemic myocardium. *American Journal of Pathology*, **102**, 262–70.

174 Chien, K.R., Pfau, R.G. & Farber, J.L. (1969). Ischemic myocardial cell injury, *American Journal of Pathology*, **97**, 505–30.

175 Balke, C.W., Lesh, M.D., Spear, J.F., Kadish, A., Levine, J.H. & Moore, E.N. (1988). Effects of cellular uncoupling on conduction in anisotropic canine ventricular myocardium. *Circulation Research*, **63**, 879–92.

176 Delmar, M., Michaels, D.C., Johnson, T. & Jalife, J. (1987). Effects of increasing intracellular resistance on transverse and longitudinal propagation in sheep epicardial muscle. *Circulation Research*, **60**, 780–5.

177 Spach, M.S., Kootsey, J.M. & Sloan, J.D. (1982). Active modulation of electrical coupling between cardiac cells of the dog: A mechanism for transient and steady state variation in conduction velocity. *Circulation Research*, **51**, 347–62.

178 Serpescu, E.H., Kinosita, K. & Tsong, T.Y. (1985). Reversible and irreversible modification of erythrocyte membrane permeability by electric field. *Biochimica et Biophysica Acta*, **812**, 779–85.

179 Tovar, O., O'Neill, R.J. & Tung. L. (1990). Membrane conductance of frog heart cells following electropermeabilization. *Proceedings of the International Conference on Electroporation and Electrofusion* (Woods Hole, Mass.), p. 27.

180 Hoffman, B.F., Cranefield, P.F., Lepeschkin, E., Surawicz, B. & Herrlich, H.H. (1959). Comparison of cardiac monophasic action potentials recorded by intracellular and suction electrodes. *American Journal of Physiology*, **196(6)**, 1297–301.

181 Sonnenblick, E.H. Myocardial ultrastructure in the normal and failing heart. In *The Myocardium: Failure & Infarction*, E. Braunwald, ed. Chap. 1, New York: HP Publishing Co.

# 19

# Skeletal muscle cell membrane electrical breakdown in electrical trauma

DIANE C. GAYLOR
DEEPAK L. BHATT
RAPHAEL C. LEE

## Introduction

Rhabdomyolysis is a characteristic clinical feature of electrical trauma. The release of large quantities of myoglobin into the intravascular space[1] and the frequent localization of technetium-99 in skeletal muscle[2] are common manifestations. It was this attribute of electrical trauma victims that caused several experienced clinicians to liken electrical trauma to the mechanical crush injury[3,4] in its clinical manifestations. More than a decade later, the pathogenic mechanisms responsible for rhabdomyolysis following electrical trauma have yet to be specifically identified by clinical studies. While heat generation by the passage of electrical current (joule heating) has commonly been believed to be the only mediator of tissue injury, over the past few decades considerable evidence has accrued suggesting that other nonthermal mechanisms may be important.

In many cases of electrical trauma, particularly when the duration of electrical contact is short, heating is predictably insignificant in some regions in the current path where skeletal muscle damage is common (see Chapter 14). This information has been the motivation to postulate that in these instances cell membrane rupture due to the induced transmembrane potential may be the important mechanism of cellular damage. This chapter describes the rationale for the hypothesis and details the results of experiments designed to test its validity.

For a given applied electric field, the magnitude of the induced transmembrane potential imposed by the field depends on the cell size and orientation in the field. In typical cases of electrical trauma, long skeletal muscle and nerve cells, oriented in the direction of the electric field, can experience transmembrane potentials large enough to lead to cell membrane rupture by electrical breakdown[5,6], a process often termed electroporation[7] or electropermeabilization[8].

## Membrane electrical breakdown

Cell membrane disruption by pure electrical stress is a well-documented phenomenon. Exposure of cells to brief intense electric field pulses has become a standard laboratory technique to produce cell fusion and to exchange genetic material between cells[8]. For artificial planar bilayer lipid membranes, rupture has been shown to occur when transmembrane potentials of 200–500 mV are applied for at least 100 $\mu$s[9,10]. A reversible electrical breakdown of both artificial and biological membranes has been shown to occur when transmembrane potentials exceeding 500 mV are applied for times of the order of nanoseconds to microseconds[8,11,12]. Permeabilization of rat skeletal muscle cells by induced transmembrane potentials has been demonstrated on the order of 500 mV applied for 4 ms[13]. Membrane electrical breakdown results in increased membrane permeability, which can lead to chemical imbalances in the cell. If not reversed, the effects can cause cell disfunction and death.

## Muscle impedance changes following electrical shock

In a study by Chilbert et al.[14], the relationship between tissue destruction and tissue resistivity was investigated. In these experiments, a current of 1 A at 60 Hz was passed between the hind legs of dogs until the temperature in the gracilis muscle reached 60°C. The changes in muscle resistivity correlated well with the severity of the damage inflicted by the applied current. Tissue exhibiting severe cellular disruption was shown to have a resistivity 70% lower than in controls. Tissue exhibiting minimal cellular damage had a resistivity 20–40% lower than in controls. This study demonstrated that a decline in the resistance to electrical current is a strong indicator of cellular disruption in electrical injury.

Field-induced changes have also been observed in muscle tissue impedance[15]. A drop in impedance has been demonstrated to occur following the application of short-duration, high-intensity electric field pulses to intact skeletal muscle explants in the absence of significant heating effects. Impedance of the muscle explant was determined using a chamber designed for two-port impedance measurements at 10 Hz. For field exposure, the explants were transferred to a separate chamber filled with a physiologic saline solution. Electric field pulses were applied which ranged from 30 to 120 V/cm to cover the range of expected tissue exposure in electrical accidents. The pulses ranged in duration from 0.5 to 10.0 ms, short enough to prevent significant joule heating. The impedance was measured within five minutes following the delivery of a total of 10, 30, and 60 pulses of a specified magnitude and duration. A decrease in impedance magnitude occurred following electric field pulses which exceeded threshold values of 60 V/cm in magnitude and 1.0 ms in duration. The field strength, pulse duration and number of pulses were all factors in determining the extent of the damage. The salient results are illustrated in Fig. 19.1. Control studies demonstrated that cell disruption was not mediated by excitation–contraction coupling. This study demonstrates the relevance of nonthermal damage mechanisms to electrical trauma.

## Induced transmembrane potential

### Electric field interaction with cells

Characteristically, at frequencies much lower than 1 MHz, mammalian cell membranes are highly resistive to electrical current passage compared with the intracellular and extracellular fluids. As a consequence, currents established in the extracellular space by such low-frequency fields are shielded from the cytoplasm by the electrically insulating cell membrane. This shielding leads to large induced transmembrane potentials in certain membrane regions. For a nonspherical cell, the maximum induced transmembrane potential depends on the cell's orientation with respect to the electric field. The largest potentials are reached when the major axis of the cell is parallel to the direction of the electric field. This results in large induced potentials in the ends of the cell.

Major electrical trauma frequently involves the upper extremity, setting up electrical current pathways as qualitatively described in Fig. 19.2. In such instances, the long axes of most skeletal muscle cells are oriented roughly parallel to the direction of the electric field lines. The potentials induced in the ends of these cells are significantly larger than those experienced by skeletal muscle cells in any other orientation or experienced by smaller cell types such as fibroblasts. Thus, skeletal muscle is expected to be particularly susceptible to damage by the mechanism of membrane electrical breakdown.

### Cable model analysis

To determine the induced transmembrane potential for the case of an elongated cell aligned parallel to an applied electric field, the traditional cable model approach[5] has been used. The cell membrane is treated as an

(a)

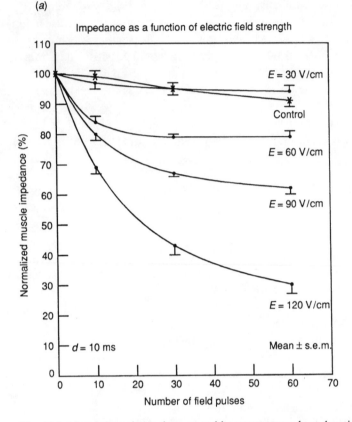

Fig. 19.1. Muscle impedance drop caused by exposure to short duration (*d*), high-intensity (*E*) electric field pulses. Pulses were separated by 10 seconds. Impedance measurements were normalized to the initial value before field pulses were applied. Each point represents the mean and standard error of the mean for five muscle samples.

electrically insulating cylindrical boundary separating two good electrical conductors, which represent the intracellular and extracellular fluids. The membrane as well as both the intracellular and extracellular fluids are assumed to be homogeneous and isotropic, and to have electrical properties that are independent of the applied fields until membrane breakdown. Electrical properties of the membrane are modelled by a series of parallel resistors and capacitors[16,17], as illustrated in Fig. 19.3. Longitudinal current in the membrane is ignored because the membrane has a negligible cross-sectional area. This lumped-parameter circuit model of the membrane is combined with the specified resistivities of the intracellular and

(b)

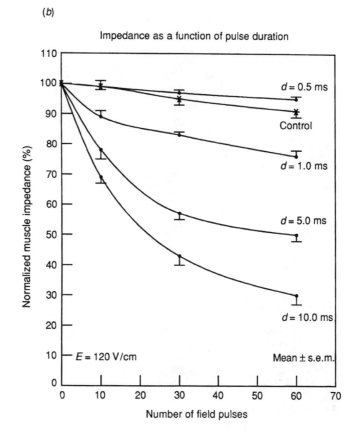

Impedance as a function of pulse duration

extracellular media to result in the cable circuit representation. In the presence of an applied uniform field $E(t)$ in the $\vec{z}$ direction, a transmembrane potential will be superimposed over the natural resting potential across the membrane. The cable equations are used to solve for the spatial distribution of the induced transmembrane potential. Because human skeletal muscle cells may have significant cross-sectional areas, this application of the cable model necessitates the use of a boundary condition which accounts for the transmembrane current through the ends of the cell. The induced transmembrane potential distribution will be solved for isolated muscle cells and then for cells within intact tissue.

Analysis of the circuit model leads to a differential equation for the induced transmembrane potential $v_m(z,t)$:

$$\lambda^2 \frac{\partial v_m(z,t)}{\partial z^2} = v_m(z,t) + \tau_m \frac{\partial v_m(z,t)}{\partial t}. \tag{1}$$

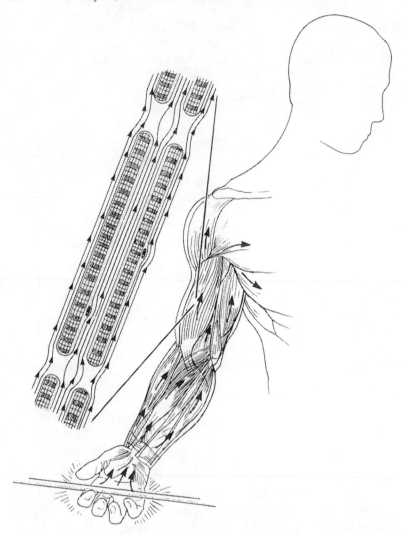

Fig. 19.2. Illustration of the current path through the upper extremity during electrical contact. Expanded view demonstrates electric field lines around muscle cells when the cells are near parallel to the major axis of the skeletal muscle cells.

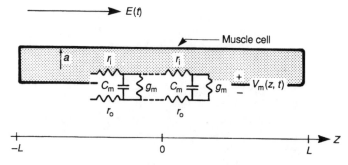

Fig. 19.3. Cable circuit model of a skeletal muscle cell aligned parallel to an applied electric field $E(t)$. $V_m(z,t)$ is the induced transmembrane potential superimposed over the natural resting potential. Cell length is $2L$; cell radius is $a$.

The space constant $\lambda$ and the time constant $\tau_m$ are given by

$$\lambda = \sqrt{\frac{1}{(r_i + r_o)g_m}}, \qquad \tau_m = \frac{c_m}{g_m}, \tag{2}$$

where $r_i$ and $r_o$ are the resistivities (ohm/cm) of the intracellular and extracellular fluids respectively, and $c_m$ and $g_m$ are the capacitance per unit length (F/cm) and the conductance per unit length (mhos/cm) of the membrane respectively. For the case of a single cell in an infinitely extending bath of extracellular fluid, $r_o$ is negligible compared to $r_i$ since the extracellular space is much greater than the intracellular space. However, when the effects of neighbouring cells are considered, this approximation is no longer valid.

For simplicity, the cable equation will be solved for the d.c. case. The analysis for powerline a.c. frequencies has been covered in Gaylor *et al*[5]. With $V_m(z)$ representing the d.c. induced transmembrane potential, the differential equation simplifies to

$$\lambda^2 \frac{d^2 V_m(z)}{dz^2} = V_m(z). \tag{3}$$

An appropriate solution is

$$V_m(z) = A \sinh(z/\lambda), \tag{4}$$

where $A$ is a constant to be determined from the boundary conditions. The boundary conditions constraining $V_m(z)$ can be determined from Kirchhoff's voltage law,

$$\frac{dV_m(z)}{dz} = -r_iI_i(z) + r_oI_o(z), \tag{5}$$

where $I_i(z)$ is the total current in the $\vec{z}$ direction inside the cell, and $I_o(z)$ is the total current in the $\vec{z}$ direction outside the cell.

At the ends of the cell ($z = \pm L$), charge conservation requires that the current through the membrane equal the current just inside the cell ($I_i(\pm L)$). If the conductance of the portion of the membrane which 'caps' the end of the cell is denoted by $G_e$ (in mhos),

$$I_i(\pm L) = \pm G_e V_m(\pm L). \tag{6}$$

It is assumed that the magnitude of the induced transmembrane potential is approximately constant over the entire ends of the cell at $|z| = L$. It is well known that electrical properties near the ends of skeletal muscle cells may differ substantially from the remainder of the cell's membrane[18]. This is generally attributed to the extensive membrane folds and invaginations which usually occur at the ends. Thus, it cannot be assumed that $G_e = \pi a^2 g_m$. Unfortunately, this difference has not been well characterized for most species.

### Isolated cell model

For the isolated cell case, it is assumed that $I_o(z)$ is much greater than $I_i(z)$ because the extracellular space is much larger than the intracellular space. Therefore, the product $r_oI_o(z)$ can be assumed to be approximately constant, leading to the condition

$$r_oI_o(z) \approx E_o. \tag{7}$$

The constant $A$ can be determined by substituting the boundary conditions (6) and (7) into Equation (5), and evaluating at $z = L$. Thus,

$$V_m(z) = \frac{\lambda E_o}{\cosh(L/\lambda)} \frac{\sinh(z/\lambda)}{1 + \lambda r_i G_e \tanh(L/\lambda)}. \tag{8}$$

This potential distribution is illustrated in Fig. 19.5. As shown, the induced transmembrane potential is greatest at the ends of the cell.

Examination of Equation (8) shows that for typical dimensions and electrical properties of human skeletal muscle cells, *the field in the membrane at the ends of the cells can be four to five orders of magnitude larger than the applied field*[5]. This induced transmembrane potential increases with an increase in cell length to a maximum value of $E_o\lambda$. The potential also increases with an increase in cell radius. Thus, large cells will have larger induced transmembrane potentials than smaller cells in the same field.

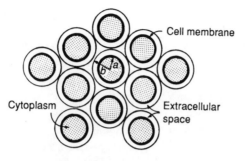

Fig. 19.4. Hexagonal array representation of a bundle of parallel skeletal muscle cells. Cell radius is $a$; extracellular fluid radius is $b$.

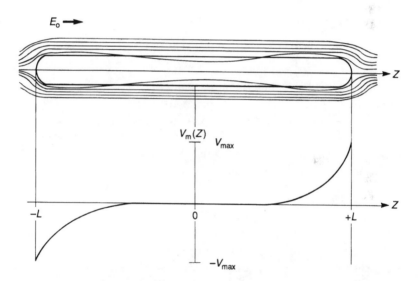

Fig. 19.5. Induced transmembrane potential distribution for an isolated elongated cell aligned parallel to an applied electric field $E_o$. The electric field and current in and around the cell are also pictured.

### Tissue model

For cells within intact tissue subjected to an electric field, the previous analysis can be modified to include the effects of neighbouring cells on the induced transmembrane potential. The cells are assumed to be ordered parallel to each other in a hexagonal array as illustrated in Fig. 19.4. To facilitate the comparison of induced transmembrane potential in tissue with the case of isolated cells, the quantity $V_c/2L$ is used as the 'source' term, where $V_c$ is the voltage drop across the full length of a cell. For the isolated cell case, $V_c/2L$ is equal to the applied field amplitude $E_o$.

In this tissue model, each cell is surrounded by a volume of extracellular fluid. By symmetry, no current crosses the boundary into the adjacent extracellular region. This conveniently isolates each cell from its neighbours for the purposes of the analysis. Here, the boundaries are modelled by cylinders of radius $b$ as indicated in Fig. 19.4. The cross-sectional area of extracellular space will determine the extracellular resistivity $r_o$. Generally, for cells that are not on the muscle surface, $r_o$ is not negligible compared to $r_i$ and significantly affects the value of the space constant in Equation (2). In addition, the extracellular electric field amplitude between muscle cells is not constant in $z$. Therefore, the approximation of Equation (7) is no longer valid. The induced transmembrane potential under these conditions has been derived in Gaylor *et al.*[5]:

$$V_m(z) = \frac{V_c}{2L} \left[ \frac{\lambda(r_o + r_i)/r_i}{\cosh(L/\lambda)} \right] \frac{\sinh(z/\lambda)}{1 + \lambda((r_i + r_o)G_e + r_o/(Lr_i))\tanh(L/\lambda)}. \quad (9)$$

Examination of Equation (9) shows that *the effect of surrounding cells is to increase the maximum transmembrane potential beyond that predicted for isolated cells* by Equation (8)[5]. With more resistance outside the cells (due to the smaller extracellular space), more current flows through the ends of the cells, resulting in the larger potential. The more closely packed the cells, the higher the induced potential.

### Charging time

Just as the voltage of a capacitor cannot change instantaneously, the transmembrane potential will not change instantaneously following a change in the applied electric field. As demonstrated by Cooper[19], a modal transient solution to the cable equation that is axisymmetric about $z = 0$ is

$$V_t(z,t) = \sum_{n=1}^{\infty} A_n \sin(a_n z/\lambda) e^{-(1+a_n^2)t/\tau_m}; \qquad a_n = \frac{n\pi\lambda}{2L} \quad (10)$$

Thus, the time-dependent terms decay with a time constant

$$\tau_n = \frac{\tau_m}{1 + \left(\frac{n\pi\lambda}{2L}\right)} \quad (11)$$

The time $\tau_1$ is the maximum time constant and is thus the time required for the cell to attain the transmembrane potential distribution predicted by the cable model analysis. For long cells, this time approaches $\tau_m$ (typically on the order of milliseconds), but decreases for cells of decreasing length. The charging time for skeletal muscle cells aligned perpendicular to the electric field and for smaller cell types such as fibroblasts is considerably less than $\tau_m$.

The fact that the charging time is on the order of milliseconds implies that, for a 60 Hz applied field, the cell may not charge to its maximum value during each excursion of the sinewave, since the duration of each excursion is about 8 ms and its magnitude is only above the r.m.s. value for 4 ms. This is reflected in the cable model solution for the sinusoidal steady state derived in Gaylor *et al.*[5]

### Imaging the induced transmembrane potential

The potentiometric dye di-4-ANEPPS has been used to measure optically induced transmembrane potentials in skeletal muscle cells[13]. This dye is taken up by cell membranes and undergoes a change in fluorescence intensity of approximately 8–10% per 100 millivolt change in transmembrane potential[20]. Di-4-ANEPPS is classified as a charge-shift dye since it undergoes a large charged shift upon excitation. The energy difference between the ground and excited states is therefore sensitive to an external electric field oriented in the direction of the shifting charge.

Rat skeletal muscle cells were harvested from adult female Sprague–Dawley rats[10,21,22]. The isolated muscle cells ranged between 500 and 1000 $\mu$m in length and between 15 and 30 $\mu$m in diameter. The characteristic striations and numerous nuclei were clearly visible, as illustrated in Fig. 19.6. The average fluorescence intensity change at the ends of cells exposed to a 5 V/cm field was measured to be $10.9 \pm 1.6\%$. This corresponds to an induced transmembrane potential of about 120 mV. This value can be compared to the cable model prediction of pp. 403–8. Nominal values for the membrane electrical properties of rat skeletal muscle cells in culture are $r_m = 1/g_m = 500$ $\Omega\text{cm}^2$ and $r_i = 100/(\pi a^2)$ $\Omega/\text{cm}$[10,21]. The cells used in the experiment had diameters ($2a$) of 15–30 $\mu$m and lengths ($2L$) of 500–1000 $\mu$m. Using these values, the expected maximum induced transmembrane potential ranged over 20 to 40 mV for each applied volt/cm. Thus, an applied field of about 5 V/cm is expected to induce a maximum potential in the range of 100–200 mV for these cells. This was in good agreement with the measured value, indicating that the cable model derived on pp. 403–8 provides a good estimate of the induced transmembrane potential for skeletal muscle cells aligned parallel to an applied electric field.

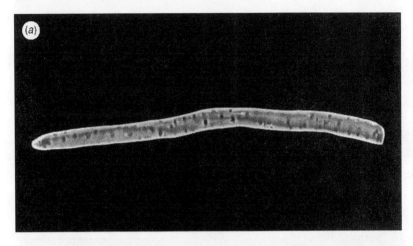

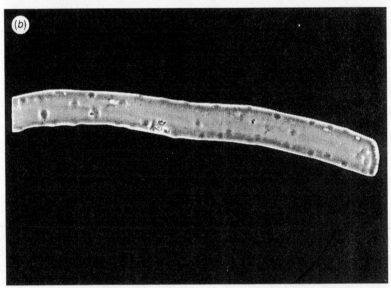

Fig. 19.6. Isolated rat skeletal muscle cell photographed using 10x and 40x phase contrast optics. Cells were typically 500 to 1000 $\mu$m in length and 15 to 30 $\mu$m in diameter. The characteristic striations and numerous nuclei are clearly visible. The two ends illustrate typical morphologies of skeletal muscle cell end regions.

## Electropermeabilization of the skeletal muscle cell membrane

The response of skeletal muscle cells to electrical stimuli[13] has been studied. The cytomorphological changes induced by intense electric field pulses were observed using cells bathed in physiological solution. The stimuli led to cell twitching and contraction. In separate experiments using cells paralysed in hypertonic solutions and loaded with the fluorescent dye carboxyfluorescein, induced changes in membrane diffusive permeability were observed and quantified. In this way, the thresholds for membrane damage due to membrane electrical breakdown were determined.

Rat skeletal muscle cells were used in these experiments, as described on pp. 411–12. Carboxyfluorescein diacetate was used to determine cell viability and to demonstrate and quantify changes in cell membrane permeability. This dye diffuses across cell membranes, where esterases of healthy cells cleave the dye molecules producing carboxyfluorescein. This is a negatively charged fluorescent molecule that does not diffuse readily across the cell membrane and thus accumulates in the cytoplasm. Only cells with cell membrane integrity will retain the dye.

In most experiments, a pulse duration of 4 ms was used. This value was chosen for its relevance to electrical injury. It is the time during which the voltage in a 60 Hz signal is above its r.m.s. value, occurring twice every cycle. Thus the 4 ms square pulse roughly models the 'pulses' of a sinusoidal signal.

### *Cytomorphological response*

Isolated skeletal muscle cells in isotonic solutions responded dramatically to the application of brief electric field pulses. Cells exhibited a strong twitch in response to all stimuli imposed (fields of 30–300 V for durations of 0.1–4.0 ms). This response was more pronounced for the stronger and longer duration pulses. Cells aligned perpendicular to the applied electric field exhibited a more forceful twitching response, in general, than those aligned parallel to the field.

In one set of experiments, a pulse of 1–4 ms duration and 100–300 V/cm magnitude was applied every 15 seconds until irreversible contraction occurred. A typical experiment is pictured in Fig. 19.7. In this case, a cell approximately 1 mm in length aligned perpendicular to the field was exposed to 1 ms, 300 volt/cm pulses. Irreversible contraction occurred after only one pulse (*b*). Several more pulses resulted in the total collapse of the cell (*c*),(*d*). Similar responses were observed in all other trials. The higher

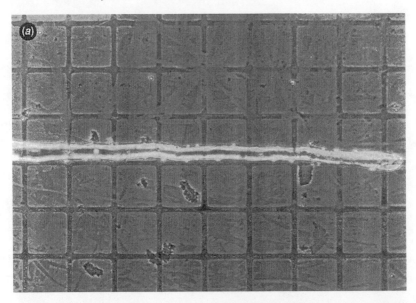

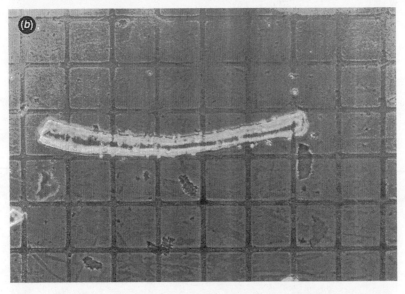

Fig. 19.7. Typical cytomorphological response to electric field pulses of 1–4 ms duration and 100–300 V/cm magnitude. In this series of photographs, the cell was exposed to a 1 ms, 300 V/cm pulse every 15 seconds. The cell was about 1 mm long (grid is 100 μm) and aligned perpendicular to the applied field (*a*). After a single pulse, an irreversible contraction occurred (*b*). Further pulses led to the eventual collapse of the cell along its long axis (*c*, *d*).

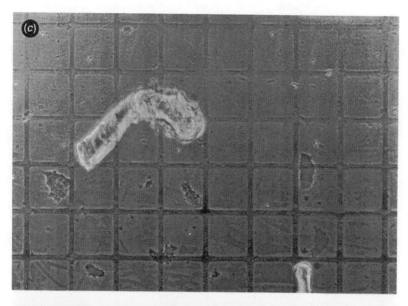

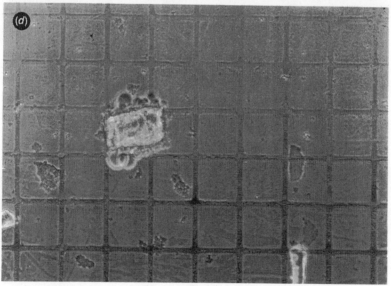

field strengths and pulse durations, in general, caused more rapid cell collapse.

The twitch response exhibited by cells in isotonic solutions was the natural cellular response to a membrane action potential. Apparently, the perpendicular field is more effective in producing a contraction in isolated cells. This observation is unexplained but may be a result of cellular structure. The T-tubules are themselves perpendicular to the long axis of the cell. These small channels transmit electrical signals to the inside of the cell, causing the release of calcium from the sarcoplasmic reticulum and triggering the contractile response. When the cells were perpendicular to the field, the current could flow through the T-tubules from one side to the other. When the cells were parallel to the field, the current in the T-tubules must have been zero along the centre axis of the cell. Thus, the contractile mechanism received a stronger electrical stimulus when the cell was perpendicular to the field, leading to a more dramatic response. The increased response may also have to do with the longer charging time of parallel cells compared to perpendicular cells.

The irreversible contraction that occurred indicated damage to the excitation–contraction coupling mechanism or to the contractile apparatus itself. The total collapse of the cell can be explained only by a breakdown of the contractile proteins, since the intact structure can only contract by about 32%[23]. It is well known that actin and myosin filaments are very sensitive to their environments and that small changes in pH or ion concentration cause their breakdown into globular form[24-26]. These changes are expected following membrane disruption.

It appeared that the cell membrane remained largely intact, but significantly permeabilized, following pulsed electric field applications and resultant cell collapse. In experiments performed with cells loaded with carboxyfluorescein in isotonic solution, no obvious dye leakage was observed, even following the collapse of the cells. However, in most cases, the overall cell fluorescence intensity appeared to the eye to decrease at a rate beyond that due to bleaching, indicating an increase in the membrane permeability to the dye molecules. Quantification of the dye leakage using this protocol was not possible due to the movements of the cells. The next section describes experiments where quantification of the rate of dye leakage was possible. It is important to note that the volume of the cell in Fig. 19.7 following its collapse is roughly the same as it was before the collapse. The length was reduced by a factor of about 6.5, but the radius was increased by a factor of about 2.5. Modelling the cell as a cylinder, the volume is proportional to the length and to the square of the radius. Thus, the volumes are approximately the same. It appears that no cytoplasm was lost in the process.

### Membrane permeability changes

In order to quantify changes in membrane permeability using fluorescent dyes, it was necessary that the cells remained absolutely stationary during the protocols. It has been shown that contractility can be completely blocked by exposure to solutions of tonicity made two to three times normal by the addition of solutes unable to penetrate the cell membrane[27,28]. Membrane properties such as the transmembrane potential are not significantly affected. Thus, for use in the following experiments, the tonicity of phosphate buffered saline (PBS) was made 3.0 times normal with either sucrose or mannitol.

The experiments performed with cells loaded with carboxyfluorescein in hypertonic solutions were designed initially to provide visual evidence of membrane disruption by making evident sites of dye leakage. However, at no time was such obvious leakage detected, indicating that the effect of the field was to permeabilize but not to grossly rupture the cell membrane. Membrane permeability changes were observed as an increased rate of dye loss from cells in hypertonic solutions. As will be seen, the induced transmembrane potential required to produce these changes is in the range known to cause membrane electrical breakdown.

The experiments demonstrating electrical breakdown were performed using cells aligned perpendicular to the applied field. Experimental conditions prohibited observation of increased permeability states induced in cells aligned parallel to the field. The hypertonic solution used to paralyse the skeletal muscle cells caused the removal of some water from the cells. It was demonstrated, using the potentiometric dye di-4-ANEPPS (see pp. 411–12), that the water loss appeared to alter the internal structure of the cells, blocking the current flow along the long axes of the cells. Cells in isotonic solution exhibited induced transmembrane potentials roughly as predicted by the cable model analysis of pp. 403–8. However, this response was nearly eliminated for cells in hypertonic solutions of 3.0-times normal tonicity[13]. The changes in the internal structure of the cells that led to these problems probably have to do with the membranes of the T-tubules and the sarcoplasmic reticulum which exist at each sarcomere. The loss of water may cause some overlap or bunching of the membranes leading to the blockages. One need not assume that this occurs at every sarcomere to explain the observations, but it must occur frequently along the cell. This is not expected to affect the results significantly when the cells are aligned perpendicular to the field because the membrane blockages are in this case parallel to the electric field, and current flow will not be appreciably altered.

Cells exposed to 20 4 ms 300 V/cm pulses spaced at 15 s lost all or nearly all fluorescence intensity in the 15 minutes following the exposure if aligned perpendicular to the applied electric field, but appeared unchanged if aligned parallel. Cells exposed to 250 V/cm pulses and aligned perpendicular to the field exhibited evidence of slow dye leakage. Large fluorescence intensity losses were usually not noticed until 30 min after exposure. It could take an hour or longer for cells to lose all intensity. When cells were exposed to 200 V/cm pulses, only slight differences between the fluorescence intensities of perpendicular and parallel cells were noted 1 hour after exposure. Cells exposed to 150 V/cm pulses showed no obvious intensity loss beyond that which occurred in cells of both alignments due to natural leakage and bleaching.

The induced changes in membrane permeability following electric field exposure were quantified for applied fields of 250, 272, and 300 V/cm. All cells were aligned perpendicular to the field. Using image processing techniques, average cell intensity as a function of time was plotted. To facilitate comparison of the responses, each intensity value in a given trial was normalized to the intensity value recorded immediately before pulse application began and the normalized plots were averaged. The results are shown in Fig. 19.8. Fluorescence intensity loss in cells occurred before the pulse application due to the combined effects of natural dye leakage and bleaching. These effects were removed from the data by subtracting the initial rate of dye loss. The results are shown in Fig. 19.8. In this figure, the fluorescence intensity drop is due solely to the effects of the electric field pulses.

The maximum induced transmembrane potential in a cell aligned perpendicular to an applied electric field $E_0$ is approximately $E_0 d$, where $d$ is the cell diameter[13]. The diameters of the cells in hypertonic solution were in the range of 15–20 $\mu$m. For this range, the predicted induced potential for an application of 250–300 V/cm is approximately 400–600 millivolts. These potentials are in the range known to cause membrane electrical breakdown for pulse widths on the order of milliseconds and a temperature of about 25°C[18]. For shorter pulse widths and/or lower temperatures, the critical potential is expected to be higher. However, for the physiological temperature 37 °C, the critical potential is expected to be lower.

The experiments were performed at room temperature. The temperature rise in the chamber due to the electric field pulses was never more than 5 °C.

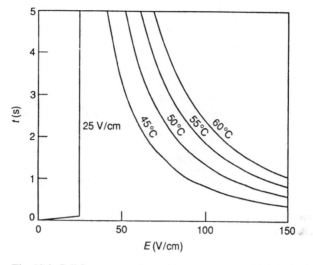

Fig. 19.8. Cell fluorescence intensity as a function of time for cells exposed to twenty 4 ms electric field pulses of the indicated magnitude between the 10 and 15 min marks. The effects of natural dye leakage and bleaching have been subtracted off. Thus, the intensity drop is due solely to the effects of the electric field pulses.

Thus, the chamber temperature never exceeded the physiological temperature of 37 °C, and thermal damage could not have contributed to the permeability changes measured.

As illustrated in Fig. 19.8, the damage incurred by the cells due to the field exposure appears to be at least partially reversible. For a field application of 300 V/cm, a complete reversal seems to occur during a 5 min period following the exposure. This effect may be due partially to non-linearities of the imaging system, as the cell intensities were significantly lower 5 min after the exposure than they were at the start. It is also likely that the cell exposure to the hypertonic solution caused some dye to become trapped in the internal membrane system due to water removal. In this case, the cell intensity cannot be expected to go to zero, and irreversible damage could lead to the results illustrated in Fig. 19.8. However, the fact that the slope began to reverse almost immediately after the exposure was completed is evidence that at least a partial reversal of the permeability increase occurred. The trials using 250 and 275 V/cm showed less evidence that a small, but steady, dye loss could proceed for as long as an hour after exposure.

Reversible electric breakdown of artificial planar bilayer–lipid membranes has been shown to occur at higher potentials than those causing irreversible breakdown[11]. The proposed reason for this is that, when higher voltages are applied, the membrane quickly breaks down and discharges, analogous to the breakdown of a capacitor. This quick phenomenon (thought to last on the order of nanoseconds) appears to cause no lasting damage to the membrane. However, lower induced potentials lead to a slower discharge, and more permanent damage to the membrane.

### Conclusions

This final section will examine the relevance of the experimental results to electrical injury. It will be assumed that the threshold determined using cells perpendicular to the applied field holds generally. That is, membrane electrical breakdown occurs for the skeletal muscle cell membrane whenever and wherever potentials of the order of $\frac{1}{2}$ volt are induced. This results in a state of increased membrane permeability which, if not promptly reversed, can lead to chemical imbalances in the cells.

Cell membrane disruption can also be caused by exposure to supraphysiological temperatures[29-32]. The kinetics of the two processes are quite different. Membrane rupture caused by temperatures of 45 °C to 60 °C occurs over minutes while rupture by electrical breakdown can occur in less than 100 $\mu$s. Thus, membrane electrical breakdown may occur long before joule heating becomes significant. These separate processes may also act synergistically; heating appears to increase the probability of membrane electrical breakdown[33].

In order to determine the applied electric field strength that puts a muscle tissue at risk of membrane electrical breakdown, the induced transmembrane potential, as a function of field strength, must be known. The cable model analysis of pp. 403–8 provides this relationship for cells aligned parallel to the applied electric field. The induced potential is largely dependent on the cell length and radius. For the isolated skeletal muscle cells used in the experiments, an applied field of only 10–25 volts/cm could lead to an induced transmembrane potential of $\frac{1}{2}$ volt in the ends of cells aligned parallel to the electric field. As shown in pp. 403–8, cells in intact muscle experience larger induced transmembrane potentials than isolated cells for a given applied field, so the required applied field for membrane electrical breakdown may be significantly less than this amount. For larger human skeletal muscle cells, which can reach lengths of 10 cm[23], the value should be lower still. Nevertheless, for the purposes of the following discussion, the critical electric field will be assumed to be 25 volts/cm. As

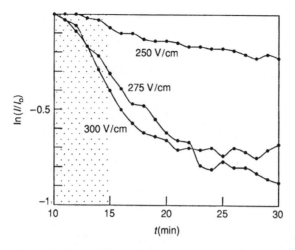

Fig. 19.9. Electric field strength and contact duration required for cellular damage by thermal and electrical mechanisms. Membrane electrical breakdown will occur for fields above 25 V/cm for any realistic contact duration. For large fields or long contact durations, thermally mediated damage will mask this effect, as indicated by the temperature curves. Thus, membrane electrical breakdown is important at low field strengths and short contact durations.

will be seen, the value is low compared to the fields generally required to produce significant heating with contact durations of interest, so a more precise value is not required for the comparison of the two mechanisms.

The heating expected to occur in muscle tissue experiencing a given field strength $E$ for a given period of time $t$ can be easily computed using

$$\Delta T = \frac{\sigma E^2 t}{\rho \Theta} \tag{12}$$

where $\sigma$ is the conductivity of the muscle, $E$ is the applied electric field, $t$ is the time of exposure, $\rho$ is the density of the muscle, and $\Theta$ is the specific heat of the muscle. Muscle tissue has a conductivity $\sigma$ of approximately $4 \times 10^{-3}$ mhos/cm and a product $\rho\theta$ of approximately 4.14 J/gm/°C[12]. Thus, the temperature rise in °C is about $E^2 T/1000$. This equation is plotted for temperature rises from 37 °C to 45 °C, 50 °C, 55 °C, and 60 °C in Fig. 19.9. The effects of these elevated temperatures on skeletal muscle cell membranes are examined in Chapter 15.

As shown in Fig. 19.9, *there is a large range of exposures having short duration and/or low intensity that can lead to membrane electrical breakdown but not to thermally mediated damage.* Typical electrical injury exposures will now be examined in order to demonstrate the relevance of this region.

According to an Edison Electric Institute 1984 report, the most common nonfatal high-voltage electrical injury experienced by electrical utility workers results from contact with a 6000–10 000 volt electric powerline. The current entry and exit sites on the body determine the strength of the electric field experienced by the tissues. A hand-to-hand contact between the line voltage and ground would lead to an average field in the arms of about 60–100 V/cm, assuming an arm length of 0.5 m. Hand-to-foot contact would lead to a similar average field in the arm, but a lower average field in the leg due to its greater length and width. Contacts separated by shorter distances can lead to much higher electrical field strengths in the tissue. Thus, in most cases of high-voltage electrical injury, the fields in the muscle tissues are great enough to cause membrane electrical breakdown.

It is interesting to compare these 'high-voltage' exposures to the 'low-voltage exposure' of a child sucking on a household extension cord. In the latter case, 120 volts is dropped across about 1 cm, setting up an electric field larger than that occurring in many cases of high-voltage electrical injury. Since it is the field strength that determines the extent of heating and membrane electrical breakdown, it is clear that the classification of injuries into 'high-voltage' and 'low-voltage' has little relevance clinically.

The duration of voltage contact in most cases of electrical injury is not known. High-voltage injuries often occur without physical contact with the voltage line since arcing through the air can establish the current flow. In these cases, the victim is quickly thrown away from the line and the contact may last only a fraction of a second. In the other extreme, victims grasping a dead line will usually find themselves unable to let go when the line is energized due to muscular contractions. In this case, the contact may last for a few seconds longer. Long contacts also can occur when victims fall on a line or a line falls on them and the victim can not easily escape. As illustrated in Fig. 19.9, for long contact durations, occurrence of membrane electrical breakdown will be masked by thermally mediated damage. However, for short contact durations, membrane electrical breakdown may be the primary mechanism of cellular damage.

The occurrence of membrane electrical breakdown may explain the clinically observed 'progressive' necrosis of muscle tissues. Damage caused by this mechanism may be initially unrecognized since the tissues will not appear to be burned. The chemical imbalances in the cytoplasm which result from the electropermeabilization may lead to a slower rate of cell death than that caused by protein denaturation and other thermal effects, particularly if the permeabilization is reversed following the exposure. By recognizing this, appropriate therapeutic treatments may help salvage tissues which are currently lost.

In summary, it has been demonstrated that electrical injury is more complicated than was previously thought. As shown, heating of tissues cannot account for all of the damage observed clinically in typical cases. The patterns of damage that occur can only be explained when the two mechanisms of joule heating and membrane electrical breakdown are considered.

### References

1 Baxter, C.R. (1970). Present concepts in the management of major electrical injury. *Surgery Clinics of North America*, **50**, 1401–18.

2 Hunt, J.L., Sato, R.M. & Baxter, C.R. (1980). Acute electric burns: current diagnostic and therapeutic approaches to management. *Archives of Surgery*, **115**, 434–8.

3 Artz, C.P. (1974). Changing concepts in electrical injury. *American Journal of Surgery*, **128**, 600–2.

4 Rouse, R.G. & Dimick, A.R. (1978). The treatment of electrical injury compared to burn injury: a review of pathophysiology and comparison of patient management protocols. *Journal of Trauma*, **18**, 43–7.

5 Gaylor, D.C., Prakah-Asante, K. & Lee, R.C. (1988). Significance of cell size and tissue structure in electrical trauma. *Journal of Theoretical Biology*, **133**, 223–37.

6 Lee, R.C. & Kolodney, M.S. (1987). Electrical injury mechanisms: electrical breakdown of cell membranes. *Plastic and Reconstructive Surgery*, **80**, 672–9.

7 Powell, K.T. & Weaver, J.C. (1986). Transient aqueous pores in bilayer membranes: a statistical theory. *Bioelectrochemistry and Bioenergetics*, **15**, 211–27.

8 Zimmermann, U. (1986). Electrical breakdown: electropermeabilization & electrofusion. *Reviews of Physiology, Biochemistry and Pharmacology*, **105**, 176–256.

9 Abidor, I.G., Arakelyan, V.B., Chernomordik, L.V., Chizmadzhev, Yu A., Pastushenko, V.F. & Tarasevich, M.R. (1970). Electric breakdown of bilayer lipid membranes I: the main experimental facts and their qualitative discussion. *Bioelectrochemistry and Bioenergetics*, **6**, 37–52.

10 Bekoff, A. & Betz, W.J. (1977). Physiological properties of dissociated muscle fibers obtained from innervate and denervated adult rat muscle. *Journal of Physiology*, **271**, 25–40.

11 Benz, R., Bechers, F. & Zimmermann, U. (1979). Reversible electrical breakdown of lipid bilayer membranes: a charge-pulse relaxation study. *Journal of Membrane Biology*, **48**, 181–204.

12 Zimmermann, U., Scheurich, P., Pilwat, G. & Benz, R. (1981). Cells with manipulated functions: new perspectives for cells biology, medicine and technology. *Angewandte Chemie International Edition English*, **20**, 325–44.

13 Gaylor, D.C. (1989). Physical Mechanisms of Cellular Injury in Electrical Trauma. PhD thesis, Massachusetts Institute of Technology.

14 Chilbert, M., Maiman, D., Scances, A. Jr, Myklebust, J., Prieto, T.E.,

Swionek, T., Heckman, M. & Pintar, K. (1985). Measure of tissue resistivity in experimental electrical burns. *Journal of Trauma*, **25**, 209–15.

15  Bhatt, D.L., Gaylor, D.C. & Lee, R.C. (1990). Rhabdomyolysis due to pulsed electric fields. *Plastic and Reconstructive Surgery*, in press.

16  Adrian, R.H. (1983). Electrical properties of striated muscle. In *Handbook of Physiology, Section 10: Skeletal Muscle*, pp. 275–300, Bethesda, Maryland: American Physiological Society.

17  Jack, J.J.B., Noble, D. & Tsien, R.W. (1975). *Electric Current Flow in Excitable Cells*, London: Oxford University Press.

18  Milton, R.L., Mathias, R.T. & Eisenberg, R.S. (1985). Electrical properties of the myotendon region of frog twitch muscle fibers measured in the frequency domain. *Biophysical Journal*, **48**, 253–67.

19  Cooper, M.S. (1986). Electrical cable theory, transmembrane ion fluxes, and the motile responses of tissue cells to external electrical fields. In *Bioelectric Interactions Symp. IEEE/Engineering in Medicine and Biology Society, 7th Annual Conference*, Chicago, Illinois.

20  Gross, D. & Loew, L.L. (1989). *Fluorescent indicators of membrane potential: Microspectrofluorometry and imaging*, volume 30, chap. 7, pp. 193–218, San Diego: Academic Press.

21  Bekoff, A. & Betz, W.J. (1977). Properties of isolated adult rat muscle fibers maintained in tissue culture. *Journal of Physiology*, **271**, 537–47.

22  Bischoff, R. (1986). Proliferation of muscle satellite cells on intact myofibers in culture. *Developmental Biology*, **115**, 129–39.

23  Mannherz, H.G. & Holmes, K.C. (1982). *Biomechanics*, chap. 14, pp. 566–640, Berlin: Springer-Verlag.

24  Laki, K., (ed.) (1971). *Contractile Proteins and Muscle*. New York: Marcel Dekker, Inc.

25  Lapanje, S. (1978). *Physiochemical Aspects of Protein Denaturation*. New York: John Wiley & Sons.

26  Tonomura, Y. (1973). *Muscle Proteins, Muscle Contraction, and Cation Transport*. Baltimore, University Park Press.

27  Caputo, C. (1983). Pharmacological investigations of excitation-contraction coupling. In *Handbook of Physiology, Section 10: Skeletal Muscle*, pp. 381–415, Bethesda, Maryland, American Physiological Society.

28  Eisenberg, R.S. (1983). Impedance measurements of the electrical structure of skeletal muscle. In *Handbook of Physiology, Section 10: Skeletal Muscle*, pp. 301–23, Bethesda, Maryland, American Physiological Society.

29  Gershfeld, N.L. & Murayama, (1988). Thermal instability of red blood cell membrane bilayers: temperature dependence of hemolysis. *Journal of Membrane Biology*, **101**, 67–72.

30  Mixter, G. Jr, Delhery, G.P., Derksen, W.L. & Monahan, T.I. (1963). The influence of time on the death of HeLa cells at elevated temperatures. In *Temperature: Its Measurement and Control in Science and Industry*, Hardy, J.D., ed., New York Reinhold.

31  Moussa, N.A., McGrath, J.J., Cravalho, E.G. & Asimacopoulos, P.J. (1977). Kinetics of thermal injury in cells. *ASME Journal of Biomechanical Engineering*, **99**, 155–9.

32  Moussa, N.A., Tell, E.N. & Cravalho, E.G. (1979). Time progression of hemolysis of erythrocyte populations exposed to supraphysiological

temperatures. *ASME Journal of Biomechanical Engineering*, **101**, 213–17.

33 Tropea, B.I. (1987). A numerical model for determining the human forearm thermal response to high voltage injury. SB Thesis, Massachusetts Institute of Technology.

# 20

# Theory of nonlinear conduction in cell membranes under strong electric fields

RAPHAEL C. LEE
KWASI PRAKAH-ASANTE

### Introduction

Many of the immediate clinical signs of electrical injury relate to neuromuscular damage. Intense muscular spasm and rigour are often described by witnesses and are frequently observed on admission to the hospital. These observations in addition to the release of myoglobin into the circulation suggest that muscle cell membranes are often ruptured by electrical trauma.

Bilayer–lipid membranes comprise 60% of cell membranes. When bilayer–lipid membranes are exposed to electric fields, their electrical conductivity and diffusive permeability increase. This process has been termed electroporation. The theory of electroporation assumes that thermally driven molecular defects or pores transiently form in bilayer–lipid membranes. These pores explain the ability of large molecules like glucose to permeate. When strong enough electric fields are imposed in the bilayer, the pores enlarge. If the pores become large enough, then the membrane ruptures.

Depending on the make-up of the membrane, the threshold transmembrane potential required to cause membrane rupture by electroporation ranges in amplitude from 300 mV to 500 mV and is 100 $\mu$s or more in duration[1,2,3]. The resultant increase in transport allows substances which cannot normally permeate the membrane (e.g. DNA), to cross. Even localized rupture may spontaneously reseal. Electroporation can, therefore, be used for sequestering proteins, DNA, and various drugs into cells[4]. During application of the voltage pulses, if the membranes of neighbouring cells are close enough, they may fuse to form a hybrid cell.

Because the membrane defects fill with water, determining the defect size is important in modelling the electrical properties of the membrane. To gain physical insight into this process, this work aims to develop a quantitative model of the conductivity of a planar bilayer membrane with a transmembrane potential imposed by a d.c. voltage source. Using the steady-state solution of Weaver's[2,3,7] statistical model of pore size distribution and the solution of Jordan's[10] model for the conductivity of an electrolyte-filled pore, the relationship between bilayer–lipid membrane conductivity and transmembrane potential is calculated.

## Distribution of pores in bilayer–lipid membranes

The statistical theory of electroporation describes the pore size distribution to be a function of the transmembrane potential[3,5,6,7] (see Fig. 20.1). For simplicity, and due to lack of detailed information about the geometry of pores, they are assumed to be cylindrical. Consider a flat, rectangular patch of bilayer–lipid membrane of thickness $\delta$ surrounded on both sides with physiologic solutions. When a pore, of radius $r$, is formed in the membrane, an area equal to $\pi r^2$ is removed from each membrane surface, and a surface of area $2\pi r\delta$ is formed within the cylindrical pore. Let $\Gamma$ be the bifacial energy per area of membrane in contact with the surrounding water.

Since the lipid molecules along the edge of a pore are squeezed closer together than those in the bulk of the membrane, extra energy is required to form an edge. Let $\kappa$ be the energy required to form a unit length of pore edge. $\nabla \xi_m(r)$, the total mechanical energy required to form a pore of radius $r$, is then given by:

$$\nabla \xi_m(r) = 2\pi r\gamma - \pi r^2 \Gamma \tag{1}$$

and

$$\gamma = \kappa + \frac{\delta\Gamma}{2} \tag{2}$$

and $\gamma$ is the total mechanical energy stored per unit length of pore edge.

With a transmembrane potential, $V_m$, across the membrane, there is a decrease in electrical energy when a pore is formed. This is because the electrolyte which fills the pore has a higher dielectric permittivity, $\epsilon_\omega$, than that of the bulk bilayer–lipid membrane, $\epsilon_m$. The decrease in electrical energy, $\nabla \xi_e(r, V_m)$, is given by:

$$\nabla \xi_e(r, V_m) = \pi r^2 a V_m^2 \tag{3}$$

where

$$a = \frac{\epsilon_\omega - \epsilon_m}{2}\delta$$

Density of pores vs. radius

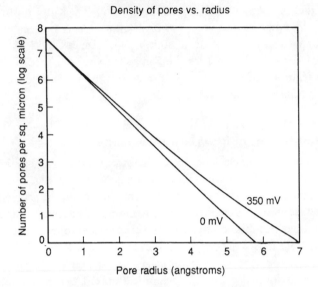

Fig. 20.1. Energy required for a pore with a radius $r$, to form a bilayer–lipid membrane.

Therefore, $\nabla \xi_e(r, V_m)$, the total increase in energy due to the formation of a pore of radius $r$ in the bilayer–lipid membrane, is

$$\nabla \xi(r, V_m) = 2\pi r\gamma - \pi r^2 (\Gamma + aV_m^2) \qquad (4)$$

The bigger the value of $\nabla \xi(r, V_m)$, the higher the energy barrier preventing the formation of pores, and, therefore, the less probable it is for pores of radius $r$ to be formed in the membrane. The radius for the peak value of $\nabla \xi(r, V_m)$ is defined as the critical radius, $r_c(V_m)$. For radii less than $r_c(V_m)$, the energy barrier increases with pore radius, and, therefore, small pores are more likely to be formed than bigger pores. When the transmembrane potential, $V_m$, increases, $\nabla \xi(r, V_m)$ decreases, and it becomes more probable for more pores of bigger radii to be formed in the membrane. Pores of radii bigger than $r_c(V_m)$ spontaneously increase in size and cause the membrane to rupture.

In the steady state, the distribution of pores in a patch of membrane is given by:

$$n(r, V_m) = n(o, o) \exp[-\beta \varDelta \xi 1 r, V_m)] \qquad (5)$$

with $n(r, V_m)\mathrm{d}r$ = the number of pores with radius between $r$ and $r + \mathrm{d}r$ of the membrane, and

$$\beta = 1/KT \tag{6}$$

$\rho(r,V_m)dr$, the number of pores with radius between $r$ and $r + dr$ per unit area, is obtained by normalizing $n(r,V_m)$ to $A_m$, the membrane area:

$$\rho(r,V_m) = \frac{n(o,o)}{A_m}\exp[-\beta\Delta\xi(r,V_m)] \tag{7}$$

## A continuum model of bilayer–lipid membrane conductivity

By considering the pores of different radii in the membrane as electrically in parallel, and assuming no conduction through the unperforated portions of the membrane, the average conductivity of a patch of bilayer–lipid membrane is estimated as a function of transmembrane potential. As the transmembrane potential increases, the numbers and sizes of pores increase and the membrane conductivity increases. The predicted membrane conductivity at zero transmembrane potential is compared with measurements to refine electroporation theory by determining the constant $\rho(o,o)$ (Fig. 20.2).

## Conductivity of a single pore in a bilayer–lipid membrane

Conduction of electrical current through a single pore of radius $r$ for a transmembrane potential $V_m$ (Fig. 20.2). is estimated from three resistances in series:

1 Resistance to current flow from the bulk solution to the pore entrance, $R_1(r)$.
2 Resistance to current flow through the pore channel, $R_2(r,V_m)$.
3 Resistance to current flow from the pore exit to the bulk solution, $R_3(r)$.

The entrance and exit resistance is equivalent to the resistance of current flow into a perfectly conducting disc on the surface of an insulating sheet which has been shown to be[8]:

$$R_1(r) = \frac{1}{4\sigma_o r} = R_3(r) \tag{8}$$

where, $\sigma_o$ is the conductivity of the surrounding physiological solution. Since the conductivity of intracellular fluid is approximately equal to that of the surrounding physiological solution, $R_1(r)$ is approximately equal to $R_3(r)$. $R_2(r,V_m)$ is estimated using Eyring rate theory with the primary

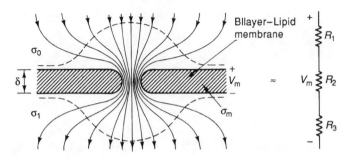

Fig. 20.2. Current through a pore in a bilayer–lipid membrane.

energy barrier being the Born energy for ion transport through a pore in a pure bilayer–lipid membrane[9].

### Estimation of the Born energy

An estimate of the Born energy barrier, $E_B(r)$, for an ion of charge, $zq$, to cross a lipid membrane of dielectric permittivity, $\epsilon_m$, through an aqueous pore with radius, $r$, is much smaller than its length, has been computed by Jordan[10] for a cylindrical pore of radius, $r$, and length, $\delta$. The maximum energy barrier to ion flow through the pore, $E_B(r)$, is given by

$$E_B(r) = \frac{z^2 q^2}{2\epsilon_w r} \Phi\left(\frac{\delta}{2r}\right) \qquad (9)$$

where $\dfrac{zq}{2\epsilon_w r}\Phi\left(\dfrac{\delta}{2r}\right)$ is the image potential for an ion at the centre of the pore.

$q$ is the charge of an electron.

$\epsilon_w$ is the dielectric permittivity of water ($\sim 80\ \epsilon_0$).

Equation (9) is plotted as a function of $r$ in Figure 20.3.

From Jordan[10] when $r > \dfrac{\delta}{32}$, $\Phi\left(\dfrac{\delta}{2r}\right)$ is well approximated by

$$\Phi\left(\frac{\delta}{2r}\right) = \Phi_\infty\left(\frac{\epsilon_m}{\epsilon_w}\right)\left[1 - \exp\left(-\frac{b\delta}{2r}\right)\right] \qquad (10)$$

where $\Phi_\infty\left(\dfrac{\epsilon_m}{\epsilon_w}\right)$ is the image potential due to an ion in an infinite pore.

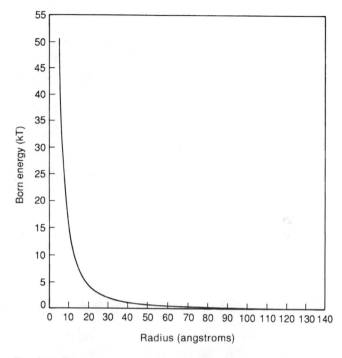

Fig. 20.3. Born energy for ion transport through a pore.

## Current density through an aqueous cylindrical channel

Assuming the rate of entry of ions into a pore is sufficiently low that ion–ion interactions or space–charge effects are eligible, the electric field within the pore is approximately uniform. Therefore, with the addition of the image potential, the constant field approximation from Eyring rate theory can be used to describe the flow of ions through such a pore. The problem is solved for the univalent case[8].

$R_2(r,V_m)$ describes the resistance to flow of ions through an aqueous cylindrical channel of radius $r$, and, in general, depends on the potential across the channel $V_{ch}(V_m)$. The conductivity is assumed to be uniform within the pore. Thus, from Ohm's law,

$$R_2(r,V_m) = \frac{\delta}{\pi r^2 \sigma_p(r,V_m)} \tag{11}$$

where the pore conductivity, $\sigma_p(r,V_m)$, is defined by

$$J_z(r,V_m) = \sigma_p(r,V_m)E_z(r,V_m) \tag{12}$$

where $J_z(r,V_m)$ and $E_z(r,V_m)$ are respectively, the current density and electric field in the channel (Fig. 20.3).

According to Eyring rate theory[8,11] the current density, $J_z(r,V_m)$, can be represented by two opposite rate constants:

$$J_z(r,V_m) = zq(c_1k_{12} - c_1k_{21}) \tag{13}$$

where

$$k_{12} = f\exp\left[\frac{-\epsilon_B(r) - \dfrac{zqV_{ch}}{2}}{KT}\right] \tag{14}$$

and

$$k_{21} = f\exp\left[\frac{-E_B(r) - \dfrac{zqV_{ch}}{2}}{KT}\right] \tag{15}$$

$f = \frac{KT}{h} = 6 \times 10^{12}\ s^{-1}$. $T$, $K$, $h$, $c_1$ and $c_2$ are the absolute temperature, Boltzmann's constant, Planck's constant, and the ionic concentrations on sides 1 and 2 of the membrane. The current density $J_z(r,V_{ch})$, as a function of $V_{ch}$, and the Born energy, $E_B(r)$ is therefore:

$$J_z(r,V_{ch}) = \frac{2\sigma_0 KT}{\delta zq}\, e^{-\frac{E_B(r)}{KT}}\, \sinh\left(\frac{zqV_{ch}}{2KT}\right) \tag{16}$$

and

$$\sigma_p(r,V_m) = \frac{2\sigma_0 KT}{zqV_{ch}}\, e^{-\frac{E_B(r)}{KT}}\, \sinh\left(\frac{zqV_{ch}}{2KT}\right) \tag{17}$$

$\sigma_p$ is plotted as a function of both $V_m$ and $r$ in Figure 20.4.

### Bilayer–lipid membrane conductivity

From the distribution of pores in the membrane, $\rho(r,V_m)$, and considering all the pores of different sizes in parallel, the average conductivity of the membrane is estimated as follows:

$$\sigma_m(V_m) = \int_0^{r_cV_m} \rho(r,V_m)\pi r^2 \sigma_p(r,V_m)dr \tag{18}$$

$\rho(r,V_m)$ and $\sigma_p(r,V_m)$ are obtained from Equations (7) and (17) respectively. The predicted membrane conductivity, $\sigma_m(V_m)$, is compared with measurements to refine electroporation theory by determining the constant $\rho(0,0)$.

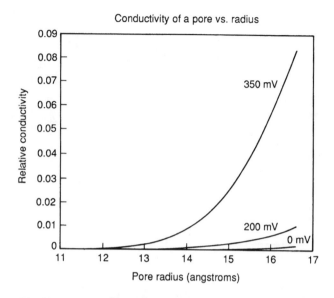

Fig. 20.4. The conductivity of a pore in a bilayer–lipid membrane at two different transmembrane potentials (0 mV, 200 mV and 350 mV). The conductivity is normalized to that of the surrounding solution.

Figure 20.5 shows a plot of the conductivity of a bilayer–lipid membrane, $\sigma_m(V_m)$, as a function of the transmembrane potential, $V_m$. Increase in transmembrane potential increases the number and average radius of pores in the membrane, and, consequently, increases both the fraction of membrane area occupied by pores and the membrane conductivity. This model predicts that the electrical properties of cell membranes are a strong nonlinear function of transmembrane potential.

## References

1 Benz, R. & Zimmermann U. (1980). Pulse-length dependence of the electrical breakdown in lipid bilayer membranes. *Biochimica et Biophysica Acta*, **597**, 637.

2 Weaver, J.C. *et al.* (1984). The diffusive permeability of bilayer membranes: the contribution of transient aqueous pores. *Bioelectrochemistry and Bioenergetics*, **12**, 405.

3 Weaver, J.C. & Mintzer, R.A. (1986). Conduction onset criteria for transient aqueous pores and reversible electrical breakdown in bilayer membranes. *Bioelectrochemistry and Bioenergetics*, **15**, 229.

4 Zimmermann, U., Vienken, J. & Pilwat, G. (1980). Development of drug carrier systems: electric field induced effects in cell membranes. *Bioelectrochemistry and Bioenergetics*, **7**, 553.

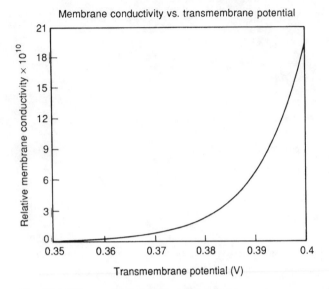

Fig. 20.5. The conductivity of a bilayer–lipid membrane normalized to that of the surrounding solution and scaled by $10^{10}$.

5 Neumann, E., Sowers, A. & Jordan, C. (eds). (1986). *Electroporation and Electrofusion in Cell Biology*, Plenum Press.
6 Powell, K.T., Derrick, E.G. & Weaver, J.C. (1986). A quantitative theory of reversible electrical breakdown in bilayer membranes. *Bioelectrochemistry and Bioenergetics*, **15**, 243.
7 Powell, K.T. & Weaver, J.C. (1986). Transient aqueous pores in bilayer membranes: a statistical theory. *Bioelectrochemistry and Bioenergetics*, **15**, 211.
8 Bertil Hille. *Ionic Chanels of Excitable Membranes*, Sunderland MA: Sinauer Associates Inc.
9 Parsegian, A. (1969). Energy of an ion crossing a low dielectric membrane: solutions to four relevant problems. *Nature*, **221**, 844.
10 Jordan, P.C. (1982). Electrostatic modeling of ion pores: energy barriers and electric field profiles. *Biophysical Journal*, **39**, 157.
11 Cooper, K., Jakobsson & E. Wolynes, P. (1985). The theory of ion transport through membrane channels. *Progress in Biophysics and Molecular Biology*, **46**, 51.

# Index